Progress in
Cancer Research and Therapy
Volume 20

LYMPHOKINES AND THYMIC HORMONES: THEIR POTENTIAL UTILIZATION IN CANCER THERAPEUTICS

Progress in Cancer Research and Therapy

Progress in
Cancer Research and Therapy
Volume 20

Lymphokines and Thymic Hormones: Their Potential Utilization in Cancer Therapeutics

Editors

Allan L. Goldstein, Ph.D.
Professor and Chairman
Department of Biochemistry
The George Washington University
School of Medicine
Washington, D.C.

Michael A. Chirigos, Ph.D.
Chief, Virus and Disease Modification Section
Division of Cancer Treatment
National Cancer Institute
National Institutes of Health
Bethesda, Maryland

Raven Press ■ New York

Raven Press, 1140 Avenue of the Americas, New York, New York 10036

Made in the United States of America

International Standard Book Number 0–89004–697–2
Library of Congress Catalog Number

Great care has been taken to maintain the accuracy of the information contained in the volume. However, Raven Press cannot be held responsible for errors or for any consequences arising from the use of the information contained herein.

Preface

Recent advances in immunology and immunopharmacology indicate that lymphokines and thymic hormones are destined to play an important role in increasing host immunity and in modifying biological responses in patients with cancer and other diseases associated with immune dysfunction. Because of the rapid expansion of scientific knowledge of these natural substances, the Biological Response Modifier Subcommittee of the Board of Scientific Advisors of the Division of Cancer Treatment, National Cancer Institute, organized a workshop to explore the potential utilization of lymphokines and thymic factors in cancer therapeutics.

Experts in the fields of lymphokine and thymic hormone research were invited to participate in this workshop to review recent developments in the chemical characterization, mechanism of action, regulation and potential utilization of these biological response modifiers in cancer therapeutics. They were asked to critically analyze the state of the art, including the intracellular mechanisms controlling lymphokine and thymic hormone action in biological response modification. They also asked to address the potential clinical applications of lymphokines and thymic hormones in cancer research therapy.

The volume is divided into three investigational categories: The first category deals with the purification and characterization of lymphokines and lymphokine stimulators. The state of the art used to define the biochemical characterization of the interleukins, lymphotoxins, transfer factors and other T-cell growth and proliferation factors, as well as lymphokines that stimulate non-lymphoid cells, is reviewed. In addition, a description of monoclonal antibodies against several of the lymphokines is presented and detailed methods for the purification of several of the biologically active molecules are discussed.

The second category is devoted to biological and molecular models of lymphokine and thymic hormone function. In this section, the role of these agents in modulating lymphocyte and monocyte populations is explored in depth, including mechanisms of cell/cell communication, pharmacological modulation, and regulatory properties. The role of several of the suppressor lymphokines is discussed and data are presented outlining their biological properties *in vivo* and *in vitro*.

The third section of the volume is devoted to the potential role and current status of lymphokines and thymic factors in cancer therapy in humans and animals. Immunotherapeutic effects of thymosin and lymphokines are reported in a number of tumor models in animals, including the use of liposomes to achieve activation of tumoricidal properties of murine macrophages. The final part of this section reviews the status and potential of using lymphokines to treat advanced cancer patients.

It is apparent from the studies presented herein that great strides and progress are being made in our understanding of the chemical nature of several of the thymic hormones, such as thymosin α_1 and thymosin β_4, as well as in the purification of several of the important lymphokines, such as T-cell growth factor, interleukin II, and the lymphotoxins. The chemistry and biological activities of a new lymphokine termed interleukin III are presented for the first time.

This collection of research efforts reveals that the biologically active molecules collectively designated as lymphokines and thymic hormones have essential roles in the regulation of the immune system and in anti-tumor immune defense mechanisms. It also becomes apparent that much of the research with lymphokines has been carried out with relatively crude preparations, and that there is a major need for further chemical characterization of the biologically active factors.

The availability of several of the purified lymphokines and thymic hormones through utilization of large scale production techniques, chemical synthesis and recombinant DNA cloning technologies are beginning to provide researchers with enough of these important biological agents to study both in laboratory and clinical settings. The results of all of these dramatic developments will hopefully provide the clinician with novel approaches to the treatment of cancer in the years to come.

This volume will be of considerable interest to basic scientists and clinicians interested in acquiring information on the state of the art of the new frontiers of immunobiology, immunopharmacology, and experimental and clinical oncology concerning lymphokines and thymic hormones.

Allan L. Goldstein
Michael A. Chirigos

Acknowledgments

The editors of this volume wish to express their gratitude to Dr. V. T. DeVita, Jr., Director of the National Cancer Institute and Dr. R. K. Oldham, Director of the Biological Response Modifiers Program, Division of Cancer Treatment, National Cancer Institute, and their staff for their invaluable support that made this Workshop possible, and to the members of the Biological Response Modifiers Subcommittee: Drs. E. Mihich, A. Fefer, E. Hersh, M. J. Mastrangelo, H. Oettgen, M. Krim, M. Mitchell, J. Whisnant, J. Betram, and A. Goldin for their encouragement and suggestions.

Contents

Biological and Molecular Models of Lymphokine Function

Utilization of Lymphokines and Thymic Factors in Cancer Therapy in Humans and Animals

Contributors

A. J. Ammann
University of California, San Francisco
The Departments of Radiation Oncology and
    Pediatrics
San Francisco, California 94143

B. Araneo
Department of Pathology
The Jewish Hospital of St. Louis
St. Louis, Missouri 63110

Thomas M. Aune
Departments of Pathology and Microbiology
    and Immunology
Washington University School of Medicine
St. Louis, Missouri 63110

S. Baron
Department of Microbiology
University of Texas Medical Branch
Galveston, Texas 77550

Jack R. Battisto
Department of Biology
Case Western Reserve University and
Department of Immunology
Cleveland Clinic Foundation
Cleveland, Ohio 44106

Elsa H. Berenstein
Laboratory of Microbiology and
    Immunology
National Institute of Dental Research
National Institutes of Health
Bethesda, Maryland 20205

Yael Bromberg
Section of Immunology
Department of Human Microbiology
Sackler School of Medicine
Tel-Aviv University
Tel-Aviv 69978, Israel

Denis R. Burger
Surgical Research Laboratory
VA Medical Center and Departments of
Microbiology and Immunology and of
    Surgery
University of Oregon Health Sciences Center
Portland, Oregon 97201

Charles Carter
Laboratory of Microbiology and
    Immunology
National Institute of Dental Research
National Institutes of Health
Bethesda, Maryland 20205

George J. Cianciolo
Laboratory of Immune Effector Function
Howard Hughes Medical Institute
Division of Rheumatic and Genetic Diseases
Departments of Medicine and Microbiology
    and Immunology
Duke University Medical Center
Durham, North Carolina 27710

G. Doyle Daves
The Oregon Graduate Center
Beaverton, Oregon 97005

Alain L. de Weck
Institute for Clinical Immunology
Inselspital, University of Berne
3010 Berne, Switzerland

Suanne F. Dougherty
Laboratory of Microbiology and
    Immunology
National Institute of Dental Research
National Institutes of Health
Bethesda, Maryland 20205

D. C. Dumonde
Department of Immunology
St. Thomas' Hospital
London SE1, England

Pamela A. Dunn
Cancer Research Center
115 Business Loop 70 West
Columbia, Missouri 65201

A. Englard
Laboratory of Immunopharmacology
Sloan-Kettering Institute for Cancer
    Research
New York, New York 10021

John J. Farrar
Laboratory of Microbiology and
*   Immunology*
National Institute of Dental Research
National Institutes of Health
Bethesda, Maryland 20205

William L. Farrar
Biological Carcinogenesis Program
Frederick Cancer Research Center
Frederick, Maryland 21701

I. J. Fidler
Cancer Metastasis and Treatment
*   Laboratory*
National Cancer Institute
Frederick Cancer Research Center
P.O. Box B
Frederick, Maryland 21701

W. R. Fleischmann, Jr.
University of Texas Medical Branch
Galveston, Texas 77550

W. E. Fogler
Cancer Metastasis and Treatment
*   Laboratory*
National Cancer Institute
Frederick Cancer Research Center
P.O. Box B
Frederick, Maryland 21701

Phillip C. Fox
Laboratory of Microbiology and
*   Immunology*
National Institute of Dental Research
National Instiues of Health
Bethesda, Maryland 20205

Maya Freund
Section of Immunology
Department of Human Microbiology
Sackler School of Medicine
Tel-Aviv University
Tel-Aviv 69978, Israel

Janet Fuller-Farrar
Laboratory of Microbiology and
*   Immunology*
National Institute of Dental Research
National Institutes of Health
Bethesda, Maryland 20205

R. C. Gallo
Laboratory of Tumor Cell Biology
National Cancer Institute
National Institutes of Health
Bethesda, Maryland 20205

Charles W. Gehrke
University of Missouri
Columbia, Missouri 65211

Frederick W. George IV
Department of Microbiology and
*   Immunology*
Duke University Medical Center
Box 3839
Durham, North Carolina 27710

C. Dean Gilliland
Cancer Research Center
115 Business Loop 70 West
Columbia, Missouri 65201

Steven Gillis
Fred Hutchinson Cancer Research Center
1124 Columbia Street
Seattle, Washington 98104

Moshe Glaser
National Cancer Institute
National Institutes of Health
Bethesda, Maryland 20034

Allan L. Goldstein
Department of Biochemistry
George Washington University School of
*   Medicine*
Washington, D.C. 20037

G. A. Granger
Department of Molecular Biology and
Biochemistry
University of California, Irvine
Irvine, California 92717

E. Hadden
Laboratory of Immunopharmacology
Sloan-Kettering Institute for Cancer
*   Research*
New York, New York 10021

J. W. Hadden
Laboratory of Immunopharmacology
Sloan-Kettering Institute for Cancer
*   Research*
New York, New York 10021

Anne S. Hamblin
Department of Immunology
St. Thomas' Hospital
London SE1, England

Andrew J. Hapel
Biological Carcinogenesis Program
Frederick Cancer Research Center
Frederick, Maryland 21701

C. Healy
Roche Institute of Molecular Biology
Nutley, New Jersey 07110

Howard T. Holden
Laboratory of Immunodiagnosis
National Cancer Institute
National Institutes of Health
Bethesda, Maryland 20205

F. den Hollander
Organon Scientific Development Group
Oss, The Netherlands

James N. Ihle
Biological Carcinogenesis Program
Frederick Cancer Research Center
Frederick, Maryland 21701

Aniela Jakubowski
Section of Immunology
Department of Human Microbiology
Sackler School of Medicine
Tel-Aviv University
Tel-Aviv 69978, Israel

J. Kapp
Department of Pathology
The Jewish Hospital of St. Louis
St. Louis, Missouri 63110

Yona Keisari
Section of Immunology
Department of Human Microbiology
Sackler School of Medicine
Tel-Aviv University
Tel-Aviv 69978, Israel

Jonathon Keller
Biological Carcinogenesis Program
Frederick Cancer Research Center
Frederick, Maryland 21701

Phillip Klesius
U.S. Department of Agriculture
SEA-AR-SR, Regional Parasite Research
* Laboratory*
Auburn, Alabama 36830

Jim Klostergaard
Department of Molecular Biology and
* Biochemistry*
University of California, Irvine
Irvine, California 92717

K. Krupen
Roche Institute of Molecular Biology
Nutley, New Jersey 07110

Lawrence B. Lachman
Department of Microbiology and
* Immunology*
Duke University Medical Center
Box 3839
Durham, North Carolina 27710

John C. Lee
Biological Carcinogenesis Program
Frederick Cancer Research Center
Frederick, Maryland 21701

Terry Lee
The Oregon Graduate Center
Beaverton, Oregon 97005

Teresa L. K. Low
Department of Biochemistry
The George Washington University School
* of Medicine and Health Services*
2300 I Street, N.W.
Washington, D.C. 20037

Mildred C. McDaniel
Ouillen-Dishner College of Medicine
East Tennessee State University
Johnson City, Tennessee 37614

John E. McEntire
Cancer Research Center
115 Business Loop 70 West
Columbia, Missouri 65201

Richard S. Metzgar
Department of Microbiology and
* Immunology*
Duke University Medical Center
Box 3839
Durham, North Carolina 27710

J. Mier
Laboratory of Tumor Cell Biology
National Cancer Institute
National Institutes of Health
Bethesda, Maryland 20205

Steven B. Mizel
Microbiology Program
The Pennsylvania State University
University Park, Pennsylvania 16802

Ruth Neta
Department of Microbiology
University of Notre Dame
Notre Dame, Indiana 46556

M. H. Neely
University of California, San Francisco
The Departments of Radiation Oncology and
  Pediatrics
San Francisco, California 94143

I. Nowowiejski
Roche Institute of Molecular Biology
Nutley, New Jersey 07110

D. O'Connell
Department of Radiotherapy
Charing Cross Hospital
London W6, England

Joost J. Oppenheim
Laboratory of Microbiology and
  Immunology
National Institute of Dental Research
National Institutes of Health
Bethesda, Maryland 20205

Ben W. Papermaster
Cancer Research Center
115 Business Loop 70 West
Columbia, Missouri 65201

F. J. Paradinas
Department of Histopathology
Charing Cross Hospital
London W6, England

Edgar Pick
Section of Immunology
Department of Human Microbiology
Sackler School of Medicine
Tel-Aviv University
Tel-Aviv 69978, Israel

Carl W. Pierce
Department of Pathology and Laboratory
  Medicine
The Jewish Hospital of St. Louis
St. Louis, Missouri 63110

Melanie S. Pulley
Department of Immunology
St. Thomas' Hospital
London SE1, England

Carol C. Rigby
Institute of Urology
London WC2, England

M. R. G. Robinson
Pontefract General Infirmary
Yorkshire, England

Ned D. Rodes
Cancer Research Center
115 Business Loop 70 West
Columbia, Missouri 65201

Jeffrey L. Rossio
Biological Response Modifier Program
Frederick Cancer Research Center
Frederick, Maryland 21701

J. R. Sadlik
Laboratory of Immunopharmacology
Sloan-Kettering Institute for Cancer
  Research
New York, New York 10021

Samuel B. Salvin
Department of Microbiology
School of Medicine
University of Pittsburgh
Pittsburgh, Pennsylvania 15261

A. Schuurs
Organon Scientific Development Group
Oss, The Netherlands

Cary M. Seals
Department of Biochemistry
George Washington University School of
  Medicine
Washington, D.C. 20037

A. K. Singh
Department of Haematology
St. Thomas' Hospital
London SE1, England

Reuben P. Siraganian
Laboratory of Microbiology and
*   Immunology*
National Institute of Dental Research
National Institutes of Health
Bethesda, Maryland 20205

Ralph Snyderman
Division of Rheumatic and Genetic
*   Diseases*
Duke University Medical School
Durham, North Carolina 27710

Clemens Sorg
Department of Experimental Dermatology
Universitats-Hautklinik
4400 Munster, West Germany

Barbara M. Southcott
Department of Radiotherapy
Charing Cross Hospital
London W6, England

Beda M. Stadler
Laboratory of Microbiology and
*   Immunology*
National Institute of Dental Research
National Institutes of Health
Bethesda, Maryland 20205

G. J. Stanton
University of Texas Medical Branch
Galveston, Texas 77550

S. Stein
Roche Institute of Molecular Biology
Nutley, New Jersey 07110

Donatella Taramelli
Laboratory of Immunodiagnosis
National Cancer Institute
National Institutes of Health
Bethesda, Maryland 20205

Gary B. Thurman
Biological Response Modifier Program
Frederick Cancer Research Center
Frederick, Maryland 21701

Arthur A. Vandenbark
Surgical Research Laboratory
VA Medical Center and Departments of
*   Microbiology and Immunology*
University of Oregon Health Sciences Center
Portland, Oregon 97201

Elenie van Vliet
Organon Scientific Development Group
Oss, The Netherlands

Luigi Varesio
Laboratory of Immunodiagnosis
National Cancer Institute
National Institutes of Health
Bethesda, Maryland 20205

H. Verheul
Organon Scientific Development Group
Oss, The Netherlands

R. Mark Vetto
Surgical Research Laboratory
VA Medical Center and Department of
*   Surgery*
University of Oregon Health Sciences Center
Portland, Oregon 97201

D. W. Wara
University of California, San Francisco
The Departments of Radiation Oncology and
*   Pediatrics*
San Francisco, California 94143

W. M. Wara
University of California, San Francisco
The Departments of Radiation Oncology and
*   Pediatrics*
San Francisco, California 94143

D. R. Webb
Roche Institute of Molecular Biology
Nutley, New Jersey 07110

K. Wieder
Roche Institute of Molecular Biology
Nutley, New Jersey 07110

Henry L. Wong
Department of Biology, Case Western
Reserve University and Department of
*   Immunology*
Cleveland Clinic Foundation
Cleveland, Ohio 44106

Robert S. Yamamoto
Department of Molecular Biology and Biochemistry
University of California, Irvine
Irvine, California 92717

Marion M. Zatz
Department of Biochemistry
George Washington University School of Medicine
Washington, D.C. 20037

Lymphokines and Thymic Hormones: Their Potential Utilization in Cancer Therapeutics, edited by A. L. Goldstein and M. A. Chirigos, Raven Press, New York © 1981.

Lymphokines and Other Immunoactive Soluble Cellular Products: Prospects for the Future

Alain L. de Weck

Institute for Clinical Immunology, Inselspital, University of Berne, 3010 Berne, Switzerland

My first contact with the initials BRM geos back to more than 30 years ago; at that time, BRM did not mean Biological Response Modifiers but British Racing Motors, a highly successful but small British company producing racing cars. In the meantime, the British BRM has gone broke and my task in this lecture should be to demonstrate why the same fate should not occur to the Biological Response Modifier Programm!

Indeed the term of Biological Response Modifier is so broad as to become almost meaningless; it may encompass substances and products as different as biologically active glycoproteins produced by lymphocytes, monocytes or various types of cells including tumor cells, hormones, corticosteroids, prostaglandins and many others. I would therefore like to restrict that discussion to those biologically active proteins produced by activated lymphocytes or monocytes and collectively known under the term of lymphokines (LKs) or monokines (MKs).

There are several possible ways to classify lymphokines, namely according to their cellular origin, their target cells, their mode of action (antigen-specific or not, MHC-restricted or not), their biological activity, their effect on the cell cycle and their physicochemical characteristics. The main biological roles of lymphokines, monokines or cytokines, as presently known, are given in Table 1.

TABLE 1. <u>Biological roles of lymphokines, monokines,</u>
<u>cytokines</u>

Maturation and differentiation of lymphoid cells
Mobilization of lymphoid and inflammatory cells
Intercellular cooperation, regulation of system
Activation of lymphoid cells and non lymphoid cells
              inflammation, growth, regeneration
Killing / inactivation of target cells

1

In attempting to define more precisely the biological role of a lymphokine and to characterize and isolate such a substance, one is repeatedly stumbling over a number of difficulties, which held the whole field in disrepute for a number of years. These are: (a) The fact that lymphokines are usually produced by a mixture of cell types and may often require cooperation (e.g. among macrophages and lymphocytes) in order to be effectively produced; (b) that correspondingly any culture supernatant from activated cells usually contains several different LKs and MKs; (c) that the target cell population used for assessing LK's biological activity is itself frequently heterogeneous and capable of producing LKs, MKs and other factors having an enhancing or inhibiting effect on the biological assay under study. Under such circumstances, attempts to ascribe molecular identity to factors exhibiting different biological activities in vitro when dealing with the "black box" of crude culture supernatants amounts to little more than wishful thinking. Unfortunately, the literature of the past 15 years is full of statements in which culture supernatants and factors with a given name are used indiscriminately as synonyms. Even in this presentation, I will not entirely avoid this bad habit. We must, however, now that technical means to purify LKs have made so much progress, become aware that the only data really worth striving for are those obtained with purified materials.

A similar thought should be given to the impurities which the experimentator is deliberately introducing into the system used either to produce lymphokines or to test their biological activity, namely the adjunction of serum. This is the more inexcusable, as it is no longer really required in most assays, especially if some new forms of defined supplemented media are used. The introduction of serum causes variability at several levels: (a) The concentration of stimulant (e.g. mitogen) available for stimulation and thereby its toxicity; (b) the stimulating event itself influenced by activators and/or inhibitors present in the serum itself; (c) the viability of the cells cultured in presence of serum or of a defined supplemented medium. Obviously, some of these supplemented media are operating better for some types of lymphoid cells than for others. While the Iscove's medium is obviously very suitable for murine B cells (6), a medium recently developed in our laboratory (8) has been found better for T cells (Fig. 1).

When considering the possible role of lymphokines or monokines in defence against tumors, one should distinguish between: (a) those factors directly involved in the immune processes leading to the destruction of the tumor cell as target; (b) those involved in the general development and regulation of the immune response as such and (c) those influencing the local environment in which the tumor cells grow and which may particularly influence the possibility of

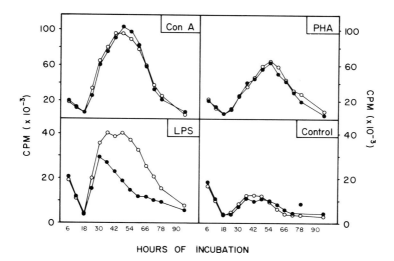

FIG. 1. Proliferation of murine spleen lymphocytes in presence of 3% fetal calf serum (o—o) or 3% serum free-defined AATSZ medium (●—●). Kinetics of ^{3}H-thymidine uptake evaluated by 6 hour pulses following stimulation by Concanavalin A, Phytohemagglutinin, E. Coli Lipopolysaccharide or in the absence of mitogen (control). For experimental details, see ref. 8.

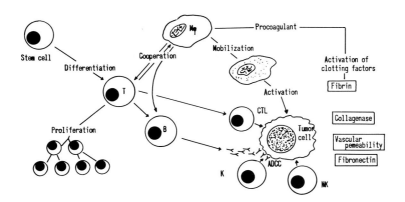

FIG. 2. Possible roles of lymphokines in the immune surveillance of tumor cells. These roles involve: (a) the differentiation and recruitment of immunologically active cells; (b) the activation of macrophages (m), cytotoxic T lymphocytes (CTL), antibody-dependent cytotoxic (ADCC)

Killers (K) cells and natural killer (NK) cells; (c) the
modification of the environment of tumor cells (fibrin de-
posits, vascular permeability, etc.)

metastasis (Fig. 2).
    In the general concept of immune surveillance of tumors,
four main possible lines of defence have been identified,
which are not mutually exclusive and which also probably
play a role at different times of a tumor's development. I
would like now to review briefly the possible role of
lymphokines in these various systems of defense.

Natural killer cells

    Natural killer cells, among lymphoid cells, have not yet
taken their final place. They may represent a heterogeneous
population of monocyte and/or T cell lineage. Several
features, however, distinguish them clearly from other better
specified cell types involved in tumor defences (Table 2).

TABLE 2. <u>In vivo relevance of mouse NK cells in rejection
of tumor cells</u>

- Correlation between in vitro NK activity and rejection of
  tumor transplants (various genotypes)
- Mice with T and/or B cell deficiency but normal or elevated NK activity resist to NK-sensitive tumors
- Lymphocyte populations enriched in NK cells delay tumor
  growth upon transfer in irradiated syngeneic recipients
- Bone marrow chimeras between NK high- or low-reactive F_1
  genotypes show same in vivo resistance as bone marrow
  donor
- Correlation between NK activity in vitro and ability to
  reject prelabelled tumor cells
- Correlation between in vitro and in vivo decline in NK-
  mediated tumor rejection with age and increasing incidence
  of spontaneous tumors
- Mouse mutant beige, selectively impaired in NK function,
  rejects tumor transplants and metastases less efficiently.

This is not the place to review the arguments pleading for
the role of NK cells in rejection of tumor cells; it suffices
to say that arguments in this direction are steadily accumulating (3,12). Natural killer cells appear to diminish in
number with age; their activity is modulated by interferons
and interferon inducers, as well as by anti-interferon antibodies (12). Although a possible role of other LKs than
interferon on NK cells cannot be entirely excluded for the

time being, I am not aware of convincing evidence in this respect. Indirectly, of course, considering the fact that a number of interferon inducers are also LK inducers, this possibility should be kept in mind. Interferon seems to affect the killing ability of NK cells, but not their number, as judged from the percentage of NK cells binding to their target (12).

Specific cytolytic T lymphocytes (CTL)

When dealing with immune T lymphocytes capable of recognizing and attacking tumor targets, a family of LKs and MKs has emerged in recent years as being probably of prime importance and which become increasingly known under the name of interleukins. I shall not at this point discuss whether that name is appropriate, justified, timely or merely esthetic. It is not to be denied that the increased sophistication of our purification techniques and the availability of monoclonal antibodies will soon justify the abolition of too many different acronyms solely based upon phenomenological biological assays (1).

Our concepts on the interplay between IL-1 and IL-2 and their requirement for the production of active CTL, on the one hand, and of an effective T helper system on the other hand, have crystallized during the past few years. It is remarkable that, on the basis of different approaches and experimental systems, several groups seem to come to very similar conclusions. Considering the past history of the lymphokine field, this is no minor achievement. From the concept of two T cell populations, one producing IL-2 and one using it for proliferation, as suggested by Smith (14) and others (2), one quickly added the requirement of macrophages and IL-1 for IL-2 production, and the requirement for all 3 types of cells involved for a stimulating signal, be it antigen or a so called "mitogen". Indeed, this IL-1/IL-2 interplay seems essential to produce active cytotoxic T lymphocytes.

In our laboratory, we have recently been interested in evaluating the effects of IL-1 and IL-2 on the lymphocyte cell cycle (9). Although these results are up to now obtained with crude supernatants, the cell populations used for generating the lymphokines (for IL-1 thioglycollate induced peritoneal cells and non adherent spleen cells for IL-2) as well as the mode of activation (no additional mitogen for IL-1), as well as the kinetic results obtained led us to believe that these two supernatants very predominantly contain the LKs for which they are labelled. On non-stimulated mouse thymocytes, kinetic experiments adding IL-2 not only at time 0 but also at $+_{18}$ and $+_{30}$ clearly show that IL-2 is not mitogenic by itself, as could have been wrongly assessed, if only the results of addition at the beginning of the culture would have been considered (Fig. 3).

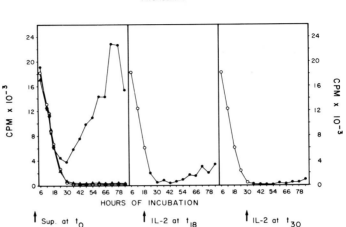

FIG. 3. Effect of interleukins on the proliferation of non-stimulated mouse thymocytes. Proliferation assessed by 6-hour pulses with ^{3}H-thymidine, following the addition of interleukin 1 (▲—▲), interleukin 2 (●—●) - containing or control (O—O) supernatant at various times. While IL-2 added at time O increases the proliferation of thymocytes apparently prestimulated in vivo, this is no longer the case after 18 and 30 hours. For experimental details, see ref. 9.

I suspect that a number of so called mitogenic factors described in the literature are in fact nothing else than IL-2-like factors susceptible of carrying through the cell cycle _in vitro_ cells which have already been stimulated _in vivo_.
    IL-1 alone, as well known, has not even this capacity. A similar picture can be seen, when the thymocytes are activated in vitro by PHA and IL-2 or IL-1 added at various times, evaluating the proliferative response with 6 hours ^{3}H-thymidine pulses (Fig. 4). Whether the relatively low increase in proliferation observed in PHA-activated cells upon the addition of IL-1 (the formerly denominated LAF effect) is due to contamination of our IL-1 by IL-2, to endogenous production of IL-2 in our thymocyte target population or to a direct proliferation-promoting effect of IL-1 on part of the thymocyte population shall not be discussed

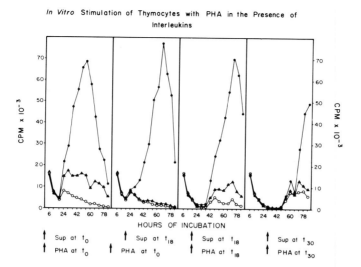

FIG. 4. Effect of interleukins on the stimulation of mouse thymocytes by PHA. Addition of PHA and of supernatants containing either IL-1 (▲—▲) or IL-2 (●—●) or control supernatants (o—o) at various times. Kinetics of proliferation assessed by 6-hour pulses with ^{3}H-thymidine. For experimental details, see ref. 9.

at this time. From close observation of the kinetics presented here, it is clear that IL-2 begins its effect approximately 10-12 hours after activation by PHA; this seems to be the time required for activation of the cells into the G_1 to S phase and the generation of the IL-2 receptor postulated and demonstrated by other groups.

Further insights on the mechanism of IL-2 action have been gained by direct observation of its effect on the cell cycle by cytofluorometry (Fig. 5). Evaluation of the increasing RNA content in thymocytes following stimulation by "mitogens", while the DNA content is not yet increased (so called G_0 - G_1 window), clearly showed that IL-2 produces a dramatic increase in RNA in a cell population which has been pushed by PHA until some stage of activation (G_{1a}), which without the additional presence of IL-2 does not pursue until DNA synthesis. IL-1, on the other hand, has no detectable stimulating effect on RNA content. This observation permits us to distinguish tentatively two stages in the G_1 phase, G_{1a} and G_{1b}. When correlating DNA synthesis, i.e. ^{3}H-thymidine uptake, with the number of cells in G_1 phase, it can be seen that the correlation is much better with cells in G_{1b} than with the totality of cells in G_1, confirming that there must be within the G_1 phase a restriction point, which is overcome by the addition of IL-2.

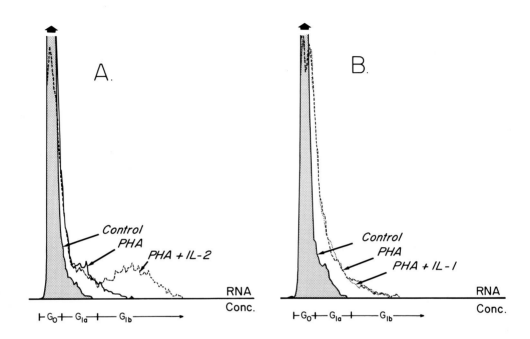

FIG. 5. Histogram of mouse thymocytes stimulated by PHA in
the absence or presence of IL-2 (A) or IL-1 (B). The assessment of RNA content of the cells is performed by flow cyto-
metry as described in ref. 9. While the addition of IL-1
does not push the cells beyond a restriction point defined
as G_{1a}, the addition of IL-2 increases RNA content still
further and promotes the cells into a G_{1b} phase of the cell
cycle.

     These conclusions are summarized in Fig. 6. Since IL-2
dependent T cell clones appear to grow continuously without
the need for further stimulation by antigen or mitogen, it
is postulated that such cells are also sensitive to IL-2
and that they bypass the G_O phase.
     Summarizing our current information on the IL-1 - IL-2
cycle we arrive to a more complex figure (Fig. 7), in which
the effect of IL-1 on B cell differentiation postulated by
some and the relationship to clonal expansion of B cells
effected by TRF should not be forgotten.

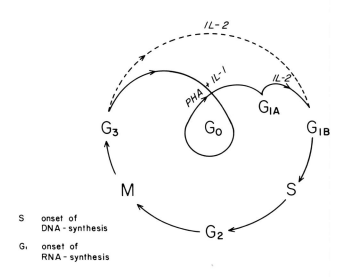

FIG. 6.   Role of interleukin 2 in the lymphocyte cell cycle.

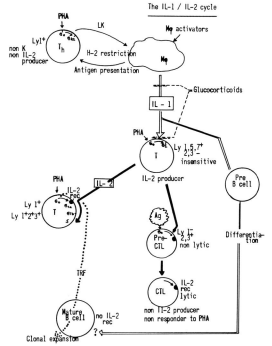

FIG. 7. The IL-1/IL-2 cell cycle. While the production of
IL-1 requires the production of some lymphokine (LK) by T
helper cells (Th) and activation of the IL-1 producing
macrophages (m), the production of IL-2 is performed by a

subset of T lymphocytes. IL-2 is required for the generation of cytotoxic T lymphocytes (CTL) and for the proliferation of non IL-2 producing T cells. IL-2 acts only on the late G_1 phase (G_{1b}), after under the stimulation by mitogen (e.g. PHA) a membrane receptor for IL-2 will have appeared. B cells may be helped in their differentiation by IL-1 and require for clonal expansion a T cell replacing factor (TRF), which appears to be distinct from IL-2.

In so far as CTL play a role in cancer, there is some evidence that IL-2 will also play a role in tumor defences, also when injected in vivo (11, 16). However, the evaluation of IL-2 as an alternative or as a competition for interferon as anti-cancer biological agent is only beginning. A word of caution is required: in preliminary experiments in collaboration with Dr. Fontana, we have shown that a human factor promoting the proliferation of mouse glial cells (4) chromatographes in the same region as human IL-2 although this by no means suffices to imply identity. We wonder whether the proliferation-promoting effect of IL-2 is really only restricted to T cells and could not also apply, at least to some tumor cells.

In aged mice, it is well known that the proliferative response of T cells to mitogens decreases (7). Is this due to a diminution of the mitogen-responding population, to a lack of required factors such as IL-2 or to both? As we observed (7), the number of cells promoted to the G_1 phase by Con A or PHA effectively decreases, while the kinetics of activation, within the cell cycle remain the same. What is interesting is that the ratio between cells in G_1 phase and proliferating cells diminish in the old, a result compatible but not yet proving a relative insufficiency in IL-2. Along similar lines goes the following observation: when cells are analyzed at time 0, without any additional stimulation, the old individuals possess a significant higher number of G_1 cells. In other words, old individuals have a higher number of G_1 cells activated in vivo and a smaller number of activatable and proliferating cells in vitro; both results compatible with a relative deficiency in IL-2. This, however, still remains to be formally tested.

Activated macrophages

Several LKs are known to act on macrophages in various ways, for example to mobilize them towards a lesion or a tumor (macrophage chemotactic factor), to immobilize them at the site of action (macrophage migration inhibiting factor) and to activate them to possible cytolytic activity for tumor cells (macrophage activating factor). The continuing arguments for identity or diversity and mode of action of these macrophage-active products will be more thorougly discussed during this conference.

Obviously, there are numerous differences between activated macrophages and natural killer cells (13) among which tissue distribution, chronologic appearance, different selectivity for targets, genotype distribution and mechanism of cytolytic action could be emphasized. The activation of macrophages by lymphokines or other means may not be a goal to be pursued indiscriminately in cancer therapy: indeed the macrophages produce prostaglandins as potent inhibitors of immune reactions, including tumor-directed cytotoxic effects. Furthermore, some macrophage products may have colony stimulating effects on some tumor cells. It seems interesting to study further the combination of lymphokine-promoting agents and of indomethacin and other prostaglandin synthesis inhibitors since this may indeed potentiate the desired cytotoxic effects of lymphokine-stimulated immune cells (10).

Antibody-producing cells

Last but not least, the cells producing antibodies against tumor antigens should not be forgotten. Much less is known still about the LKs directly acting on B cells, either as differentiation promoters or as favoring the proliferation and clonal expansion of B cells, in analogy to the role played by IL-2 for T cells. In how far, LKs directed to promote or inhibit B cell function will ultimately have a beneficial or detrimental effect on the evolution of tumors brings us back to the eternal discussion about cytotoxic versus blocking antibodies.

Prospects for the future

Can lymphokines be contemplated as therapeutic agents in cancer? The answer is probably a qualified yes. Indeed the fact that so many of the cells and mechanisms possibly involved in one way or another in tumor defences are directly producing and/or affected by LKs pleads for a continued evaluation of their role and use in cancer therapy. It should be clear from the preceding discussion, however, that LKs actions have many facets and that these substances should not be used indiscriminately. In particular, the negative feedback loops present in all the immune circuits must be carefully evaluated. Just to name one, LKs have recently been shown to raise steroid levels (15) and steroid levels appear to influence both IL-1 production and activity (14).

In terms of concrete suggestions for continued progress, the following should be emphasized:

(a) Progress must be achieved in the standardization of LK biological assays
(b) Large scale production of several human LKs is an essential condition for progress
(c) Production of monoclonal antibodies against LKs is the key to rapid advances in the field, including
    - identification and quantitative evaluation of LKs in pathological conditions
    - structural caracterization and mass-scale production
    - evaluation of LK functions in vivo and selective access to immunological regulation

At present, a number of anti-LK hybridomas are growing in various laboratories and I have little doubt that they will signal the advent of a new aera in LK research. Only through an integrated effort, which surpasses the capacity of individual scientists will it be possible to make true the promises clearly lying ahead of us. If indeed, the BRM programm can contribute to foster this integration, it will have rendered a great service to immunology certainly and to cancer therapy hopefully.

REFERENCES

1. Aarden, L.A. et al. (1979): J. Immunol., 123: 2928.

2. Bonmard, G.D., Yasaka, K., Jacobson, D. (1979): J. Immunol., 123: 2704.

3. Djen, J.Y., Heinbaugh, J.A., Holden, H.T., Herberman, R.B. (1979): J. Immunol., 122: 175.

4. Fontana, A., Grieder, A., Arrenbrecht, S., Grob, P. (1980): J. Neurol. Sci., 46: 55.

5. Herberman, R.B., Nunn, N.E., Lavrin, D.H. (1975): Int. J. Cancer, 16, 216.

6. Iscove, N.N., Melchers, F. (1978): J.Exp.Med., 147: 923.

7. Joncourt, F., Bettens, F., Kristensen, F., de Weck, A.L. Immunology, in press.

8. Kristensen, F., Joncourt, F., de Weck, A.L.. Defined serum-free media for human and murine T lymphocyte cultures. Submitted.

9. Kristensen, F., Bettens, F., de Weck, A.L.. Effect of interleukins 1 and 2 on lymphocyte cell cycles. Submitted.

10. Lynch, N.R., Salomon, J.C. (1979): J. Natl. Cancer Inst., 62: 117.

11. Paetkau, V., Shaw, J., Mills, G., Caplan, B. (1980): Immunol. Rev., 51: 157.

12. Roder, J.C., Karre, K., Kiessling, R. (1981): Progr. Allergy, 28: 66.

13. Schultz, R.M. (1981): Cancer Immunol. Immunother., 10: 61.

14. Smith, K.A. (1980): Immunol. Rev., 51: 337.

15. Sorkin, E., Del Rey, A., Besedovsky, H.O. (1981): J. Immunol., 126: 385.

16. Wagner, H., Hardt, C., Heeg, K., Röllinghof, M., Pfizenmaier, K. (1980): Nature, 284: 278.

Lymphokines and Thymic Hormones: Their
Potential Utilization in Cancer Therapeutics,
edited by A. L. Goldstein and M. A. Chirigos,
Raven Press, New York © 1981.

Purification to Homogeneity of Interleukin 1

Steven B. Mizel

Microbiology Program, Pennsylvania State University, University Park, Pennsylvania 16802

INTRODUCTION

The generation of antigen-specific cytotoxic T cells and antibody forming B cells involves a shared cascade of cellular interactions that are regulated, in large part, by extremely potent peptide mediators. Evidence from a number of studies indicate that the initiating signal in these activation pathways emanates from the macrophage and is dualistic in nature (1,2,4,7,8). The activation of the primary T cell target of the macrophage is dependent on not only the presentation of antigens in an immunogenic form, but also on the synthesis and secretion of a peptide termed interleukin 1 (IL 1). This conclusion is supported by the data presented in Table 1. In this experiment,

TABLE 1. Dualistic nature of the macrophage signal for T cell activation[a]

LNL[b]	PC$_x$[c]	Additions	CPM [^{3}H]-TdR Incorporation[d]
Untreated	–	None	1929± 602
		OVA	3903± 803
		IL 1	2420± 881
		OVA + IL 1	15733±2258
Anti-macrophage serum treated[e]	–	OVA + IL 1	3310±1628
Anti-macrophage serum treated	+	OVA	1167±469
		OVA + IL 1	15082±1227

[a]Adapted from Reference 4.

[b]T cell-enriched lymph node lymphocytes (4x10^5) from OVA primed mice.

[c]Irradiated peritoneal cells (1x10^4) from unprimed mice.

[d][^{3}H]-TdR incorporation was measured after 72 hrs of culture.

[e]Anti-macrophage serum was obtained from rabbits immunized with P388D$_1$ cells. The antiserum was absorbed with thymocytes prior to use.

CS7B1/6J mice were primed with ovalbumin (OVA). After 10-12 days, a T cell enriched population of popliteal lymph node cells (93% Thy 1.2 positive) was prepared and the cells were incubated in vitro with OVA in

the presence or absence of IL 1. In the absence of IL 1, the LNL did
not respond to OVA, whereas cells incubated with both OVA and IL 1 exhibited a proliferative response that was of comparable magnitude to
that of unfractionated lymph node cells. The ability of IL 1 to restore
the antigen responsiveness of the cells was completely lost, however,
when the T cell-enriched LNL were first treated with a specific anti-
macrophage serum prepared by immunizing rabbits with the murine macrophage cell line, $P388D_1$. Of critical importance was the observation
that the antigen responsiveness could be restored by the addition of
IL 1 and small numbers of irradiated peritoneal cells from unprimed
syngeneic mice. Since the added PC_x by themselves were unable to restore responsiveness, we concluded that PC_x were present in sufficient
numbers to present antigen, but were unable to produce the level of
IL 1 that was necessary to initiate a proliferative response. Studies
on the activation of helper and cytotoxic T cells have also provided
evidence in support of the dualistic nature of the signal required for
macrophage-mediated T cell activation (1,2).

In addition to its stimulatory effect on T cell activation, IL 1
may also participate in the macrophage-mediated regulation of non-
lymphoid cells that are involved in inflammatory responses. For
example, IL 1 has been shown to markedly enhance the production of
collagenase and prostaglandins by human rheumatoid synovial cells (5).
Furthermore, IL 1 may stimulate the proliferation of human dermal
fibroblasts (J. Schmidt, S. B. Mizel, and I. Green, manuscript in
preparation). In view of the possibility that IL 1 may be a major
regulatory mediator for a variety of cell types that are under the
influence of the macrophage, it is of obvious importance to purify this
peptide and define its mechanism of action as well as the factors that
regulate its production. In this report, I shall review our recent
studies on the purification of murine IL 1.

Superinduction of IL 1

Lymphokine research has been plagued by the problem of producing
sufficient quantities of an active mediator for purification and
characterization studies. Most investigators have assumed that it is
necessary to grow cells in large fermentors to obtain reasonable
quantities of material. Volume is not, however, the only variable
that can be manipulated to yield microgram-milligram quantities of a
mediator. Studies on interferon production by fibroblasts clearly
revealed that protocols could be designed to greatly enhance the
interferon production capacity of the cells. In view of the success
achieved with a superinduction protocol for interferon production, we
explored the use of a similar protocol to augment IL 1 production (6).
We used the murine macrophage cell line, $P388D_1$, as a source of IL 1 and
phorbol myristic acetate (PMA) as our primary stimulant. When $P388D_1$
cells were incubated with PMA (10 μg/ml) for 5 hr, washed, and incubated
for an additional 24 hr, little if any supernatant IL was detected
(Table 2). In contrast, incubation of the cells with cycloheximide and
PMA for 4 hr, followed by a 1 hr incubation with actinomycin D, resulted
in the production of approximately 900 units of IL 1. This value is to
be compared with the 11 units of IL 1 produced when $P388D_1$ cells were
incubated with PMA for 6 days (3). The production of IL 1 can be further enhanced if cells are also supplemented with sodium butyrate
throughout the entire incubation.

TABLE 2. Superinduction of IL 1

Additions	Time in Culture	Units of Interleukin 1
	hr	
None		<1
10 µg/ml phorbol myristic acetate	0-5	<1
10 µg/ml phorbol myristic acetate + 10 µg/ml cycloheximide	0-5	903
+ Actinomycin D	4-5	
10 µg/ml phorbol myristic acetate + 10 µg/ml cycloheximide + 2 mM sodium butyrate	0-5	
+ 10 µg/ml actinomycin D	4-5	1393
+ 2 mM sodium butyrate	5-29	

[a] 2×10^6 P388D$_1$ cells/ml were incubated in RPMI 1640 + 1% fetal calf serum in Costar TC$_{24}$ tissue culture plates (1 ml/well). After a 1 hr incubation to permit the cells to adhere to the plates, the various drugs were added.

[b] After 5 hr, the cells were washed 2 times with RPMI 1640 and were then incubated for an additional 24 hr in 1 ml of RPMI 1640 containing 1% fetal calf serum ± sodium butyrate. From Reference 6.

TABLE 3. Purification of Interleukin 1[a]

Purification Step	Amount	Protein	Units of interleukin 1	Units of Interleukin 1 / mg protein	Yield
	ml	mg			%
Crude supernatant	4780	1262	4.4×10^6	3490	100
Ammonium sulfate precipitation	69	431	3.0×10^6	7000	69
Phenyl Sepharose	5	49	5.4×10^5	10930	12
Ultrogel AcA54	63	6	2.8×10^5	49040	6
Isoelectric-focusing	4	0.064	6.6×10^4	1037000	2

[a] From Reference 6.

Purification of IL 1

Having developed a protocol for the production of relatively high
levels of IL 1, we prepared large scale culture of superinduced P388D$_1$
cells. The cell-free supernatant was concentrated using ammonium sulfate fractionation. The material that precipitated with 65% ammonium
sulfate was sequentially chromatographed on phenyl Sepharose and Ultrogel AcA54 and then isoelectrofocused in a pH 4-7 gradient using the LKB
Multiphor flat-bed focusing apparatus. The final product had a specific
activity of approximately 1 x 10^6 units/mg protein (Table 3). Sixty-
four micrograms of protein was obtained from 5 liters of starting
culture fluid. The yield of IL 1 was relatively poor, however, being
about 2 percent of the starting material.

The purity of the final product was assessed using Tris-glycinate
polyacrylamide gel electrophoresis (Fig. 1). The IL 1 activity co-
migrated with two closely spaced bands that were easily detected using
Coomassie Blue stain. When the IL 1 was electrophoresed for an
additional hour, a third band of IL was detected (Figure 2). Using

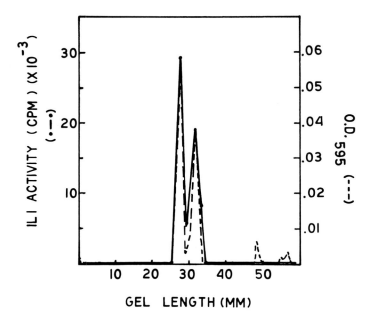

Figure 1. Tris-glycinate polyacrylamide gel electrophoresis of the
purified interleukin 1. The purified interleukin 1 (approximately 8 μg)
obtained after isoelectrofocusing was electrophoresed in 10% Tris-
glycinate discontinuous gels (0.5 mA/0.5 hr, 1 mA/hr, 2 mA/2hr). One
gel was stained with Coomassie Brilliant Blue and scanned at 595 μm to
detect the protein bands. A second identical gel was sliced into 2-mm
fragments and the interleukin 1 was eluted and assayed for thymocyte
proliferative activity. From Reference 6.

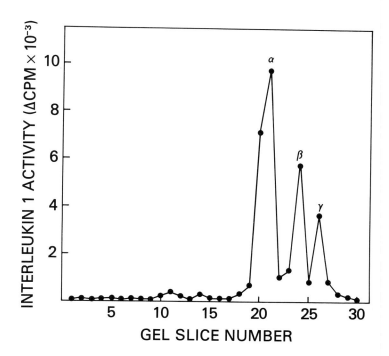

Figure 2.   Resolution of three charge species of purified interleukin
1.   The purified interleukin 1 was electrophoresed as described in
Figure 3 except that the gels were electrophoresed at 2 mA for 3 hr.
instead of 2 hr.   The charge species have been termed α, β, and γ.
From Reference 6.

   two-dimensional gel electrophoresis and a highly sensitive silver
stain, three proteins of molecular weight 14,000 that differed slightly
in charge (pI range 4.8-5.2) were detected.   Thus, we were able to
associate biologic activity with each detectable band, the activity
being proportional to protein content.   One unit of IL 1 was found to
equal 1 ng of protein; fifty percent of the maximal thymocyte proliferation being obtained with approximately 3.5×10^{-10} M IL 1.   In one liter
of superinduced $P388D_1$ cell culture fluid, we have detected as much as
1-2 mg of IL 1.
   The results of these studies clearly indicate that sufficient IL 1
can now be obtained for biologic and biochemical studies.   If the
purified IL 1 can be radiolabeled without loss of biologic activity, it
should now be possible to define and isolate the receptor of IL 1.
Monoclonal antibodies to such a receptor may prove to be of great
value in the treatment of various disorders, eg., rheumatoid arthritis,
that may involve an overproduction of IL 1.

References

1. Farrar, J. J., and Koopman, W. J. (1978): In <u>Biology of the Lymphokines</u>, edited by S. Cohen, E. Pick, and J. J. Oppenheim, pp. 325–346. Academic Press, New York.

2. Farrar, W. L., Mizel, S. B., and Farrar, J. J. (1980): <u>J. Immunol</u>. 124:1371–1377.

3. Mizel, S. B. (1980): <u>Mol. Immunol</u>. 17:571–577.

4. Mizel, S. B., and Ben-Zvi, A. (1980): <u>Cell. Immunol</u>. 54:383–389.

5. Mizel, S. B., Dayer, J. M., Krane, S. M., and Mergenhagen, S. E. (1981): <u>Proc. Natl. Acad. Sci. (USA)</u>, in press.

6. Mizel, S. B., and Mizel, D. (1981): <u>J. Immunol</u>. 126:834–837.

7. Oppenheim, J. J., and Rosenstreich, D. L. (1976): <u>Prog. Allergy</u> 120:1991–1995.

Lymphokines and Thymic Hormones: Their
Potential Utilization in Cancer Therapeutics,
edited by A. L. Goldstein and M. A. Chirigos,
Raven Press, New York © 1981.

Human Interleukins 1 and 2: Purification and Characterization

Lawrence B. Lachman, Frederick W. George IV,
and Richard S. Metzgar

*Department of Microbiology and Immunology, Duke University Medical Center,
Durham, North Carolina 27710*

INTRODUCTION

Monocytes and Lymphocytes release soluble mediators when stimulated in vitro by lectins and bacterial products. Although studied for many years, these mediators have been difficult to purify. A lymphocyte or monocyte culture medium exhibiting biological activity in vitro may contain less than 1ng/ml of the lymphokine or monokine. This exceptional biological activity indicates the importance of these mediators and may demonstrate the rapid, short range effect of these factors upon the immune response.

The observation by Morgan et.al.(15) that conditioned medium from PHA-stimulated human lymphocytes could support continuous growth of human T cells stimulated intense research into the nature of this factor. Now known as Interleukin 2 (IL 2), this factor also stimulated the generation of cytotoxic T cells, the induction of antibody response to heterlogous erythrocyte antigens in nude mice and allowed dilute cultures of thymocytes to respond to lectins (5). The release of IL 2 from lymphocytes was demonstrated to require lectin stimulation and the presence of macrophages. The macrophages could be replaced by macrophage culture medium and the active component of this medium was identified as Interleukin 1 (IL 1) previously known as Lymphocyte Activating Factor (12,17,18). IL 1 is also able to stimulate the generation of cytotoxic T cells and increase the number of antibody forming cells, but cannot sustain continuous growth of T cells (2).

The Interleukins are distinct molecules which may have significant clinical value for the treatment of immunodeficiency diseases. Also, the Interleukins may be useful as non-specific immunostimulants in cancer therapy. In this paper we discuss our recent progress which has led to the purification to homogeneity of human IL 1 and preliminary characterization of human IL 2. Also, biological properties of the factors are discussed.

MATERIALS AND METHODS

Most materials and methods used in this paper have been previously described (10). IL 1 containing medium was prepared from acute monocytic leukemic cells following LPS stimulation. IL 1 was assayed as increased (^{3}H)thymidine incorporation by CD-1 thymocytes (without lectin stimulation. IL 2 containing medium was prepared from ficoll-hypaque purified peripheral blood cells stimulated with PHA and an allogeneic human B cell line (1). IL 2 was assayed as increased (^{3}H)thymidine incorporation by 10-21 day old continuous T cell lines (CTC) established from PHA-stimulated human blood using IL 2 containing growth medium. Units of IL 1 and IL 2 activity were calculated according to the procedure of Gillis, et.al.(3)

RESULTS AND DISCUSSION

Production of IL 1 from Acute Monocytic Leukemia Cells

Leukemic cells from Acute Monocytic Leukemia (AMoL) or non-specific esterase positive Acute Myelomonocytic Leukemia (AMML) release IL 1 into the culture medium (8). The leukemic cells, like peripheral blood monocytes, release IL 1 into the culture medium following LPS stimulation. The blood and serum of our most recent AMoL patient was screened for IL 1 activity and found to be negative. Blood and serum of earlier patients were not tested.

Leukemic cells offer a valuable source of IL 1 and other factors since the cells can often be obtained in great quantity (10^{11} - 10^{12}) when patients require therapeutic leukophoresis. The leukemic cells can be frozen or used at once to prepare very large quantities of IL 1 from a single donor. Also, the cells can be cultured at high densities to result in extremely active conditioned medium.

AMoL cells, 2×10^{10} frozen at -60° in 50 ml tubes, were slowly thawed and added to a spinner flask containing six liters of MEM, 5% normal human serum and 10 µg/ml E.coli LPS. The cells were stirred for 48 hrs. at 37° at which time the cells were discarded following centrifugation and the conditioned medium was frozen in 500 ml aliquots. The conditioned medium exhibited IL 1 activity in the thymocyte assay at a final dilution of 1:1,000.

Purification of AMoL Cell IL 1

Hollow Fiber Diafiltration and Ultrafiltration. This procedure has been recently described in detail (10). Briefly, 1 liter of conditioned medium was extracted with 10 L of 0.85% NaCl using a 50,000 MW cut off hollow fiber device. IL 1 activity was found in both the <50,000 MW diafiltrate and the >50,000 MW extracted medium. The diafiltrate (10 L) was concentrated overnight using three ultrafiltration cells with YM10 membranes, a reservoir and an automatic shut-off device. In the morning the 10,000-50,000 MW pool (500 mls) was ultrafiltered using the same hollow fiber device used initially. The purpose of this procedure was to remove the small quantities of >50,000 MW serum proteins which were able to pass through the hollow fiber cartridge during diafiltration. The ultrafiltrate (450 mls) was concentrated to 40 mls using a stirred cell with YM10 membrane and further purified by isoelectric focusing (IEF).

Isoelectric focusing of the 10-50,000 MW Fraction. The 40 mls sample was isoelectrically focused for 20 hrs. at 4° in a pH 4-8 Ampholine and sucrose gradient (10). The pH 6.8-7.2 region was found to contain the IL 1 activity (Figure 1).

Preparative Gel Purification of the IEF Activity. Previous experiments (7) have demonstrated IEF purified IL 1 could be further purified by non-denaturing polyacrylamide gel electrophoresis (PAGE). Unfortunately, this procedure did not result in homogeneous IL 1. Analytical PAGE of the gel purified activity demonstrated the presence of transferrin as well as IL 1. For this reason we decided to take advantage of the low MW of IL 1 (about 12,000 as determined by gel filtration) by performing preparative SDS-PAGE. The IEF purified IL 1 was dialyzed against water for 1 day and lyophylized. The lyophylized sample was hydrated in 25 microliters of sample buffer (not containing sulfhydryl reducing agents) and heated for 2 hrs. at 37°. SDS-PAGE of the sample was performed at 10° using a 15% gel of 100 X 5.5 mm with a 5mm 3% stacking gel (11). Identically prepared gels containing prestained MW standards and standards to be stained following the run were used to calibrate the gels. Following electrophoresis, the IL 1 containing gel was sliced into 100 1mm slices and eluted overnight to recover the IL 1 activity. The SDS was removed from the fractions by dialysis for 48 hrs. against 0.85% NaCl, and the fractions assayed in the thymocyte assay for IL 1 activity.

In Figure 2 is seen the results of such an assay, as compared with an analytical slab gel of the IEF purified activity. The IL 1 activity was found to correspond with a darkly staining band of approximately 11,000 MW. Analytical SDS-PAGE of the gel purified IL 1 activity demonstrated a single protein band. The recovery of biological activity following preparative SDS-PAGE was quite low but this

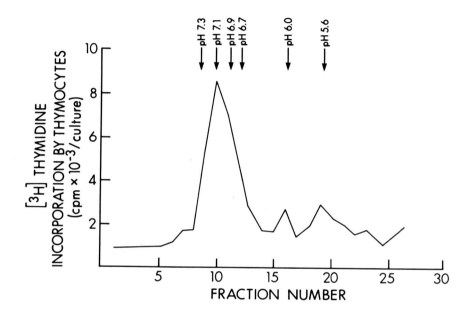

Fig. 1.   Isoelectric Focusing of the 10-50,000 MW IL 1
Activity.   The 10-50,000 MW fraction of IL 1 activity was
further purified by sucrose gradient IEF in a pH 4-8
Ampholine gradient.   At the conclusion of the IEF (18 hrs.
at 4°, 1600 V constant power), 1.5 ml fractions were
collected, the pH determined, and each fraction dialyzed
for 24 hrs. at 4° against 0.85% NaCl.   The amount of IL 1
activity in each fraction was measured in the (^{3}H)thymidine
incorporation assay using mouse thymocytes.   The profile
of activity shown above was obtained using the IEF fractions
at a final concentration of 1% (V/V) in the thymocyte
assay.

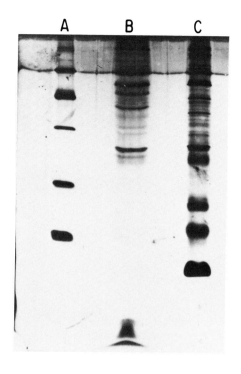
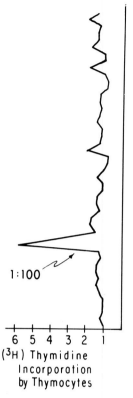

1:100

6 5 4 3 2 1
(^{3}H) Thymidine
Incorporation
by Thymocytes

Fig. 2.   SDS-Polyacrylamide Gel Electrophoresis of
IEF Purified IL 1.   The pH 6.7-7.3 fraction from IEF
(Figure 1) were pooled (7 ml) and dialyzed against deion-
ize water for 24 hrs.   The sample was divided into seven
1 ml aliquots and lyophylized.   One aliquot was applied
to a 15% analytical slab gel and another aliquot was
applied to a 15% tube gel.   The IEF purified IL 1 activity
(C) contained many protein bands, but in particular three
bands of <20,000 MW which were not found in an identically
purified sample of control medium (B) which contained
medium and serum but no cells.   The MW standards (A) are
94K, 67K, 43K, 30K, 20.1K and 14.4K.   A (^{3}H)thymidine
incorporation assay of the tube gel slices of the IEF
purified activity demonstrated a single peak of IL 1
activity which corresponded with the darkly staining band
of ~11,000 MW.   The recovered IL 1 was active at a final
concentration of 1% (V/V) and when tested again by SDS-
PAGE in an 18% gel, demonstrated a single protein band.
The AgNO$_3$ staining procedure is described in (10).

material should be suitable for protein characterization studies, including sequence determination and preparation of hybridoma antibody.

Recovery of IL 1 Following the Complete Purification. The overall recovery of IL 1 activity was quite poor and exemplifies the necessity of beginning purifications with extremely active medium. The recovery of units of IL 1 activity following the hollow fiber procedure was about 40% and recovery following IEF was usually about 4%. The IEF procedure results in a poor overall recovery of activity but very efficiently separates IL 1 from albumin, the major protein present in the hollow fiber fraction. Various techniques such as performing the IEF in the presence of non-ionic detergents and reducing agents did not increase the recovery of IL 1. It should be noted that the extremely hydrophobic nature of IL 1 probably accounts for much of the loss of IL 1 activity during purification. IL 1 binds to most sterile filters and must be filtered with hydrophobic filters (Gelman Acrodiscs) or in the presence of serum (9). Also, IL 1 binds irreversibly to many ultrafiltration membranes (not YM series of hydrophobic membranes) and to many types of gel filtration media.

As noted above, preparative SDS-PAGE of the IEF activity results in poor recovery of biological activity, but significant recovery of homogeneous protein. The amount of protein recovered from the preparative gel can be estimated by comparing the intensity of silver staining with known amounts of protein. Conventional protein determinations such as Lowry or Bradford would require that the entire SDS-PAGE purified sample be used for a single protein determination. The amount of protein recovered from the preparative gel was estimated to be 3 μg per liter of starting conditioned medium. The amount of IL 1 in the original conditioned medium can be estimated from the IEF purified material (Fig. 2). The amount of IL 1 in the IEF purified sample from 1 L of conditioned medium is about 3 μg and the yield is 4%. This implies that one liter of conditioned medium used for the purification contained approximately 75 μg of IL 1 or 75 ng of IL 1 per ml.

Biological Properties of IEF Purified IL 1. Table 1 summarizes some biological properties of IEF-purified IL 1.

TABLE 1. Biological Properties of IEF Purified Human
IL-1

1. Induces a non-endotoxin fever in rabbits
    following IV administration ($\Delta 1^{\circ}$/ml)[a]
2. Induces the appearance of neutrophils in the
    circulating blood of rats following IV
    administration ($\Delta 7,500$/mm^3 1 hr. post injection
    of 0.1 ml)[b]
3. Increase plasma levels of fibrinogen in rats
    24 hrs. following IV injection ($\Delta 43$ mg% per 0.25
    ml injected)[b]
4. Non-specific protease free[c]
5. Mitogenic for both peanut agglutinin + and -
    mouse thymocyte subpopulations[d]
6. Mitogenic for lectin-stimulated human T cells
    and thymocytes[e]

[a]Experiments performed by Elisha Atkins, Yale
University Medical School. The IL 1 preparations are
negative for the endotoxin as tested by the Limulus
lysate assay.
[b]Experiments performed by Ralph Kampschmidt, Nobel
Foundation.
[c]Experiments performed by Gerald Lazarus, Duke
University Medical Center using (^{3}H) cassein as substrate.
[d]Otterness et.al.(16) for lectin-stimulated subpopulations and unpublished data for direct stimulation of subpopulations.
[e]Maizel, et.al. (13).

Purification of Human IL 2

Hollow Fiber Diafiltration and Ultrafiltration. One
liter of IL 2 containing medium was diafiltered with 10L of
0.85% NaCl as described for IL 1. The 10L diafiltrate was
concentrated to 500 mls using ultrafiltration cells with
YM 10 membranes. Concentration of the sample to volumes of
less than 500 mls was found to greatly reduce the recovery
of IL 2. The 500 ml sample was concentrated to 40 mls by
dehydration using dialysis tubing and solid polyethylene
glycol (2X10^7 MW) flakes. The concentrated sample was
dialyzed overnight in the same bag against 4 liters of 0.85%
NaCl.

IEF of the 10-50,000 MW Fraction. The dialyzed fraction
was further purified by sucrose gradient IEF in a pH 6-9
gradient. The fractions were dialyzed against 0.85% NaCl
containing 0.1% PEG (6,000 MW) for 1 day. The PEG does not
effect the IL 2 assay. IL 2 activity was recovered as two
sharp peaks of average isoelectric points pH 6.8 and 8.0

and a minor peak of pH 7.4 (Fig. 3A). Human 10-14 day old
continuous T cell lines (CTC) were used for the (^{3}H) thymidine incorporation assay. Previous experiments using pH
3-10 gradients demonstrated only these three peaks of
activity.

The Effect of IEF Purified IL 2 on Various Human and
Mouse Cells. The IEF fractions were tested in (^{3}H) thymidine incorporation assays using unstimulated human thymocytes (Fig. 3B) and peripheral blood cells with and without a submitogenic amount of PHA (0.004%) (Fig. 3C). The
results indicate that the same fractions which were mitogenic for human CTC were also mitogenic for unstimulated
human thymocytes. The fractions were very weakly mitogenic
for peripheral blood cells in the absence of lectin but
were mitogenic in the presence of suboptimal PHA.

The same IEF fractions were tested in (^{3}H)thymidine
incorporation assays using mouse CTC (Fig. 4B) and unstimulated mouse thymus (Fig. 4C) and spleen cells (Fig. 4D).
The results demonstrated that all three peaks were mitogenic
for mouse CTC, but that the pH 8.0 peak was not mitogenic
for mouse thymocytes or spleen cells.

The Hetergeneity of Human IL 2. The pH 6.8 peak for
human IL 2 has been previously described (5,6,14) but the
pH 8.0 and pH 7.4 peaks have not. There are many possible
explanations for the heterogeneity of our IL 2 preparations.
It is possible that serum proteases may degrade the IL 2
molecule releasing biologically active fragments with different specificity for certain cell types. If this is the
case, these molecules may be used to study the IL 2
receptor(s) as well as the appearance of new IL 2 receptors
following lectin stimulation. For example, mouse thymocytes
will not incorporate (^{3}H)thymidine following stimulation
with the pH 8 peak alone, but will following Con A stimulation (data not shown). This observation may imply the
induction of a new receptor specific for the pH 8 IL 2.

Sephadex chromatography of the 10-50,000 MW fraction
demonstrated a single sharp peak of IL 2 activity with an
average MW of 15,000. No activity of lower MW was observed.
IEF of this 15,000 Sephadex peak revealed the pH 6.8, 7.4
and 8.0. Thus, these activities appear to have the accepted
MW for IL 2. IL 2 prepared according to the procedure of
Mier and Gallo (14) uses bovine serum album (BSA) as a
serum substitute. This technique does not eliminate the
possibility of cellular protease release during the 72 hr.
incubation period. Mier and Gallo (14), Hirano et.al. (6)
and Gillis et.al. (5) observed the pH 6.8 peak as the only
peak following IEF. All three purification procedures used
ammonium sulfate (AS) precipitation as an early step in
purification. Several times we concentrated the 500 ml 10-
50,000 MW fraction by 75% AS precipitation and recovered
comparable activity to experiments using PEG dehydration
but as noted by Mier and Gallo (14), we found that IEF of

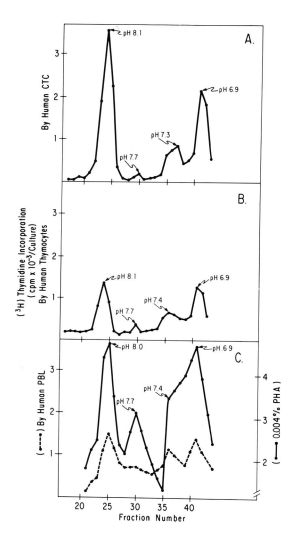

Fig. 3. Isoelectric Focusing of 10-50,000 MW IL 2
Activity. IEF of the 10-50,000 MW fraction of IL 2
activity was assayed using human CTC (A), human thymocytes
(B) and human peripheral blood cells (C) in a (^{3}H)thymidine
incorporation assay. Human CTC were cultured at a cell
density of 5 X 10^5/ml, human thymocytes at 1 X 10^7/ml and
ficoll-hypaque purified peripheral blood cells were
cultured at a cell density of 1 X 10^6/ml. The conditions
for the (^{3}H)thymidine incorporation assays were the same
as described for IL 1 assays (10).

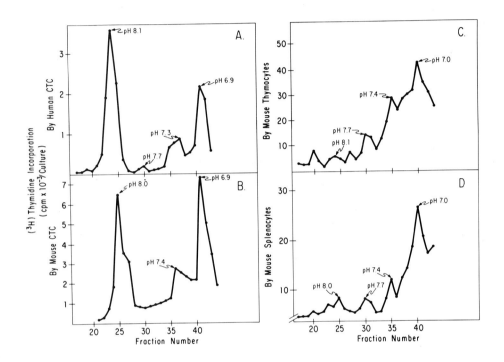

Fig. 4. Isoelectric Focusing of 10-50,000 MW IL 2 Activity. The IEF fractions from Figure 3 were assayed using human CTC (A, same as Figure 3A), mouse CTC (B), mouse thymocytes (C) and mouse spleen cells (D) in a (^{3}H) thymidine incorporation assay. The mouse CTC assay was kindly performed by Dr. Kendall A. Smith. The mouse thymocyte and spleen cell culture conditons were the same as described for IL 1 assays (10) except that spleen cells were cultured at 1 X 10^6/ml.

the AS precipitate resulted in extremely poor recovery of
activity. The pH 8 peak is probably not soluble in 75% AS
since the dialyzed supernatant did not contain IL2 activity.
The pH 8 peak may be irreversibly denatured by AS or may be
less stable than the pH 6.8 peak and thus explains its
absence following IEF.

Recovery of IL 2 Activity Following IEF. The recovery
of IL 2 activity following IEF is extremely poor. The
overall yield of the pH 7 activity is 0.6% and the pH 8
activity is 0.3%. The 10-50,000 MW PEG concentrated sample
prior to IEF contained 35% of the original activity. The
inclusion of PEG in the IEF solutions, as also noted by
Mier and Gallo, did not increase the recovery of IL 2
activity. Neither Gillis et.al.(5) nor Hirano et.al. (6)
calculated their recovery of the pH 6.8 peak following IEF.
Thus, the IEF procedure is of very low yield, but does
separate the biologically and biochemically distinct IL 2
activities.

SUMMARY

Human Interleukin 1 (IL 1), prepared in large quantities
from acute monocytic leukemia cells, has been purified to
homogeneity. Purification of human Interleukin 2 (IL 2) has
progressed more slowly due to the lack of a cell source
which releases large amounts of activity. IL 2 exhibits an
interesting biochemical and biological heterogeneity not
exhibited by IL 1.

ACKNOWLEDGEMENTS

The authors wish to sincerely thank Mrs. Stella O. Page
for careful technical assistance. Also, we wish to thank
Mr. Ralph Willet, Ms. Grace Wojno and Ms. Michelle
Pallidino for laboratory assistance. Finally, we wish to
thank Ms. Karen King for the careful preparation of this
manuscript.

REFERENCES

1. Bonnard, G.D., Yasaka, K. and Maca, R.D. (1980):
   Cell. Immunol., 51: 390-398.

2. Farrar, J.J., Simon, P.L., Farrar, W.L., Koopman,
   W.J. and Fuller-Bonar, J. (1979): Ann. N.Y. Acad.
   Sci., 332: 303-315.

3. Gillis, S., Fern, M.M., Ov, W. and Smith, K.A.
   (1978): J. Immunol., 120: 2027-2036.

4. Gillis, S., Scheid, M. and Watson, J. (1980): J.
   Immunol., 125: 2570-2577.

5. Gillis, S., Smith, K.A. and Watson, J. (1980): J. Immunol., 124: 1954-1962.

6. Hirano, T., et.al., (1981): J. Immunol., 126: 517-522.

7. Lachman, L.B., Hacker, M.P. and Handschumacher, R.E. (1977): J. Immunol., 119: 2019-2023.

8. Lachman, L.B., Moore, J.O. and Metzgar, R.S. (1978): Cell. Immunol., 41: 199-206.

9. Lachman, L.B. and Metzgar, R.S. (1980): J. Reticuloendothelial Soc., 27: 621-629.

10. Lachman, L.B., Page, S.O. and Metzgar, R.S. (1980): J. Supramol. Struct., 13: 457-466.

11. Laemmli, V.K. (1970): Nature, 277: 680-685.

12. Larsson, E.L., Iscove, N.I. and Coutinho, A. (1980): Nature, 283: 664-666.

13. Maizel, A.L., Mehta, S.R., Ford, R.J. and Lachman, L.B. (1981): J. Exp. Med., 153: 470-475.

14. Mier, J.W. and R.C. Gallo., (1980): Pro. Nat. Acad. Sci., 77: 6134-6138.

15. Morgan, D.A., Roscetti, F.W. and Gallo, R.C. (1978): Science, 193: 1007-1008.

16. Otterness, I.G., Lachman, L.B. and Bliven, M.L. (1981): Immunopharmacology, 3: 61-69.

17. Shaw, J.P., Caplan, B., Paetkav, V., Pilarski, L.M., Delovitch, T.L. and McKenzi, I.F.C. (1980): J. Immunol., 124: 2231-2239.

18. Smith, K.A., Lachman, L.B., Oppenheim, J.J. and Favata, M.F. (1980): J. Exp. Med., 151: 1551-1556.

Lymphokines and Thymic Hormones: Their
Potential Utilization in Cancer Therapeutics,
edited by A. L. Goldstein and M. A. Chirigos,
Raven Press, New York © 1981.

The Characterization of Human T-Cell Growth Factor and Its Role in the Proliferation of Malignant T-Cells

J. Mier and R. C. Gallo

Laboratory of Tumor Cell Biology, National Cancer Institute, National Institutes of Health,
Bethesda, Maryland 20205

Several years ago, Morgan et al (12) reported the discovery of a factor termed T-cell growth factor (TCGF) which is released into the tissue culture media by human peripheral blood mononuclear cells after stimulation with PHA. The stimulation of T-cells with antigens or lectins such as PHA routinely leads to the growth of these cells for only a few days. The cultured cells inevitably terminate their growth and shortly thereafter lose viability. However, the periodic addition of the factor present in the media conditioned by PHA-stimulated lymphocytes (LyCM) to antigen or lectin-stimulated bone marrow or peripheral blood lymphocytes led to the reproducible, continuous propagation of cultured T-lymphocytes for extended periods. The proliferating cells were unequivocally identified as normal T-cells by several cytochemical, immunological, and functional criteria (20). Even after months in culture, these cells remained absolutely dependent on the factor for continuous growth and retained a normal karyotype. These observations have been repeatedly confirmed in human systems and subsequently duplicated in several other species (4,18).

Recently, the mitogenic effects of TCGF were distinguished from those of lectins (8,11). TCGF has clearly been shown to induce proliferation only of T-cells that have been previously activated by a lectin or allo-antigen, whereas PHA induces blast transformation in resting T-cells. This specificity for activated T-cells has been exploited by several investigators who have used media containing TCGF at various levels of purification to sustain in tissue culture T-cells with specific cytotoxic functions (19,22).

Recently, studies from our laboratory have shown that malignant T-cells from patients with a variety of T-cell lymphoproliferative diseases can be regularly grown in culture with the addition of partially purified, lectin-free, TCGF to the culture media (13). This observation has suggested a previously unsuspected relationship between lectin or alloantigen-primed normal T-lymphoblasts and those resulting from malignant transformation. The longterm growth of several T-lymphoblastoid cell lines from patients with acute T-cell lymphoblastic leukemia and cutaneous T-cell lymphoma has been reported (13). These lines have been maintained in culture for several months and have been characterized as Epstein-Barr virus nuclear antigen negative and sheep erythrocyte rosette positive. Three lines have become independent of exogenous growth factor and have been shown to elaborate small quantities of TCGF detectable in the conditioned media. At present, there appears to be a concordance between the constituitive production of TCGF (i.e.

without lectin or alloantigen stimulation) and the presence of a novel type C retrovirus isolable from such cell lines (14).

Human T-cell growth factor has been purified to apparent homogeneity from serum-free lymphocyte conditioned media by utilizing ion exchange chromatography with DEAE-Sepharose, gel filtration with Ultrogel AcA54, and preparative $NaDodSO_4$-polyacrylamide gel electrophoresis (SDS-PAGE)(11). This mitogenic protein has a molecular weight of 13,000 as determined by SDS-PAGE and 20,000 to 25,000 by gel filtration, an isoelectric point of 6.8, and, based upon its failure to adhere to any of several lectin-sepharoses, may not be glycosylated. The material extracted from acryl-amide gels is a single homogeneous band when analysed on analytical SDS gels. The highly purified material is unstable even at -70° and requires the addition of bovine serum albumin or polyethylene glycol to maintain biological activity. It is sensitive to proteolytic digestion but resistant to nucleases and thiol reducing agents such as dithiothre-itol. Human TCGF can be reversibly denatured with urea or sodium dodecyl sulfate. The purified factor has been shown to sustain T-lym-phoblasts in tissue culture and to lack other lymphokine activities, including colony stimulating activity (CSA), interferon, and B-cell mitogenic activity. In contrast to lectins such as PHA, certain anti-gens, and crude lymphocyte conditioned media, purified TCGF does not initiate lymphocyte blastogenesis, but is a highly selective mitogen for T-cells previously activated by exposure to lectins or antigens.

PURIFICATION OF HUMAN TCGF

TCGF Bioassay

Target T-cells for the bioassays were prepared from the heparinized blood of normal laboratory personnel. Mononuclear cells, obtained with the use of Lymphocyte Separation Media (Pharmacia), were incubated at 10^6 cells/ml in RPMI 1640 with 20% fetal calf serum and PHA-P (10 ug/ml) at 37° in a humidified incubator adjusted to maintain 5% CO_2. The cell cultures were fed every 5 days with media supplemented with a dilution of an $(NH_4)_2SO_4$ precipitate of LyCM as described previously (11,12). When these cells have been maintained in culture for several days, they no longer respond to PHA and depend exclusively on the periodic addition of TCGF for further growth (11). The cells intended for use in bio-assays were kept 5-7 days without reexposure to fresh TCGF in an effort to minimize the effect of the TCGF used to maintain the culture on sub-sequent assays. All samples to be assayed were dialysed against physio-logic buffers. Briefly, 0.2 ml of the fraction to be assayed, 0.2 ml of the T-cell suspension containing 2×10^5 cells, and 1.6 ml of a mixture of RPMI 1640 media and 20% FCS were incubated at 37° for 48 hrs. After the addition of 0.2 ml ^{3}H-thymidine (10 uC/ml, 0.36 C/mmole), the cells were incubated overnight, washed, and precipitated with TCA. The pre-cipitates were collected onto glass fiber filters, dried, and the radio-activity determined in a scintillation counter. Serial dilutions were assayed as described previously to quantitate the TCGF in the assayed samples (4). Bioassays based upon estimates of DNA synthesis in cultured T-cells as described above directly correlated with growth as determined by counting the number of cells daily after exposure to the test sample.

Production of Lymphocyte Conditioned Media.

Human mononuclear cells obtained from buffy coats of multiple (3-20) normal donors were processed over nylon wool columns and incubated at 10^6 cells/ml in RPMI 1640 containing 10 ug/ml PHA-P, 0.25% BSA and no serum at 37° for 72 hrs. The cells were then removed by centrifugation and the media kept frozen until used for purification.

Ammonium Sulfate Precipitation.

With the exception of SDS-PAGE, all purification steps were carried out at 4°. The crude LyCM was clarified by centrifugation at 1,000 x g for 10 min and the supernatant subsequently filtered to remove gross cellular debris. Ammonium sulfate in sufficient quantity to produce a 50% saturated solution was slowly added to the LyCM, and after stirring for 1 hr, the precipitate was removed by centrifugation at 10,000 x g for 10 min. Ammonium sulfate was again added to the supernatant to produce an 80% saturated solution, and after stirring for 3 hrs, the suspension was centrifuged as above and the supernatant discarded. The precipitate was dissolved in a minimal amount of 10 mM tris-HCl buffer, pH 8.0, containing 0.1 mM phenylmethyl sulfonyl fluoride, 0.01% polyethylene glycol (6,000), and 1.0 mM dithiothreitol, (henceforth designated buffer A), and the solution was dialysed thoroughly against this buffer.

Chromatography with DEAE-Sepharose

The dialysed precipitate was subsequently placed on a 100 ml column of DEAE-Sepharose equilibrated with buffer A and the column was rinsed with buffer to eliminate unbound protein. The TCGF was eluted in 10 ml fractions with a 500 ml NaCl/buffer A gradient ranging from 0 to 0.15 M NaCl as shown in FIG. 1.

Ultrogel AcA54 Chromatography.

The active fractions from ion exchange chromatography, numbers 31-40, were pooled, concentrated to 5 ml on an Amicon UM – 05 membrane, and placed on a column of Ultrogel AcA54 (2.5 x 170 cm), previously equilibrated with phosphate buffered saline/1 mM dithiothreitol/0.1 mM phenylmethyl sulfonyl fluoride/0.1% polyethylene glycol (6,000), (henceforth designed buffer B). The chromatography was run at a flow rate of 15 ml/hr, and 10 ml fractions were collected. As shown in FIG. 2, the TCGF activity emerged between 550 and 650 ml, which corresponded to a molecular weight range of approximately 20,000 to 25,000. The active fractions were pooled, dialyzed against buffer A, and passed over a 10 ml column of DEAE-Sepharose. The proteins were concentrated by a step elution from the ion exchanger using buffer B as the eluant followed by a further reduction to 5 ml, achieved by dialysis against unswollen Sephadex G-100 (Pharmacia). The resulting material was again chromatographed on Ultrogel AcA54, and the TCGF-containing fractions pooled and concentrated as before on a small DEAE-Sepharose column.

Preparative SDS-PAGE

Preparative SDS-PAGE was performed with a BioRad Model 221 gel apparatus using a 1.5 mm, 13% acrylamide gel, polymerized with riboflavin (21). The acrylamide gel and reservoir buffer contained 0.1% SDS. The TCGF concentrate was dialysed against buffer A and denatured by incubation with 1% SDS (no mercaptoethanol) for 2 hrs at 37°. Bromphenol blue and glycerol were added and the sample layered onto a 3% acrylamide spacer gel. The electrophoresis was carried out at 120 volts for approximately 16 hrs. The gel matrix was subsequently sliced into 0.5

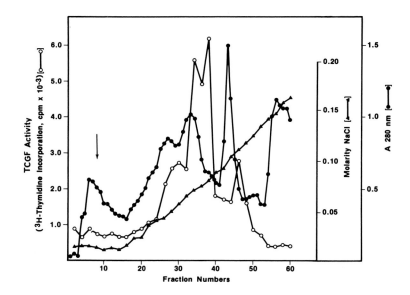

FIG. 1, Ion exchange chromatography with DEAE-Sepharose. Proteins were eluted with a tris-buffered NaCl gradient. TCGF activity is represented by (0-0), the absorbency of the protein solutions at 280 nm by (●-●), and the molarity of NaCl, determined by conductivity, by (▲-▲). The arrow signifies the beginning of the gradient. Fraction numbers 31-40 were pooled for further purification.

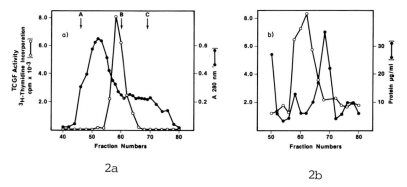

FIG. 2, Gel filtration with Ultrogel AcA54. TCGF activity is represented by (0-0). Post-ion exchange material was concentrated and chromatographed by gel filtration with Ultrogel AcA54, as shown in (2a). Protein concentrations are represented by absorbence at 280 nm (●-●). The TCGF-containing fractions were concentrated and chromatographed again by gel filtration, as shown in (2b). In the second gel filtration, protein concentrations were determined by the Lowry method. Arrows A, B, and C locate the elution points of the molecular weight standards BSA, chymotrypsinogen, and lysozyme respectively.

cm horizontal strips which were macerated through a syringe. Seven ml of buffer B were added, and the proteins extracted by gentle agitation at room temperature for 16 hrs. The SDS was removed by passing the extract over AG-1x8 resin (BioRad) (24), and after the pH was adjusted by dialysis against phosphate buffered saline, the fractions were filter sterilized and assayed as described previously. The TCGF activity was consistently associated with a fraction corresponding to a molecular weight of 13,000. A stained SDS gel of this fraction and an autoradiogram of this protein are shown in FIG.3.

Specific Activity Determinations.

Serial dilutions of pooled fractions at various stages in the purifi-

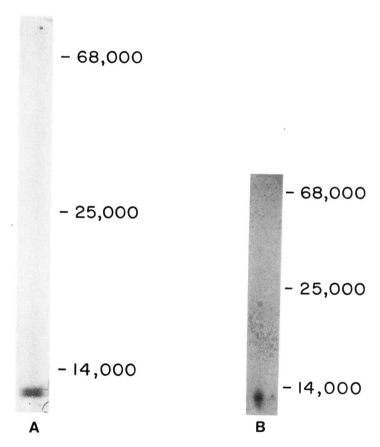

A   **B**

FIG. 3, Analytical SDS-PAGE of purified TCGF. Purified TCGF extracted from preparative SDS-polyacrylamide gels was rerun on an analytical SDS gel and the proteins visualized with the silver stain described previously (10). This is shown in gel (A). Similarly, a portion of the gel extract was iodinated with I^{125}, and an autoradiogram of this material is shown in (B). In both studies a band of molecular weight 13,000 was visualized.

cation sequence were quantitatively assayed as shown in Table I. An absolute, functional definition of TCGF activity based upon the ability of the factor to effect a predictable, reproducible response in T-cells is not possible due to target cell variability. One unit of TCGF activity was therefore arbitrarily defined as the amount present in one ml of unprocessed LyCM, and the activities of other preparations were defined by comparison with this standard. Assays of serial dilutions of partially purified TCGF fractions give rise to a series of parallel, negatively sloped lines which allow calculation of the relative potencies and total activities of the samples assayed (4). Protein determinations used in the computation of the specific activities were obtained by utilizing a modification of the Lowry method (9).

TABLE I. PURIFICATION OF HUMAN TCGF

	PROTEIN (mg)	TOTAL ACTIVITY	YIELD (%)	SPECIFIC ACTIVITY	PURIFICATION (fold)
Crude lyCM	11,760	4000	100	.34	1.0
$(NH_4)_2SO_4$ ppt.	9,750	3800	95	.39	1.14
DEAE – Sepharose	500	1440	36	2.88	8.47
1st Ultrogel	52	1080	27	20.7	60.9
2nd Ultrogel	1.49	369	9.2	255	750
Preparative SDS-PAGE	0.11	32	0.8	275	808

One unit of TCGF was defined as the amount present in one ml of crude LyCM. The total activity of the different fractions was calculated by multiplying the fraction volume by its potency relative to crude LyCM, as determined by assaying serial dilutions.

BIOCHEMICAL CHARACTERIZATION OF TCGF

Isoelectric Point Determination

Partially purified TCGF obtained by anion exchange chromatography with DEAE-Sepharose was dialysed against 10 mM Tris-HCl, pH 8.0, and after the addition of 2% ampholines (LKB) and 0.1% PEG, was focused overnight at 8.0 watts using an LKB Multiphor unit. The Ultradex gel matrix was sliced and the pH of the individual slices determined. The gel slices were suspended in PBS/0.1% PEG, poured into 5 ml syringe columns, and rinsed with the same buffer. Ampholines were removed by passing the protein solutions over AG-501 resin (BioRad), and the fractions were sterilized and assayed as described previously. The results of the focusing experiment are shown below in FIG.4. TCGF focused as a single peak at pH 6.5 with a trace component at pH 7.2. SDS-PAGE of the fractions generated by isoelectric focusing has shown a clustering of contaminant proteins in the same pH range as TCGF when the sample undergoing focusing was first subjected to ion exchange chromatography, thus rendering redundant the focusing step. However, if the crude LyCM was processed through gel filtration without ion exchange chromatography as a preliminary purification step, isoelectric focusing removed several proteins and in particular provided a quantitative resolution between TCGF and the granulocyte-macrophage colony stimulating activity present in the starting material (11).

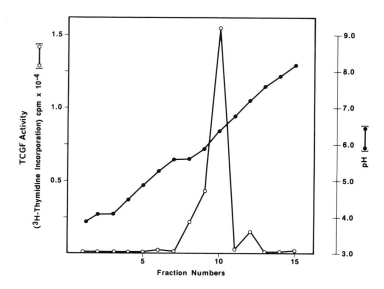

FIG. 4, Isoelectric focusing of TCGF. TCGF activity is denoted by (0-0) and the pH of the fractions assayed by (●-●). The TCGF focused as a sharp peak at pH 6.5,

Stabilization of Purified Factor.
  Human TCGF was extremely unstable at low protein concentrations. Preparations purified with ion exchange and molecular sieve chromatography without the benefit of specific buffer additives became inactive after storage at 4° for two weeks. This loss of activity could be prevented by the addition of bovine albumin or PEG (6,000) after partial purification. Freezing at -70° and the addition of other substances, including non-ionic detergents, protease inhibitors, reducing agents, and alcohols failed to maintain biological activity. The stabilizing agents tested are listed in Table II. Although the necessity of including a protease inhibitor and a sulfhydryl reagent in the chromatography buffers remains unproven, these have been empirically added with PEG to all buffers employed in the purification of the lymphokine.

TABLE II.   EFFECT OF VARIOUS BUFFER ADDITIVES ON TCGF STABILITY

ADDITIVE	RECOVERY (%)
None (4°C)	0
None (-70°C)	0
Mercaptoethanol (BME) 1 mM	0
Phenylmethyl Sulfonyl Fluoride (PMSF) 0.1 mM	0
BME, PMSF (-70°C)	0
Triton X-100 .01%	0
Triton X-100 .001%	0
Glycerol 10%	0
Ethylene Glycol 10%	0
PEG (6,000) 0.1%	100
Bovine Serum Albumin (BSA) 0.25%	65

TCGF, purified by sequential ion exchange chromatography and gel filtration, was kept for two weeks at 4°C in the presence of the above
additives. After dialysis, the samples were assayed for residual activity. The PEG-preserved material was arbitrarily selected as a 100%
control and the activities of the other samples expressed in relation to
this standard. PEG (6,000) and BSA were the only additives capable to
stabilizing TCGF activity. Freezing at -70°C had no protective effect.

Molecular Weight Determination.

The molecular weight of TCGF as determined by preparative SDS-PAGE is
considerably less than that predicted by gel filtration. This discre-
pancy is thought to be secondary to aggregation of the TCGF molecules,
which is illustrated below in FIG. 5. TCGF, purified by SDS-PAGE (13,000
molecular weight band), and labelled with I^{125} was applied to a column
of Ultrogel AcA54 (2.5 x 90 cm), equilibrated with phosphate buffered
saline/0.1% PEG.   Several radioactive peaks were generated, two of
which corresponded to the monomeric and dimeric molecular weights predicted by SDS-PAGE. Bioassay results of fractions obtained by gel filtration in the presence of 4.0 M urea were essentially identical to
those shown in FIG.2, in which the major activity peak corresponded to
the 20,000 to 25,000 molecular weight range. Exposure to 1 mM DTT did
not alter the biological activity of the growth factor nor have any dis-
cernible effect on molecular weight as determined by gel filtration or
SDS-PAGE, suggesting that the molecular structure of TCGF does not com-
prise several peptide chains linked through disulfide bonds. The aggregation is presumably due to the hydrophobicity of the growth factor.

THE PROLIFERATIVE EFFECTS OF TCGF ON NORMAL AND MALIGNANT T-CELLS

The growth of T-Lymphoblasts with Purified TCGF

Sufficient purified growth factor has been recovered from acrylamide
gels to demonstrate its proliferative effect on activated T-cells after

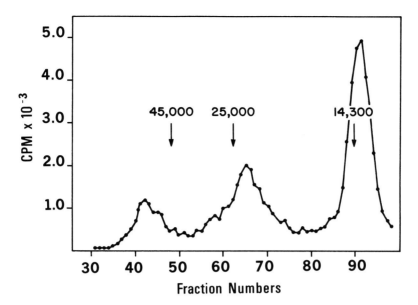

FIG. 5. Aggregation of purified TCGF. TCGF extracted from the 13,000 molecular weight region of an SDS-polyacrylamide gel was iodinated with I^{125} and chromatographed on an Ultrogel AcA54 column equilibrated with phosphate-buffered saline, and the radioactivity of the various fractions recorded. The arrows represent molecular weight standards.

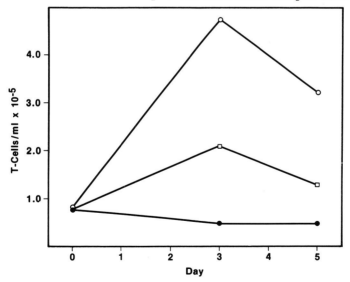

FIG. 6. The proliferative effect of purified TCGF on cultured T-cells. Crude LyCM (□-□) and TCGF purified through preparative SDS-PAGE (0-0) were both shown to induce T-cell proliferation in suspension culture. The cell counts obtained when cells were cultured without exogenous TCGF are represented by (●-●).

reversible SDS-denaturation. In FIG. 6, the mitogenic effects of the
extracted, purified factor, crude LyCM, and media alone are compared.
The purified material obtained from SDS-PAGE clearly induced an increase
in the number of T-lymphoblasts in culture. This material induced levels
of ^{3}H-thymidine incorporation well above background at protein concentration as low as 40 ng/ml. A dose response plot generated with a Multiple
Automated Sample Harvester (MASH unit) using 10^4 cells/microtiter well
is shown in FIG. 7.

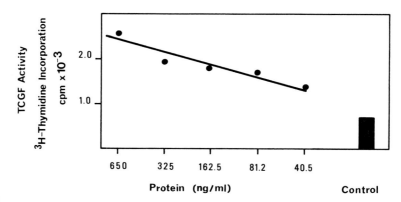

FIG. 7. Dose-response plot for TCGF. Serial dilutions of TCGF, purified
through preparative SDS-PAGE, were assayed in microtiter wells with 10^4
cultured T-cells/well. Above background levels of ^{3}H-thymidine incorporation were induced with nanogram/ml concentration of TCGF.

Specificity for Activated T-Cells

The removal of PHA with an immobilized antibody column has been shown
to augment the potency of crude TCGF preparations in assays using T-
lymphoblasts as the target cells while virtually eliminating the ability
of the preparation to induce thymidine incorporation in fresh peripheral
blood lymphocytes (8).   T-cells that had undergone blast transformation by exposure to lectins or alloantigens proliferated in response to
the lectin-free growth factor, whereas fresh peripheral blood lymphocytes did not. In addition to the affinity column described above, thy-
roglobulin - Sepharose has been utilized specifically to bind PHA and
remove it from LyCM. TCGF obtained by this method is free of any mitogenic capacity for peripheral blood lymphocytes (3).   Similarly, the
TCGF obtained from human LyCM after DEAE-Sepharose chromatography is
capable of discriminating between fresh nonactivated peripheral blood
lymphocytes and activated T-cells (11).   A comparison of the effects
of PHA and TCGF at various stages of purification on resting lymphocytes
and T-blasts obtained after a 1 week culture in the presence of an optimally mitogenic concentration of PHA is shown in FIG. 8. It is clearly
evident that T-lymphoblasts are unresponsive to further exposure to PHA
and proliferate only when incubated with TCGF. Conversely, partially
purified growth factor has no effect on resting, nonactivated lymphocytes .

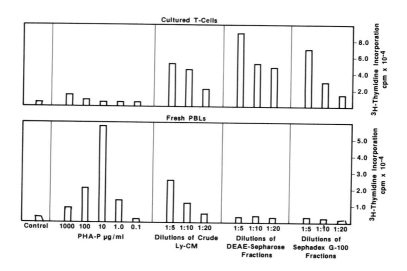

FIG. 8. The effects of PHA, crude LyCM, TCGF from DEAE-Sepharose chromatography, and more purified factor obtained after ion exchange and molecular sieve chromatography on fresh peripheral blood lymphocytes and lectin-activated, cultured T-cells. The resting T-cells respond to PHA but not TCGF, whereas the T-blasts are sensitive only to TCGF.

The Growth of Malignant T-Cells with TCGF

Partially purified, lectin-free, TCGF has been used to grow malignant T-cells in long term suspension culture (13).   Whereas only transient proliferation has been noted with the use of crude LyCM, the more purified preparations have yielded long term growth. These cells respond directly to TCGF and, unlike normal resting T-cells, do not require initial activation with an antigen or lectin. Although there are several established lymphoblastic leukemia cell lines that proliferate in culture without the addition of exogenous growth factor to the media, these cells are for the most part immature, terminal transferase positive, and E-rosette negative. The use of TCGF has permitted the long term growth of E-rosette positive, malignant T-cells from patients with more differentiated neoplasia of T-cell lineage. Several lines from patients with cutaneous T-cell lymphoma (mycosis fungoides and Sezary Syndrome) and T-cell acute lymphoblastic leukemia (ALL) have been sustained in culture for periods of at least four months with the use of TCGF purified from LyCM with DEAE-Sepharose chromatography. These are displayed in Table III. With rare exceptions (see below), they have retained their absolute dependency on the presence of exogenous TCGF for continuous growth. They have normal human karyotypes and morphologic features similar to freshly isolated cells from affected patients. The cultured cutaneous

TABLE III.   MALIGNANT T-CELL LINES ESTABLISHED WITH TCGF

Sample Designation	Diagnosis	Source*	Age,Yr, Sex	Clinical Status
CTCL-1	Sezary syndrome	PB	60;F	Untreated
CTCL-2	Sezary syndrome	PB	60;F	Untreated
CTCL-3	Mycosis fungoides	PB	28;M	Remission+
CTCL-4	Mycosis fungoides	BM	69;M	Untreated
CTCL-5	Mycosis fungoides	PB	69;M	Remission
CTCL-6	Mycosis fungoides	PB	66;F	Relapse+
ALL-1	ALL	BM	47;M	Untreated
ALL-2	ALL	BM	19;M	Untreated
ALL-3	ALL	PB	16;F	Untreated
ALL-4	ALL	PB	65;M	Untreated
ALL-5	ALL	PB	69;M	Untreated
ALL-6	ALL	PB	30;M	Untreated

*PB, peripheral blood; BM, bone marrow. The samples designated ALL-3, -4, and -5 were obtained by leukophoresis.
+After systemic chemotherapy and electron-beam radiation therapy.

T-cell lymphoma lines (CTCL) contained occasional multinucleated giant cells with florid cytoplasmic projections suggestive of hairy cell leukemia. These cells persisted even after repeated cloning. The cell lines established from patients with CTCL, T-cell ALL, and normal T-cells each had distinctive cytochemical features when stained for acid phosphatase and nonspecific esterase, the details of which are reviewed elsewhere (13).

One cell line established from a patient with mycosis fungoides became independent of exogenous growth factor. This particular line had an abnormal karyotype in which the metaphases showed marked variability in chromosome number. A deficient chromosome 16 was the most consistent aberration. This line was shown to be a constituitive (i.e., in the absence of PHA) producer of TCGF, although preliminary data has suggested that the molecule produced by this malignant line may be biochemically distinct from that produced by normal T-cells (5). Although this line grows without the addition of TCGF to the culture media, its growth in nutritionally suboptimal media can be accelerated with exogenous factor. The transient exposure of these cells to an acid glycine buffer results in the release of a significant quantity of TCGF, suggesting that a substantial portion of what the cell synthesizes is immobilized on the plasma membrane. Furthermore, these cells have the capacity to absorb TCGF from the incubating media in a fashion similar to that reported for activated normal T-lymphoblasts, implying that these cells, as is the case with their normal counterparts, have receptors for the lymphokine (2,5). It is tempting to conclude that the elaboration of an autostimulatory substance is vitally connected with the rapid proliferation of these cells in vitro and in vivo.

The Production of Hematopoietic Stem Cell Factors by Cultured T-Cells

The growth and differentiation of hematopoietic stem cells in soft agar is dependent on the presence of soluble factors, some of which are known to be macrophage secretory products (1,7). Recent evidence has suggested that T-lymphocytes also play a role in the growth and maturation of marrow blood cell precursors (17). The ability to sustain normal and malignant T-cells in tissue culture with partially purified TCGF has provided an opportunity to examine pure T-lymphoidal cell populations for their ability to produce colony stimulating activity (CSA), burst-promoting activity (BPA), and other mediators of growth and differentiation (23). Peripheral blood and marrow samples from patients with T-cell ALL and CTCL were placed in culture and cell lines established as described previously using media supplemented with TCGF purified from crude LyCM with DEAE-Sepharose. The TCGF used to propagate these lines was shown to be devoid of both CSA and BPA, whereas the media conditioned by these lines frequently contained easily detectable hematopoietic stem cell growth promoting factors. These media were assayed for the presence of CSA and BPA using previously published methods with human marrow provided by normal donors as the target cells (6). In some instances these cell suspensions were depleted of adherent cells prior to their innoculation into agar. This had no deleterious affect on the plating efficiency of the sample, and in fact, slightly augmented the number of colonies formed. There is therefore, little doubt that the marrow stem cells responded to factors in the T-cell conditioned media rather than substances released by monocyte-macrophages in the marrow sample. A summary of the data on CSA and BPA secretion by malignant and activated normal T-cells is shown in Table IV. Both TCGF-dependent and independent established T-cell lines produce CSA, whereas to date BPA has been detected only in the conditioned media of TCGF-dependent lines.

The Isolation of a Unique Retrovirus From TCGF-Secreting CTCL Lines

The isolation of a novel human Type-C retrovirus (designated HTLV) from a karyotypically abnormal CTCL line has been recently reported (14). The cell line from which the virus was isolated was derived from a patient with mycosis fungoides, and although it subsequently became TCGF-independent, it was initiated into culture with TCGF as described previously. Although 5-Iodo-2-Deoxyuridine (IUDR) was initially required for the production of the virus, the cell line subsequently became a constituitive producer. The DNA polymerase associated with this virus has template preferences typical of a viral reverse transcriptase in that much greater incorporation of labeled nucleotides resulted with the synthetic template-primers $poly(A) \cdot dT_{12-18}$ and $poly(C) \cdot dG_{12-18}$ than with $poly(dA) \cdot dT_{12-18}$. Neutralizing antibodies directed against cellular DNA polymerases and purified reverse transcriptases from several sources including primate retroviruses failed to interact with the HTLV polymerase. This enzyme showed considerably greater activity in the presence of magnesium than with manganese. An SDS-PAGE of the disrupted virus showed several protein bands ranging in molecular weight from 10,000 to 70,000 Daltons. The sizes of some of the proteins are clearly distinct from those of known type-C RNA tumor viruses, especially those of primate origin. The size of the component proteins, the atypical divalent cation preference of the polymerase, and its lack of neutralization with antibodies against reverse transcriptases from several retroviruses suggest that HTLV is not a close relative of known

TABLE IV. PRODUCTION OF CSA AND BPA BY CULTURED T-LYMPHOBLASTS

Cell Type	Time in Culture* (days)	TCGF Dependency	CSA (N pos)	BPA (N pos)
T-cell ALL	15-90	+	6/8	3/5
T-cell ALL	NA	−	0/2	0/2
CTCL	15-150	+	7/12	4/6
CTCL	NA	−	3/4	0/4
NBP	15-90	+	5/5	3/3

CSA and BPA activity in T-cell conditioned media. *Time in culture refers to the duration of time in which the cells were tested for CSA and BPA production. NA(not applicable) refers to established lines.

primate isolates.

HTLV is clearly immunogenic, and antibodies against disrupted virus as well as specific core proteins have been detected in sera from patients with mycosis fungoides and related disorders(16). A virus closely resembling if not in fact identical to the original isolate has been found in malignant T-cell lines derived from several patients with CTCL(15). These cell lines as well as clones of the original line show an absolute concordance between the production of mature virus particles and the secretion of TCGF without lectin stimulation. The role of HTLV in disease causation and its relationship to spontaneous lymphokine production are currently being studied in our laboratory.

SUMMARY

TCGF is a 13,000 molecular weight protein released into the incubating media by T-cells exposed to mitogenic lectins such as PHA. This factor specifically stimulates T-cells that have undergone blast transformation secondary to exposure to a lectin or alloantigen. The proliferative effect on antigen-primed T-cells has permitted the clonal expansion of T-lymphocytes with specific cytotoxic functions. We have recently shown that certain malignant T-cells, in particular those from patients with T-cell ALL and CTCL, can be sustained in suspension culture with lectin-free TCGF in a fashion analogous to the growth of activated normal T-cells. As was the case with lectin-primed but not resting lymphocytes, the malignant cells and their membrane derivatives can reversibly absorb TCGF activity from the culture fluid, presumably due to the presence of specific receptors. After several weeks in culture, some of these lines have become independent of exogenous TCGF. These cells can be shown to harbor a novel retrovirus and to secrete modest amounts of TCGF into the culture fluid without PHA stimulation. Despite the fact that they do not need exogenous TCGF, the cells proliferate more quickly in nutritionally deficient media when additional growth factor is supplied. These findings raise the possibility that the secretion of TCGF is not merely an epiphenomenon related to the transformed state but is, in fact, the mechanism by which these malignant cells have become immortalized in tissue culture. The role of the virus in catalysing these events remains to be clarified.

REFERENCES

1. Chervenick, P., LoBuglio, A. (1972): Science 178: 164-180.
2. Coutinho, A., Larson, E., Gronvik, K., and Anderson, J. (1979) Eur. J. Immunol. 9: 587-591.
3. Fagnani, R., and Braatz, J. (1980): J. Immunol. Meth. 33: 313-317.
4. Gillis, S., Ferm, M., Ou, W., and Smith, K. (1978): J. Immunol. 120: 2027-2032.
5. Gootenberg, J., Ruscetti, F., Mier, J., Gazdar, A., and Gallo, R. (1981): Submitted.
6. Iscove, N., and Sieber, F. (1975): Exp. Hematol. 3: 32-36.
7. Kurland, J., Meyers, P., and Moore, M. (1980): J. Exp. Med. 151: 839-846.
8. Kurnick, J., Gronvik, K., Kimura, A., Lindblom, J., Skoog, V., Sjoberg, O., and Wigzell, H. (1979): J. Immunol. 122: 1255-1260.
9. Lowry, O., Rosenbrough, N., Farr, A., and Randall, R. (1951) J. Biol. Chem. 193: 265-270.
10. Merrill, C., Switzer, R., and Van Keyren, M. (1979): Proc. Natl. Acad. Sci. 76: 4335-4339.
11. Mier, J., and Gallo, R. (1980): Proc. Natl. Acad. Sci. 77: 6134-6138.
12. Morgan, D., Ruscetti, F., and Gallo, R. (1976): Science 193: 1007-1008.
13. Poiez, B., Ruscetti, F., Mier, J., Woods, A., and Gallo, R. (1980): Proc. Natl. Acad. Sci. 77: 6815-6817.
14. Poiesz, B., Ruscetti, F., Gazdar, A., Bunn, P., Minna, J., and Gallo, R. (1980): Proc. Natl. Acad. Sci. 77: 7415-7419.
15. Poiesz, B., Ruscetti, F., Reitz, M., Kalyanaraman, V., and Gallo, R. (1981): Submitted.
16. Posner, L., Robert-Guroff, M., Kalyanaraman, V., Poiesz, B., Ruscetti, F., Bunn, P., and Gallo, R. Submitted
17. Prival, J., Paran, M., Gallo, R., and Wu, A. (1974): 53: 1583-1588.
18. Rosenberg, S., Spiess, P., and Schwarz, S. (1978): J. Immunol. 121: 1946-1950.
19. Rosenberg, S.A., Schwarz, S., and Spiess, P. (1978): J. Immunol. 121: 1951-1955.
20. Ruscetti, F., Morgan, D., and Gallo, R. (1977): J. Immunol. 119: 131-138.
21. Shuster, L. (1971): Methods in Enzynology 22: 412-414.
22. Strausser, J.L., and Rosenberg, S.A. (1978): J. Immunol. 121: 1491-1495.
23. Tarella, C., Ruscetti, F., Poiesz, B., and Gallo, R. (1981) Submitted.
24. Weber, K. and Kuter, D. (1971): J. Biol. Chem. 246: 4504-4510.

*Lymphokines and Thymic Hormones: Their
Potential Utilization in Cancer Therapeutics,*
edited by A. L. Goldstein and M. A. Chirigos,
Raven Press, New York © 1981.

Progress in the Purification of Murine Thymoma-Derived Interleukin 2

John J. Farrar and Janet Fuller-Farrar

*Laboratory of Microbiology and Immunology, National Institute of Dental Research,
National Institutes of Health, Bethesda, Maryland 20205*

INTRODUCTION

Interleukin 2 (IL 2), which was formerly known as T cell growth factor, has been implicated as an immunoregulatory molecule in T cell dependent immune responses. The factor is produced by T lymphocytes and has been shown to augment the induction of alloantigen-specific cytotoxic T cell responses (4,14,17,18) and enhance T cell-dependent antibody forming cell responses (4,18). This latter activity is presumably due to an activation of residual helper T cells within the responding B cell population. Aside from its role as a modulating factor in immune responses to antigens, IL 2 has also been shown to enhance the mitogenic response of thymocytes to either PHA or Con A (3,4,14,18). This latter assay for IL 2 has been designated the co-stimulator assay (12).

In all of these assay systems for IL 2, the macrophage product, IL 1, has also been shown to be active. In contrast, IL 2 but not IL 1 supports the proliferation of factor-dependent long term T cell lines (9). Therefore, this T cell growth activity has become the definitive assay for IL 2.

Despite the considerable biological data which has been accumulated on murine IL 2, relatively little is known about the biochemistry of the factor. From early characterization studies, we know that the factor is a protein (based on proteolytic enzyme sensitivity studies) (3,15) with an apparent molecular weight of 30,000 (as estimated by gel filtration) and isoelectric point heterogeneity between pH 3.8 and 5.0 (6,18). However, IL 2 has not been purified principally because the amount of factor produced is relatively small and because it has been prohibitively expensive and difficult to prepare the requisite large volumes of mouse spleen cell culture supernatants. We therefore, initiated a survey of various murine T cell lines to determine if any of the cell lines produced IL 2 either constitutively or following stimulation. This report presents: 1) a brief descriptive review of a subline of the EL-4 mouse thymoma that we have found to produce extremely high titers of IL 2 and 2) a progress report on the purification of the IL 2 produced by this cell line.

RESULTS AND DISCUSSION

We previously reported that Con A and phorbol myristic acetate (PMA) act synergistically to stimulate IL 2 production in unfractionated mouse spleen cells (6) and further that PMA was able to replace the requirement for macrophages in the production of IL 2 by Con A stimulated purified splenic T cells (5). Therefore, in our survey of T cells lines, we examined the ability of these agents, alone and in combination, to stimulate IL 2 production. A subline of the C57BL/6-derived EL-4 thymoma was, in fact, found to produce very high titers of IL 2 when stimulated with either PMA alone or with PMA in conjunction with non-toxic doses of Con A (6,7). The EL-4 cells produced IL 2 in response to Con A alone only when the dose of Con A had reached toxic levels. As shown previously (6) the molecular weight of the EL-4-derived IL 2, as estimated by gel filtration on AcA-54 columns, was approximately 30,000 a value which is very similar to what has been observed for spleen-cell-derived IL 2. The EL-4-derived IL 2 also exhibited the same isoelectric point heterogeneity between pH 3.8 and 4.8 as spleen cell-derived IL 2 (see 1 for reference list). Additionally, the EL-4 derived IL 2 exhibited the same spectrum of biological activities as splenic IL 2 in that the thymoma-derived factor: 1) maintained the long term growth of cloned T cells, 2) augmented the cytotoxic T cell response of alloantigen-stimulated thymocytes or splenic T cells, 3) enhanced the IgM anti-sheep erythrocyte plaque-forming cell response of nude mouse spleen cells, and 4) synergized with PHA in the thymocyte proliferative response (6). The EL-4 derived IL 2 was, therefore, biologically and biochemically indistinguishible from splenic-derived IL 2.

Following stimulation with PMA, EL-4 cells produce high titers of colony stimulating factor (CSF) in addition to IL 2 (10). Therefore, in terms of the purification of IL 2, our first concern was to separate these two proteins. Although the CSF exhibits a nearly identical molecular weight and isoelectric point heterogeneity as IL 2, it can be clearly separated from the IL 2 by phenyl sepharose hydrophobic chromatography. Figure 1 shows the results of an experiment in which a crude EL-4-derived culture supernatant was concentrated, precipitated with ammonium sulfate between 20-80% saturation, applied to a phenyl sepharose column, and eluted with a gradient of increasing concentration of ethanediol and decreasing concentration of ammonium sulfate. All of the IL 2 eluted within the gradient, whereas all of the CSF activity was found to elute in the column breakthrough (data not shown). The fractions from the phenyl sepharose column which were active for IL 2 were pooled and further purified by tris glycinate 7.5% polyacrylamide gel electrophoresis (Figure 2) in which it was found that the IL 2 eluted at an R_f of 0.63 which is considerably beyond where approximately 95% of the applied protein eluted (R_f 0.2 to 0.55). The tris-glycinate PAGE system, therefore, provided a significant purification step.

Splenic IL 2 has been reported to be resistant to treatment with 10% SDS and exhibits an apparently reduced molecular weight when analyzed by gel filtration conducted on a column equilibrated in SDS-containing

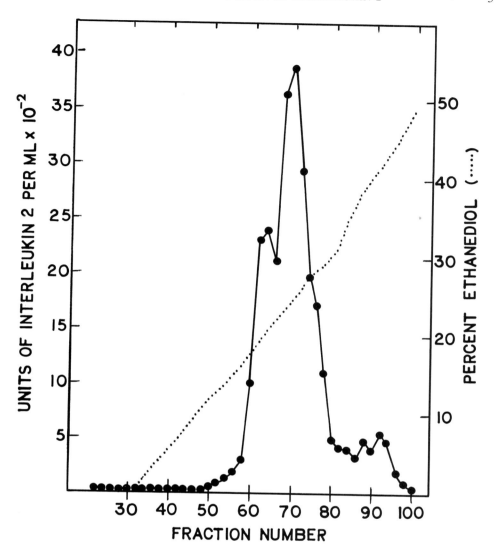

FIG. 1. Hydrophobic chromatography of EL-4 thymoma-derived IL 2 on phenyl sepharose CL-4B. A PMA-stimulated serum-free EL-4 culture supernatant was precipitated with 20%-80% $(NH_4)_2SO_4$ saturation, dialyzed to 0.8M $(NH_4)SO_4$ in 0.02 M phosphate buffered saline and applied to the phenyl sepharose column equilibrated in the same buffer. Fractions (2.0 ml volume per fraction) were collected through the breakthrough volume and following the initiation of the ethanediol gradient. The fractions were dialyzed against RPMI-1640 and assayed for T cell growth activity. The number of units of IL 2 activity is the reciprocal of the dilution yielding a CPM response which is 50% of the maximal CPM response obtained with a standard preparation of IL 2.

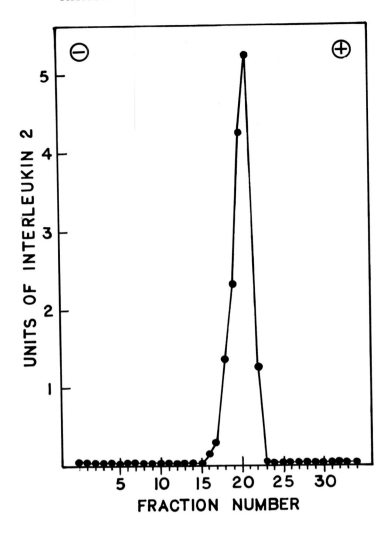

FIG. 2. Tris glycin polyacrylamide gel electrophoresis
of IL 2. The active fractions from the phenyl sepharose
column shown in Figure 1 were pooled and a portion of
the material applied to a pH 8.9 tris glycine buffered
7½% polyacrylamide cylindrical gel and electrophoresed.
The gel was sliced, each slice eluted, and assayed for
T cell growth activity. The anode and cathode orienta-
tion is shown in the figure. The activity eluted as a
single peak with an R_f of 0.63.

buffer (2). We therefore utilized SDS gels to analyze the factor obtained from the EL-4 cells. Figure 3 shows the results of an SDS PAGE
experiment with the EL-4-derived IL 2 purified by ammonium sulfate precipitation and phenyl sepharose chromatography. Similar to what Caplan
et al. have reported (2) we found the IL 2 to exhibit a molecular weight

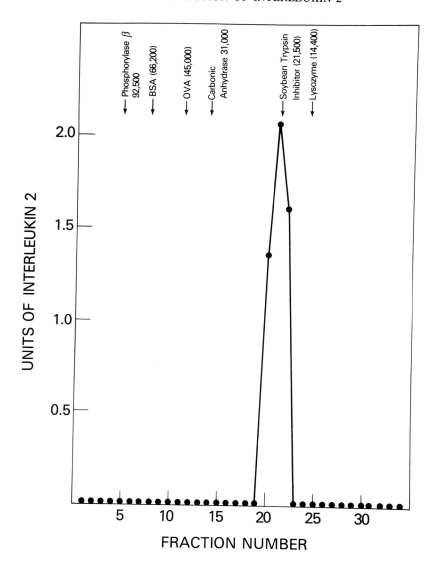

FIG. 3. SDS gel electrophoresis of IL 2. The active gel
slices from the tris glycine gel shown in Figure 2 were
pooled and a portion of the material diluted in 10% SDS
buffer and heated to 70°C for 10 minutes. The SDS-and heat-
treated sample was then electrophoresed on 12% SDS cylindrical gels, sliced, and each slice eluted in 0.02M PBS.
The SDS was then removed from each eluate by cold precipitation as described by Caplan et al. (2). The samples were
then assayed for T cell growth activity. The position of
the molecular weight markers from a parallel gel are shown.
The T cell growth activity of the IL 2 eluted as a single
peak with a molecular weight of 21,000.

lower than what is obtained by conventional gel filtration. However, our molecular weight estimate for IL 2 of 21,000 is somewhat higher than that reported by Caplan et al. (2), who showed a molecular weight of 16,000-18,000. This difference might be attributable to experimental variation or to technical differences between gel filtration and SDS gel electrophoresis. This SDS-PAGE purification step also proved to be a valuable purification procedure since greater than 90% of the applied protein exhibited molecular weights greatly in excess of 21,000.

We have also taken IL 2-containing fractions from the tris-glycinate PAGE and isoelectric focused the material in 5% acrylamide gels containing 4.0 M urea and an ampholine gradient from pH 3.5 to 7.0. In contrast to what was reported by Schimpl et al. (13) we were unable to detect a shift upward (to pH 7.0) in the isoelectric point of IL 2. Rather the biological activity continued to elute in the lower pI range (pH 4.6) (data not shown). Finally, in an effort to resolve a stainable protein band in association with IL 2 biological activity we have run 2-dimensional gels on material that had been partially purified by ammonium sulfate precipitation, phenyl sepharose chromatography, and tris-glycinate PAGE. This material was focused in a cylindrical 5% acrylamide gel for the first dimension and then run in a 12% acrylamide SDS slab gel in the second dimension. In the quadrant corresponding to an isoelectric point of 4.6 and a molecular weight of 21,000, two stainable bands were resolved using a highly sensitive silver nitrate staining procedure (11) which can detect less than 1 ng of protein per mm^3 of gel. Experiments are currently in progress to more clearly resolve these two bands in order to determine which of the proteins exhibit IL 2 biological activity. It is possible that one of the proteins is IL 2 and the other is the late-acting terminal differentiation factor (T cell replacing factor; TRF) as described by Schimpl and Wecker (13). If this separation and purification of IL 2 and TRF is achieved, it will be of interest to determine the B-cell activating and T cell-activating potentials of the two proteins. Of particular interest will be a determination of which factors are able to synergize with each other during B cell activation as has been shown by Swain et al. (16) using TRF and IL 2 preparations from independent sources.

CONCLUSIONS

In conclusion, we have utilized PMA-stimulated EL-4 thymoma cells as a source of large quantities of IL 2. Through the use of sequential ammonium sulfate precipitation, phenyl sepharose chromatography, tris glycine PAGE, and two-dimentional electrophoresis (isoelectric focusing followed by SDS gel electrophoresis) we have purified IL 2 to approximately 4,000,000 units per mg protein with only one possible contaminant which may be TRF. The final purification of IL 2 will allow more precise investigations into the nature of the interaction between this factor and its receptor and ultimately to the purification of the receptor itself. Additionally, the large amounts of factor obtainable from the EL-4 thymoma should allow in vivo studies on possible therapeutic applications for IL 2.

ACKNOWLEDGEMENTS

The authors would like to thank Drs. Joost Oppenheim and William Benjamin for their critical reviews of this manuscript and Mrs. Darleen Tenn for her excellent secretarial assistance.

REFERENCES

1. Aarden, et al. (1979): J. Immunol., 123: 2938-2929.
2. Caplan, B., Gibbs, C., and Paetkau, V. (1981): J. Immunol., 126: 1351-1403.
3. Chen, D.M., and DiSabato, G. (1976): Cell. Immunol., 22: 211-224.
4. Farrar, J.J., Simon, P.L., Koopman, W.J., and Fuller-Bonar, J. (1978) J. Immunol., 121: 1353-1360.
5. Farrar, J., Mizel, S.B., Fuller-Farrar, J., Farrar, W.L., and Hilfiker, M.L. (1980): J. Immunol., 125: 793-798.
6. Farrar, J., Fuller-Farrar, J., Simon, P.L., Hilfiker, M.L., Stadler, B.M., and Farrar, W.L. (1980): J. Immunol., 125: 2555-2558.
7. Farrar, J.J., Fuller-Farrar, J., Simon, P.L., Hilfiker, M.L. and Farrar, W.L. (1980): Behring Inst. Mitt., 67: 58-60.
8. Fuller-Farrar, J., Hilfiker, M.L., Farrar, W.L., and Farrar, J.J. (1981): Cell. Immunol., 58; 156-164.
9. Gillis, S., Ferm, M., Ou, W., and Smith, K. (1978): J. Immunol., 120: 2027-2032.
10. Hilfiker, M.L., Moore, R.N., and Farrar, J.J. (1980): (submitted for publication).
11. Oakley, B.R., Kirsch, D.R., and Morris, N.R. (1980): Anal. Biochem., 105: 361-363.
12. Paetkau, V., Mills, G., Gerhart, S., and Monticone, V. (1976): J. Immunol., 117: 1320-1324.
13. Schimpl, A., Hübner, L., Wong, C.A., and Wecker, E. (1980): Behring Inst. Mitt., 67: 221-225.
14. Shaw, J., Monticone, V., Mills, G., and Paetkau, V. (1979): J. Immunol., 122: 1633-1639.
15. Shaw, J., Caplan, B., Paetkau, V., Pilarski, L.M., Delovitch, T.L., and McKenzie, I.F.C. (1980): J. Immunol., 124: 2231-2239.
16. Swain, S.L., Dennert, G., Warner, J.F., and Dutton, R.W. (1980): Proc. Nat. Acad. Sci. (USA), (in Press).
17. Wagner, H. and Röllinghoff, M. (1978): J. Exp. Med., 148: 1523-1538.
18. Watson, J., Aarden, L.A., Shaw, J., and Paetkau, V. (1979): J. Immunol., 120: 2027-2032.

*Lymphokines and Thymic Hormones: Their
Potential Utilization in Cancer Therapeutics,*
edited by A. L. Goldstein and M. A. Chirigos,
Raven Press, New York © 1981.

New Reagents for Interleukin 2 Production and Detection

Steven Gillis

Fred Hutchinson Cancer Research Center, Seattle, Washington 98104

ABSTRACT

Although the capacity of Interleukin 2 (IL-2) to influence in vitro assays of cell-mediated immunity has been well-documented, demonstration of IL-2 regulation of in vivo immune reactivity has been difficult to establish. Attempts to study the in vivo effects of IL-2 have been hampered by two recurrent problems; the first being, the necessity to produce hundreds of liters of conditioned medium to purify sub- microgram quantities of IL-2. The second shortcoming has been the inability to assess the presence of IL-2 using a criterion other than its induction of activated T cell proliferation. In order to follow development of IL-2 production and/or response capacities in vivo it would be of benefit to use an assay which recognized the physical presence of a lymphokine in vivo as opposed to monitoring biological activity associated with its presence.

The data summarized below reviews the identification of tumor cell line sources for both human and murine IL-2. The identification of IL-2 producer tumor reagents (yielding several times the amount of IL-2 normally generated by conventional mitogen stimulated leukocyte protocols) has greatly aided further biochemical characterization of this lymphocyte regulatory molecule. We have also summarized results of fusion experimentation which produced hybrid cell lines whose soluble products significantly neutralized IL-2 dependent T-cell replication. Several lines of evidence suggested that the inhibitory activity was associated with a monoclonal IgG antibody directed against IL-2 determinants. First, passage of cloned hybrid cell culture supernatants through a Protein A-coupled Sepharose column, yielded purified immunoglobulin G fractions which inhibited mouse, rat, and human IL-2 activity. Secondly, hybridoma-derived IgG, in concert with lyophilized Staphylococcus aureus, was capable of precipitating both "cold" and intrinsically labeled IL-2 activity. We hope that identification and use of these reagents will foster the application of recombinant DNA technology to investigate the possibility of producing IL-2 in sympathetic bacteria. In the interim, we are confident however, that use of IL-2 producer tumor lines in concert with monoclonal anti-IL-2 antibody will allow definitive experimentation to document the ability of IL-2 to control in vivo T-cell proliferation and reactivity.

Special Fellow of the Leukemia Society of America, supported by NCI Grant CA 28419, and grant 1-724 from the National Foundation.

INTRODUCTION

During the past five years several laboratories have confirmed the integral role that the single class of lymphokine activities plays in affecting in vitro cell mediated immune responses (1,2,5,13,14). Biochemical fractionation of conventionally prepared, mitogen-stimulated spleen cell conditioned medium revealed that activities previously ascribed to T-cell growth factor (TCGF); killer assisting factor (KAF), killer helper factor (KHF) and thymocyte stimulating/mitogenesis factors were all mediated by biochemically identical protein moieties. In fact, all activities were found to co-migrate following sequential concentration by ammonium sulfate precipitation, gel filtration, and ion exchange chromatography, and as a final step, preparative flatbed isoelectric focusing (IEF) (5,14). For the sake of clarity, the term Interleukin 2 (IL-2) was adopted as a single factor designation serving to replace each of the above listed acronymns which had been named solely for their biological effects in single immune response assays (1).

Our interest in the area of IL-2 research continues to be split between efforts directed toward the biochemical and molecular characterization of the lymphokine and attempts at detailing its physiological role in in vivo normal and aberrant immune responses. Early after completion of initial biochemical characterization of conditioned medium derived human and murine IL-2, it became obvious to us that in order to approach the molecular basis of IL-2 action or its capacity to influence in vivo immune responses more potent sources of crude IL-2 containing conditioned medium had to be identified. Using standard, preparative isolation procedures, several hundred liters of normal murine spleen or human leukocyte mitogen-conditioned medium would have to be processed to yield even microgram quantities of IL-2. We have therefore taken considerable pains to determine optimum conditions for producing initial high titer IL-2 activity.

Tumor Cell Line IL-2 Production

Although active in a number of immune response assays, the most unequivocal test for the presence of IL-2 remains the ability of the lymphokine to trigger cloned T-cell proliferation. Using this approach the IL-2 microassay quantifies IL-2 dependent T-cell replication by measuring tritiated thymidine (^{3}H-Tdr) incorporation in replicate 4 hour pulsed, 200 microliter cultures of 3,000 cloned T-cells following overnight incubation in the presence of samples suspected of containing IL-2 (4). Probit analysis of IL-2 dependent ^{3}H-Tdr incorporation profiles allows for quantitative delineation of the amount of IL-2 activity present in a given sample. The ability of different mitogen/antigen stimulated leukocyte culture populations to produce IL-2, is reviewed in Table I. Harvest of conditioned medium with peak IL-2 activity was clearly cell concentration and culture duration dependent. This was most likely due to the observation that IL-2 supernate titer was dependent upon two competing reactions, the first being IL-2 production by a subpopulation of T-cells, and the second being the binding/absorbtion and consumption of IL-2 by proliferating ligand activated T-cells present in the same culture (12). To obtain maximal IL-2 concentration in the supernate, it was imperative that conditioned medium be harvested after a majority of the IL-2 had been produced, prior to the time when activated T-cells had proliferated to the extent where they had begun to exhaust the IL-2 supply.

Optimal murine IL-2 titer was obtained in culture supernates harvested after 24 hour Con-A stimulation of normal spleen cells (10^7 cells/ml). Greater than ten fold increases in IL-2 titer were routinely witnessed when rat spleen cells were substituted. Optimal production of human IL-2 activity was achieved either by PHA stimulation of human spleen cells or by PHA and allogeneic B-

TABLE I. RELATIVE CAPACITY OF RAT, MOUSE, AND HUMAN LYMPHOCYTE POPULATIONS TO PRODUCE IL-2

Lymphocyte Source	Mitogen	Cell Concentration[1]	Units/ml Interleukin-2 (TCGF) Activity in Filtered Medium	
			24 hr Supernate	48 hr Supernate
Mouse spleen	Con-A (1.25 µg/ml)	10^6/ml	0.10	0.35
Mouse spleen	Con-A (2.5 µg/ml)	10^7/ml	1.60	0.75
Rat spleen	Con-A (5 µg/ml)	10^6/ml	0.68	1.0 (Standard)
Rat spleen	Con-A (5 µg/ml)	10^7/ml	13.60	7.20
Human PBL	PHA 1%	10^6/ml	2.30	4.30
Human PBL	[2]B-LCL (Daudi or AR-77 2-5 x 10^5/ml live or irradiated)	10^6/ml	0.63	1.20
Human PBL	B-LCL + 1.0% PHA	10^6/ml	8.60	10.70
Human PBL	Na-GO[3]	10^6/ml	3.60	0.73
Human spleen	1% PHA	10^7/ml	25.00	12.60
Mouse Lymphoma LBRM 5A4	1% PHA	10^6/ml	535.00	520.00
Human T Cell leukemia Jurkat-FHCRC	1% PHA + 10 µg/ml PMA	10^6/ml	306.00	285.00

1.   50 ml volumes in 250 mm^2 flasks, lying flat in a humidified atmosphere of 5% CO_2 and air.

2.   B-lymphoblastoid cell line.

3.   Neuraminidase-galactose oxidase treatment (see reference 8).

lymphoblastoid cell line stimulation of peripheral blood mononuclear cells. Use of human spleen cells to produce IL-2 was of considerable advantage given the ability to recycle human splenocytes in multiple 24 hour repetitive rounds of mitogen induced IL-2 production. It should be stressed that an excellent source of mitogen free IL-2 could be obtained via neuraminidase/galactose oxidase (NaGO) treatment of human peripheral blood cells (10).

In hopes of establishing systems in which to produce initial conditioned medium with significantly higher IL-2 titer, we screened several murine and human T-cell leukemia and lymphoma cell lines for both constitutive and mitogen induce IL-2 production. Of the cell lines tested only two (one each in both human and murine systems) were found to produce high titer IL-2 upon mitogen stimulation. 1% PHA stimulation of cloned LBRM-33 cell lines resulted in culture supernates which contained several times the amount of biologically active IL-2 which was routinely generated by identical numbers of optimally stimulated rat or mouse spleen cells (6, Table I). Similarly only PHA and phorbol myristate acetate stimulation of the human leukemia T-cell line Jurkat-FHCRC produced between 100 and 300 times the amount of human IL-2/ml normally generated by identical of numbers of mitogen stimulated human PBL or spleen cells (7).

Finally, due to higher yields observed when IL-2 is produced from cloned LBRM-33 or Jurkat-FHCRC cells, we have been able to carry purification further than preparative IEF. The conditions which permit the efficient recovery and detection of IL-2 activity from SDS-polyacrylamide gel electrophoresis (PAGE) have now been determined (9). IEF pure, LBRM-33 derived IL-2 when fractionated on 7% and 10% PAGE using a mono-tris bicine modified Wiley system revealed that both pI 4.3 and 4.9 IL-2 fractions contained some 9-13 stainable protein species between the molecular weights of 35,000 and 15,000 daltons (9). Electrophoretic elution of single bands revealed that 90-95% of all biological activity resided in 2 bands corresponding to 24,000 and 21,000 m.w. (9).

Identical SDS-PAGE electrophoretic elution analysis of IEF pure human IL-2 (derived from the Jurkat-FHCRC cell line) revealed that 75-90% of all IL-2 reactivity resided in a single protein band of approximately 14,000 m.w. (15). We feel confident that SDS-PAGE eluted fractions are truly molecularly homogeneous, in that amino acid sequence analysis now underway appears to confirm the presence of only single N-terminal amino acid residues in gel band eluted samples.

The Development of IL-2 Monoclonal Antibodies

Using the gel electrophoresis and elution techniques mentioned above it is now possible to isolate microgram quantities of IL-2 corresponding to biological activities in excess of 50,000 units. Although these biochemical advances will allow more detailed molecular analysis of IL-2 (amino acid composition, sequence and determination of the molecule's active site) studies to probe the capacity of IL-2 to influence in vivo immunity would benefit from the capacity to trace biologically active lymphokine after in vivo administration. Although the microassay detailed earlier (which monitors the capacity of IL-2 to induce cloned T-cell line ^{3}H-Tdr incorporation) remains as the most rapid and unambiguous assay for IL-2 activity; it is not necessarily appropriate for analysis of in vivo IL-2 concentration. For example, in situ fluids, which would be prime assay milieux (serum and intraperitoneal exudates) have extremely inhibitory effects on IL-2 dependent T-cell proliferation even when tested in IL-2 microassays in the presence of a constant, saturating amount of purified IL-2. Therefore, studies aimed at dissection of the in vivo relevance of IL-2 would clearly benefit from development of reagents which could detect the presence of the molecule serologically, as opposed to monitoring its biological effect. In addition, development of antibodies which react with IL-2 might provide useful reagents for further examination of the molecular properties of this lymphocyte regulatory molecule, and foster biochemical comparisons between IL-2 and other lymphokine activities. Given the recent advances in cell fusion technology, we undertook an experimental program aimed at the generation of monoclonal antibodies with reactivities directed against IL-2 determinants.

BALB/c female mice were immunized once weekly for four weeks with 3,000 U of iso-electrically focused rat IL-2 (2). IL-2 (1,000 U/site) was mixed with complete (first immunication) or incomplete (last three immunizations) Freund's adjuvant and injected in 0.2 ml volumes, intradermally in both hind legs. On each occasion, 1,000 U of rat IL-2 was additionally injected in 0.5 ml of 0.9% NaCl intraperitoneally.

Two days prior to fusion, spleens from IL-2 immunized mice were removed and single cell suspensions prepared. Splenocytes were then cultured for 48 hrs in the presence of 100 μg/ml E. coli lipopolysaccharide (LPS) in Click's medium supplemented with 10% heat-inactivated (56° for 30 mins) fetal calf serum (FCS), 25 mM HEPES buffer, 15 mM NaHCO$_3$, 50 μg/ml streptomycin, 50 U/ml penicillin and 300 μg/ml fresh L-glutamine. 8×10^7 LPS-activated "IL-2 immune" splenocytes were fused with 2×10^7 SP2/D.AG14 (SP2) BALB/c myeloma cells (a derivative of the SP2/HLGK myeloma line which does not constitutively produce immunoglobulin light chain) by addition of polyethylene glycol. The fused cell solution was added to 160 ml of hypoxanthine, aminopterin and thymidine containing (HAT) medium supplemented with 8×10^8 thymocytes harvested from six week old BALB/c female mice. The entire cell suspension was mixed gently and dispersed in 200 μl aliquots to each of ten 96-well flat bottom microtiter plates (3596, Costar Inc., Cambridge, MA). The resultant microwell cultures were maintained at 37°C in a humidified atmosphere of 7% CO_2 and air.

After one week in culture, the microwells were examined microscopically for cultures containing single clusters of hybrid cell growth. These cultures were identified and fed every three days with 100 ul of fresh HAT medium. Once the hybrid cell population reached 50-70% confluence, supernate samples were assayed for anti-IL-2 reactivity.

Because sufficient quantities of purified rat IL-2 were not available, it was necessary to screen hybridoma supernate samples for their capacity to inhibit IL-2 in standard factor-driven T-cell line ^{3}H-Tdr incorporation assays. Furthermore, because hybridoma antibodies are usually incapable of forming large precipitating complexes, we chose to screen both in the presence and absence of an additional complexing agent. In this manner, we felt confident that we could detect both neutralizing antibodies (reactive against determinants present on, or near, the active site of IL-2) as well as antibodies that might be directed against determinants elsewhere on the molecule. Therefore, screenings were conducted by adding 50 ul aliquots of hybridoma microwell culture supernate to replicate microwell cultures containing: (i) 4×10^4 IL-2 dependent CTLL cells (3) (harvested from long-term culture) suspended in 100 μl of 10% FCS-supplemented Click's medium; (ii) 50 μl of rat IL-2 containing conditioned medium and (iii) either 50 ul of FCS-supplemented Click's medium (neutralizing screening cultures) or 50 μl lyophilized Staphylococcus aureus (Igsorb, Enzyme Center Inc., Boston, MA, precipitating screening cultures).

Using the above methods, each CTLL screening culture contained a 1/5 dilution of hybridoma supernate and 0.5 U/ml IL-2 activity. Precipitating screening cultures contained a 1/200 final dilution of the Igsorb reagent. Following 24 hrs of culture (37°C, 5% CO_2 in air) screening cultures were pulsed for 4 hrs with 0.5 μCi of ^{3}H-Tdr (20 Ci/mM specific activity, New England Nuclear, Boston, MA) and harvested with the aid of a multiple automated sample harvester. ^{3}H-Tdr incorporation was determined by liquid scintillation counting.

Of the 1,000 wells tested, 2 were found to produce supernate which inhibited (>50%) IL-2 dependent CTLL proliferation in either of the two screening cultures. Of the 24 putative anti-IL-2 antibody producing cultures , all but five neutralized IL-2 activity in the absence of the Igsorb reagent. Of the nineteen hybridoma supernates which significantly neutralized IL-2 dependent cell proliferation, the addition of Igsorb markedly increased the inhibitory capacity of the supernate in all but one case.

Figure 1 reviews the results of experimental screening assays (8). In initial screening of the plate 4 culture only cells in microculture 4E12 produced a supernate which significantly inhibited IL-2 dependent CTLL ^{3}H-Tdr incorporation. HAT medium or supernates harvested from SP2 myeloma cultures mediated no inhibition of CTLL cell proliferation in either neutralizing or precipitating screening trials. Limiting dilution cloning (2 hybrid cells/ml) resulted in the establishment of several new hybrid cultures which, (since they formed single clusters), appeared to be monoclonal in origin. Of these, supernates from the culture identified as 4E12B2 inhibited almost 90% of the IL-2 dependent CTLL proliferation observed in control (HAT medium or SP2 supernate) experiments. Although we were confident that the hybrid culture 4E12B2 was a true clone, subsequent subcloning (2 hybrid cells/ml) and rescreening experimentation was conducted to provide additional functional data to confirm the hybrid line's origin from a single cell. All 4E12B2 daughter clones produced supernates which significantly inhibited IL-2 activity. Of the resultant hybridoma clones, the line designated 4E12B2D10 was observed to produce the most inhibitory supernate and

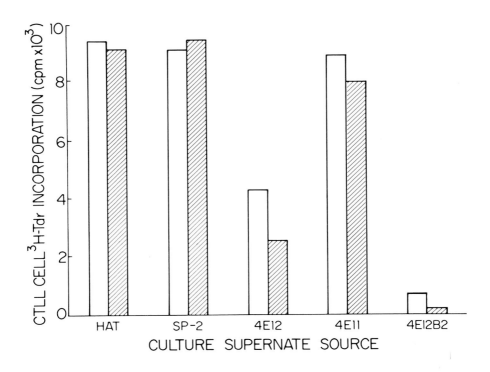

FIG. I.   Results of neutralization (□) and precipitating (▨) screening trials monitoring the isolation of anti-IL-2 producer hybridomas. In the initial plate 4 culture only microwell culture 4EI2 produced supernate which significantly inhibited IL-2 dependent T-cell replication.   Replicate rounds of sub-cloning together with visual inspection revealed that all 4EI2B2 daughter clones produced supernates which markedly inhibited the effects of IL-2. Control HAT medium or medium conditioned by the parent SP2 myeloma had no effect on IL-2 dependent CTLL cell ^{3}H-Tdr incorporation.

was selected for further analysis and was consequently expanded in *in vitro* culture.

Purification and Use of Hybridoma Anti-IL-2 Immunoglobulin.

Of the putative anti-IL-2 hybridomas detailed above, we were particularly interested in those which demonstrated markedly enhanced anti-IL-2 activity in the presence of the precipitating complex, Igsorb. As the complexing component of Igsorb is a *Staphylococcus aureus* membrane glycoprotein (Protein A with high affinity for the Fc portion of immunoglobulin G molecules, we reasoned that if the anti-IL-2 activity present in hybridoma supernates was indeed a monoclonal antibody, we would be able to purify the antibody by taking advantage of its affinity for Protein A.

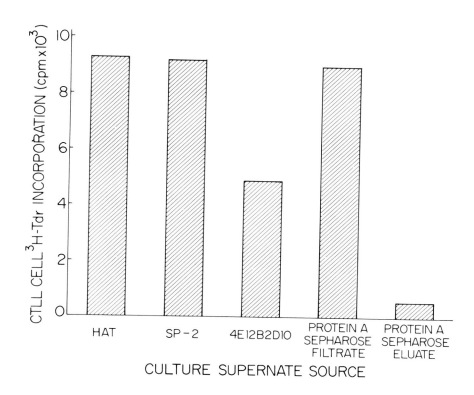

FIG. 2. Igsorb precipitation screening cultures monitoring the anti-IL-2 effects of HAT medium, SP-2 conditioned medium and supernate harvested from the cloned hybridoma 4E12B2D10. The capacity of 4E12B2D10 supernate to inhibit IL-2 dependent CTLL cell ^{3}H-Tdr incorporation was lost by passge over Protein A conjugated Sepharose. However enhanced anti-IL-2 activity could be recovered from the column by standard acid elution and subsequent dialysis.

To test this hypothesis, protein present in 25 ml of 24 hr supernate harvested from cultures of the 4E12B2D10 hybridoma was precipitated by the slow addition of solid ammonium sulfate, to a final saturation of 50% (w/v). After overnight stirring at 4°C, the precipate was pelleted by a 20 min, 10,000xg centrifugation and was dialyzed for an additional 24 hrs against 1,000 volumes of 0.9% saline. The resulting dialyzed protein solution (3 ml) was applied to a column of Protein A Sepharose previously equilibrated in 0.9% saline (pH 7.2) and subsequently washed with additional 0.9% saline. The filtrate was retained and tested for anti-IL-2 activity. The column was then washed with 0.2 M glycine HCl (pH 3) buffer to elute whatever IgG present in the hybridoma product might have been bound to the protein A Sepharose matrix. The column acid wash (eluate) was then dialyzed sequentially against 1,000 volumes each of 0.9% NaCl (pH 7.2) and Hank's buffered salt solution prior to testing for anti-IL-2 activity. Figure 2 displays the results of precipitating anti-IL-2 tests using both Protein A Sepharose filtrate and acid eluate solutions. As was detailed earlier (Figure 1), CTLL microwell cultures containing IL-2 and Igsorb were unaffected by the addition of either HAT medium or tissue culture medium conditioned by SP2 myeloma cells. In contrast, crude supernates from 24 hr cultures of 4E12B2D10, significantly inhibited CTLL cell proliferation. Furthermore, no inhibitory activity was found to be associated with the Protein A Sepharose filtrate sample, whereas enhanced anti-IL-2 activity was found in the acid eluate from the same column. Collectively considered, the data detailed in Figure 2 suggested that the anti-IL-2 inhibitory activity present in 4E12B2D10 hybridoma supernates was due to the presence of a monoclonal (IgG) antibody which could be bound and eluted from a Protein A Sepharose column (8).

Based on the capacity of the 4E12B2D10 hybridoma antibody to markedly inhibit IL-2 biological activity in the presence of Igsorb, we were interested to determine whether identical protocols might be effective in the immune precipation of radio- labeled IL-2. Because the 4E12B2D10 antibody demonstrated the ability to inhibit LBRM-33 derived mouse IL-2 activity (data not shown) we chose to use, as an initial source of antigen, biosynthietically radio-labeled IL-2 prepared from LBRM-33 cells. Previous experiments had shown that although I^{125} labeling of iso-electrically focused murine IL-2 resulted in a product of high specific activity, the biological activity was diminished and markedly unstable. With the demonstration of an IL-2 producing tumor cell line (6), we developed a protocol which would biosynthetically label IL-2. ^{3}H-labeled IL-2 activity was prepared by growing the IL-2 producing tumor cell line LBRM-33-5A4 in the presence of five amino acids bearing ^{3}H-label (leucine, lysine, phenylalanine, proline, and tyrosine, Catalog #TRK550, Amersham Corp., Arlington Heights, IL). LBRM-33 cells (7 X 10^5 cells/ml) were cultured in 25 ml volumes of 2% FCS-supplemented RPMI 1640 medium selectively deficient (20% of normal concentration) for leucine, lysine, phenylanaline, proline, and tyrosine. Tritium-labeled amino acids (those listed above) were added to the culture at time zero, (final composite concentration of 10μCi/ml) and the cells were cultured for 2 days prior to the addition of 1% PHA (by volume). Twenty-four hrs after mitogen stimulation the IL-2 rich supernate was harvested, concentrated by 85% ammonium sulfate precipitation and fractionated by sequential DEAE cellulose ion exchange and Sephadex G-100 gel exclusion chromatography (3). This procedure reulted in the preparation of IL-2 active fractions (20-100 U/ml) which contained considerable radioactivity (approximately 100,000 cpm/ml).

In immune precipitation experiments, ^{3}H-IL-2 (approximately 1,200 cpm in 20 μl) was incubated at 37°C in the presence of serial $\log_2$ dilutions (50 μl) of test supernate. After a 30 min incubation, 20 μl of Igsorb was added to the reaction and the incubation continued for an additional 45 mins. Resultant Igsorb-immune complexes were pelleted by 450xg centrifugation and were washed three times in 2 ml of 0.9% NaCl. The washed pellet was then resuspended in 3.5 ml of Biofluor scintillation cocktail, placed in mini scintillation vials and, tritium label associated with the pellet counted by liquid scintillation. The results of immune precipitation of ^{3}H labeled IL-2 activity are detailed in Table II. Precipitation tests using either HAT medium or SP2 conditioned medium resulted in immobilization of only 100-150 cpm of ^{3}H label. Identical tests using a 1/5 dilution of tissue culture medium obtained from the 4E12B2D10 hybridoma revealed precipitation of 856 cpm (70% of the label added to the reaction mixture). The capacity of the 4E12B2D10 supernate to precipitate radio-labeled IL-2 remained high (794 cpm in the washed pellet) even when a 1/20 dilution of the hybridoma supernatant was tested. The precipitation of radio-labeled IL-2 was totally inhibited by the presence of a ten-fold excess of unlabeled IL-2. Purification of the 4E12B2D10 IgG in 25 ml of hybridoma conditioned medium (as detailed above) resulted in an antibody solution which precipitated peak levels of radio-labeled IL-2 when tested at a dilution of 1/80.

TABLE II. IMMUNE PRECIPITATION OF RADIOLABELED IL-2 ACTIVITY

Culture Supernate	CPM of ^{3}H-IL-2 Associated with Igsorb Pellet[1]				
	Supernate Dilution				
	1/5	1/10	1/20	1/40	1/80
HAT medium	80	110	75	95	86
SP-2	123	116	135	117	110
4E12B2D10 (anti-IL-2 hybridoma)	856	737	794	544	244
4E12B2D10 + XC Cold-IL-2	172	134	136	121	129
4E12B2D10 Protein A Sepharose-Acid Eluate (anti-IL-2 IgG)	186	245	615	775	892

1. 1200 cpm added to each reaction mixture.

Based on the ability of anti-IL-2 IgG to inhibit IL-2 dependent T-cell proliferation and precipitate radiolabeled IL-2, we questioned whether similar addition of 4E12B2D10 IgG to mixed lymphocyte cultures (MLC), would result in decreased generation of cytolytic effector cell (CTL) reactivity. The effect of anti-IL-2 on the generation of CTL was tested in 2 ml MLC (RPMI 1640, 2% FCS) containing 5×10^6 C57Bl/6 responder cells and 10^5 BALB/c irradiated (1500R) splenic stimulator cells. Replicate MLC were conducted containing various concentrations of anti-IL-2 IgG or an irrelevant monoclonal IgG (anti gp70) in the presence of Igsorb (1/400 dilution). After five days of culture (37°C in a humidified atmosphere at 5% CO_2 in air) viable effector cells were harvested and tested for their ability to lyse ^{51}Cr-labeled P815 (H-2^d) mastocytoma target cells. Methods for performance of ^{51}Cr release assays in 200 µl V-bottom microculture wells have been described in detail elsewhere (11). As shown in Table III, the addition of anti-IL-2 IgG had a markedly deleterious effect on the recovery and strength of viable effector CTL. Not only did anti-IL-2 serve to depress the lytic efficiency of CTL generated in MLC, its addition to allo stimulated spleen cell cultures significantly curtailed proliferation and recovery of responsive CTL. In contrast to the results when cultures were supplemented with anti-IL-2 IgG, addition of an irrelevant anti gp70 immunoglobulin had no effect either on the number or lytic reactivity of the alloresponsive CTL generated (even when tested at antibody concentrations as high as 40 µl/ml).

TABLE III. EFFECT OF ANTI IL-2 ON MLC GENERATION OF ALLO-REACTIVE CTL.

Effector Cells	Anti IL-2 Present	% Yield	% Specific Lysis (P815) 50:1	25:1	10:1
C57BL/6 x BALB/c$_{X-irr}$	none	45	54	43	34
"	5 ug/ml	7	0	0	0
"	2 ug/ml	9	1	0	0
"	1 ug/ml	15	30	23	8
"	0.5 ug/ml	19	32	25	10
"	0.25 ug/ml	24	38	31	12

Effector Cells	Anti Gp 70 present	% Yield	% Specific Lysis (P815) 50:1	25:1	10:1
C57BL/6 x BALB/c$_{X-irr}$	none	50	56	41	27
"	40 ug/ml	40	49	40	27
"	20 ug/ml	49	54	38	32
"	10 ug/ml	42	48	42	29
"	5 ug/ml	56	49	44	25
"	2 ug/ml	59	48	41	24

5 day MLC, 50/1 Responder/Stimulator Ratio containing a 1/400 dilution of Igsorb.

SUMMARY

The data displayed above have reviewed (i) the identification of tumor cell lines which produce high titer IL-2 containing conditioned medium and (ii) the development of monoclonal antibodies which recognize determinants present on IL-2. These two advances have fostered considerable progress with regard to biochemical characterization of this lymphocyte regulatory molecule. Indeed, now that tumor cell line sources of conditioned medium can be generated which contain hundreds of units of IL-2 activity per ml, it has been possible to generate sufficient quantities of IEF pure IL-2 to foster further molecular separation by SDS polyacrylamide gel electrophoresis (with retention of biological activity). The capacity to produce and purify molecularly homogeneous IL-2 together with the production of monoclonal anti IL-2 IgG provides a sufficient armamentarium with which to approach the in vivo physiological relevance of IL-2. Not only will anti-IL-2 be of great value for use as an affinity sorbent, the capacity of hybridoma IgG to precipitate biologically active, radiolabeled IL-2 forms the basis of a competitive radioimmunoassay which can be used to assess in vivo IL-2 concentration either during the course of an on-going immune reaction or after passive administration. Finally, as indicated by its ability to limit alloantigen induced T-cell replication and CTL differentiation, it is conceivable that antibody directed against determinants present on the IL-2 molecule may function as a potent immunosuppressive drug.

REFERENCES

1. Aarden, L.A. (1979): J. Immunol. 123,2928.
2. Farrar, J.J., P.L. Simon, W.J. Koupman, and J. Fuller-Bonar. (1978): J. Immunol. 121:1353.
3. Gillis, S., and Smith, K.S. (1977): Nature 268:154.
4. Gillis, S., Ferm, M.M., Ou, W., and Smith, K.A. (1978): J.Immunol., 120:2027.
5. Gillis, S., Smith, K.A., and Watson, J.D. (1980): J. Immunol., 124:1954.
6. Gillis, S., Scheid, M. and Watson, J. (1980): J. Immunol., 125:2570.
7. Gillis, S. and Watson, J. (1980): J.Exp.Med., 152:1709.
8. Gillis, S. and Henney, C.S. (1981): J. Immunol., 126:1978.
9. Mochizuki, D., Watson, J., and Gillis, S. (1980): J. Immunological Methods, 39:185.
10. Novogrodsky, A., Suthanthiran, M., Saltz, B., Newman, D., Rubin, A.L. and Stenzel, K.H. (1980): J.Exp.Med.,151:755.
11. Okada, M., Klimpel, G.R., Kuppers, R.C. and Henney, C.S. (1979): J. Immunol., 122:2527
12. Smith, K.A., Gillis, S., Baker, P.E., McKenzie, D., and Ruscetti, F.W. (1979): Proc. N.Y. Acad. Sci., 332:423.
13. Watson, J., Aarden, L.A., Shaw, J., and Paetkau, V. (1979): J. Immunol., 122:1633.
14. Watson, J.D., Gillis, S., Marbrook, J., Mochizuki, D., and Smith, K.A. (1979): J.Exp.Med., 150:849.
15. Watson, J., Mochizuki, D.M., Frank, M.B., and Gillis, S. (1981): In Pharmacology of the Reticuloendothelial System, edited by D. Webb, Marcel Dekker, Inc., New York.

Lymphokines and Thymic Hormones: Their Potential Utilization in Cancer Therapeutics, edited by A. L. Goldstein and M. A. Chirigos, Raven Press, New York © 1981.

Monoclonal Antibodies Against the Interleukins

Beda M. Stadler, Suanne F. Dougherty, Charles Carter, Elsa H. Berenstein, Philip C. Fox, Reuben P. Siraganian, and Joost J. Oppenheim

Laboratory of Microbiology and Immunology, National Institute of Dental Research, National Institutes of Health, Bethesda, Maryland 20205

INTRODUCTION

The generation of monoclonal antibodies against Interleukin 1 (IL 1; the lymphocyte activating factor) and Interleukin 2 (IL 2; the T cell growth factor) is of potential interest. Macrophage derived IL 1 in conjunction with a mitogen or antigen activates T cells to produce IL 2 (9). Thus, these mediators act as amplifying signals in the afferent limb of immunity. IL 1 and IL 2 have a number of biologically similar effects; therefore, antibodies might be helpful in dissecting the actions of these mediators as well as in affinity purification of these factors. Aside from these very practical *in vitro* applications of specific monoclonal antibodies it can be speculated that specific anti-Interleukin antibodies may even prove to be helpful in the *in vivo* treatment of diseases that may involve participation by Interleukins. This certainly would include neoplastic diseases. The Interleukins might either be involved in the host immune response to tumors or alternatively could even conceivably support the growth of some tumors. Insofar as the Interleukins can be considered potential biological response modifiers, antibodies to these cytokines also potentially may be useful modifiers of biological responses.

MATERIAL AND METHODS

Preparation of Interleukins

IL 1 was obtained from culture supernatants of human mononuclear cells (4×10^6/ml) by stimulating with 25 μg/ml lipopolysaccharide (LPS) for 48 hr (13). To obtain human IL 2, cells (5×10^6/ml) were stimulated with 10 μg/ml Concanavalin A (Con A), 10 ng/ml phorbol myristate acetate (PMA) in the presence of 2 mM hydroxyurea as recently described (12, 11). The production of rat and EL 4 thymoma derived IL 2 is also described elsewhere (3) and in this volume (Farrar et al.).

Bioassays

IL 2 activity was determined from the ^{3}H-TdR uptake by the IL 2 dependent murine CT6 cell line (2,11), while IL 1 activity was determined from the enhancement of ^{3}H–TdR uptake by PHA stimulated C3H/HeJ thymocytes (13). The in vitro proliferative response of human lymphocytes was determined as described earlier (11).

Partial Purification of the Interleukins

A summary of the purification of IL 2 is described in the results section, details will be reported elsewhere (10). IL 1 was partially purified by concentrating the culture supernatants using an Amicon UM 10 membrane followed by gel filtration on a calibrated Sephacryl S–200 column.

Production of Monoclonal Antibodies

Immunization of BALB/c mice was as described in the results section. The procedure for the adoptive transfer of spleen cells was performed as described by Fox et al. (4). The technique of spleen cell hybridization has also been previously described (5). Interleukin specific hybridomas were cloned by a limiting dilution method in the presence of a mouse thymocyte feeder layer (1).

Monoclonal Antibodies from Ascitic Fluid

Ascitic monoclonal antibody was obtained by transferring 8×10^6 hybridoma cells into pristane primed BALB/c mice. The antibody was precipitated from clarified ascitic fluid by the gradual addition of ammonium sulfate to 45% saturation. The antibodies were dissolved in the original volume and dialyzed against several changes of phosphate buffered saline and then against culture medium before use.

Monoclonal antibodies were coupled to CNBr activated Sepharose 4B under standard conditions as recommended by the manufacturer (Pharmacia Fine Chemicals, Uppsula, Sweden).

RESULTS

Production of Human Interleukins

Human Interleukin 2 was obtained from supernatants of cells cultured in the presence of Con A, PMA and hydroxyurea. We have recently shown that this method yields higher IL 2 supernatant activity (12,11). Con A activates lymphocytes to leave the resting phase (G_0) and enter the cell cycle. PMA partially arrests the cells in the G_1 phase which serves to prolong the phase during which the cells produce much of the growth factor IL 2. The utilization of IL 2 is maximal during S–phase and is reduced by the addition of hydroxyurea which blocks the cells at the G_1/S interphase. Table 1 shows that PMA in the absence of prior stimulation of the cells with Con A has no effect on the IL 2 production, but has a synergistic effect in the presence of Con A. Therefore, PMA has a most profound effect on stimulated cells or on cells that are already in the cell cycle such as proliferating cell line cells (3,11). The experiments shown in Table 1 show optimal IL 2 production in the presence of FCS. To facilitate purification and to obtain IL 2 with higher specific activity for immunization purposes, large scale pro- duction of IL 2 was performed under serum free culture conditions.

TABLE 1. Production of human Interleukin 2

Culture Conditions	Units of Interleukin 2	
	hydroxyurea	
	0	2mM
Control[a]	0.3 + 0.3[b]	0.5 + 0.3[b]
PMA 10 ng/ml	0.4 + 0.2	1.8 + 0.6
Con A 10 ug/ml	12.7 + 9.6	38.2 + 12.4
PMA + Con A	221.1 + 132	530.0 + 143

[a]Human PBL were cultured at 2×10^6 cells/ml for 46-48 hr in RPMI 1640 containing 2% FCS.
[b]Mean + standard error units/ml IL 2 of 4 normal donors.

The relative pattern of IL 2 production with Con A, PMA and hydroxyurea are unchanged by the absence of serum but the levels of supernatant IL 2 activity were 2-5 times lower than in comparably treated serum containing cultures.

Immunization With Partially Purified IL 2

Human IL 2 was partially purified by sequential chromatography using: a) stepwise elution with 40% ethanediol from phenyl sepharose; b) gradient elution from DEAE sephacel and c) gel filtration by Sephacryl S-200. As Table 2 shows this purification resulted in a 70 fold increase in specific activity of the serum free IL 2. BALB/c mice were

TABLE 2. Partial purification of Interleukin 2 for immunization

Sample	Units/ml	ml	Total Units	Protein (mg)	Spec.Act. U/mg	Yield (%)
Crude supernatant	100	4900	490,000	331.7	1,480	100
Phenyl sepharose	490	347	170,000	48.9	3,330	33
DEAE sephacel	2,850	84	240,000	32.7	7,410	49
Amicon UM 10 conc.	18,520	8.6	160,000	2.4	65,970	32
Sephacryl S-200	37,040	3.2	120,000	1.1	100,080	24

injected 3 times with 12,000 units of partially purified IL 2 (specific activity 1×10^5 units/mg protein; see Table 2) in complete Freund's adjuvants over a period of 6 weeks. Ten days after the last injection, spleen cells from an immunized mouse were injected IV into 2 mice (1 day post x-irradiation of the recipient with 500 rads) along with 12,000 units of IL 2 IP. Four days after this adoptive transfer the spleen cells of the recipients were used for hybridization. This adoptive transfer procedure has been shown to increase the frequency of antigen reactive clones ∿ 10 fold (4).

Hybridization of Spleen Cells

The BALB/c plasmacytoma non-immunoglobulin producing cell line, P_3-X63-Ag8-653 was used for hybridization (6) by the procedure described by Gefter et al. (5). The hybridized cells were placed in 24 well Costar plates at 0.5×10^6 spleen cells/well with a thymocyte feeder layer. Selection with HAT medium (7) was started 24 hr later and cultures were fed periodically by a 50% change of medium. After 2 weeks, the growth of HAT resistant cells was apparent in all 24 culture wells. These hypridoma culture supernatants were tested for their capacity to inhibit IL 2 supported proliferation of a murine IL 2 dependent T cell line (CT6). Ten culture supernatants were found to inhibit this bioassay. Four cultures (A,B,C,D) were selected and cloned by limiting dilution (1). Single cell clones from all the cultures were expanded; out of 168 clones 28% were inhibitory in the bioassay. Six clones were selected for the *in vivo* antibody production. Table 3 shows that the antibodies obtained from these ascitic fluids consisted of either IgM or IgG_1 immunoglobulins as determined by immunodiffusion.

TABLE 3. Inhibition of cell proliferation by monoclonal antibody

| Clone | Antibody class | Antibody titer that inhibits IL 2 induced CT6 proliferation by 30% | |
		Hybridoma culture supernatant[a]	$(NH_4)_2SO_4$ ppt. ascitic fluid[b]
B-1	μ,L	1/9[c]	1/110[c]
A-1	μ,K	1/15	1/70
C-1	μ,K	1/6	1/105
D-1	μ,K	1/4	1/160
D-2	μ,K	1/2	1/560
A-2	γ1,K	1/1	1/210
C-2	γ1,K	0	1/2

[a] CT6 cells were cultured with 5 units/ml of IL 2.
[b] CT6 cells were cultured with 10 units/ml of IL 2.
[c] Inhibition by serial dilutions of antibody was assessed and 30% inhibition was determined by linear regression and lysis.

Inhibition of CT6 Cell Line Proliferation by Monoclonal Antibody

Table 3 compares the IL 2 inhibitory capacity of hybridoma culture supernatants with that of ammonium sulfate precipitated ascitic monoclonal antibody. The 30% inhibitory titer was increased up to 250 fold by ascitic fluid antibody. The results demonstrate that there was no correlation between the degree of inhibition obtained with the supernatants as compared with that of the ascitic fluid. However cloned C-2 antibody, a negative hybridoma supernatant, remained non-inhibitory in the ascitic fluid form.

Absorption of IL 2 by Sepharose Bound Monoclonal Antibody

As shown in Table 4 antibodies coupled to CNBr-activated-Sepharose absorbed IL 2 to a variable degree. The capacity of a bound monoclonal antibody to absorb IL 2 activity was directly related to its potency in inhibiting the bioassay. Thus antibody from clone D-2 that previously inhibited the bioassay maximally also absorbed IL 2 to the greatest degree (96.4%). Uncoupled sepharose or sepharose coupled to the non-inhibitory antibody of clone C-2 did not absorb significantly super-natant IL 2 activity. These results indicate that reaction of the mono-clonal antibodies with the IL 2 molecule rather than with the lymphocyte surface is responsible for their capacity to inhibit the bioassay.

TABLE 4.   Absorption of IL 2 by sepharose bound monoclonal antibody

| Antibody from clone[a] | Absorbed Interleukin 2[b] | |
	Units/ml	%
None	906	7.5
C-2	79	0.7
B-1	8,760	73.0
A-1	3,822	31.8
C-1	5,454	45.5
D-1	5,946	49.5
D-2	11,571	96.4
A-2	9,792	81.6

[a]5 mg of protein from $(NH_4)_2SO_4$ ppt ascitic fluid was coupled to 1 ml of CNBr activated sepharose gel.
[b]0.8 ml of antibody coupled gel was incubated with 3 ml of IL 2 supernatant (12,000 units) for 18 hr in 0.4 M NaCl buffered with 0.02 M phosphate, pH 7.2.

Inhibition of Human Mononuclear Cell Proliferation
by Ascitic Monoclonal Antibody

The capacity of antihuman IL 2 antibody to inhibit human PBL as well as murine CT6 cell line proliferation was investigated. Table 5 shows that the antibodies inhibit the proliferation of human cells induced by unpurified IL 2 or by lectins such as phytohemagglutinin (PHA) and Con A. This indicates that monoclonal anti IL 2 directly inhibits human lymphoproliferative responses to both added IL 2 and to lectin induced endogenously generated IL 2. One can conclude not only that IL 2 participates in lectin induced lymphocyte proliferation, but that since endogenous IL 2 is accessible to the inhibitory antibody it presumably is not delivered in a cell contact dependent manner but must be avail-able to react with antibody in the intercellular environment.

TABLE 5.   Inhibition of human mononuclear cell proliferation by
           ascitic fluid containing monoclonal antibody

Antibody of Clone	Dilution that inhibits proliferation by 30%[a]		
	Crude IL 2 (10 units/ml)	PHA (1 ug/ml)	Con A (1 ug/ml)
B-1	1/40	1/12	1/550
A-1	1/43	1/11	1/1200
C-1	1/71	1/18	1/65
D-1	1/120	1/19	1/1100
D-2	1/280	1/74	1/1400
A-2	1/5	1/2	1/20

[a] 2×10^6 human mononuclear cells were cultured for 3 days in the
presence of various dilutions of the different ascitic fluids and IL 2,
PHA or Con A.   Cultures were pulsed on the 3rd day for 4 hr with ^{3}H-TdR.
The titer of 30% inhibition was calculated by linear regression analysis.

Non Species Specificity of Anti-IL 2 Antibody

    The inhibitory effect of antibody (D-2), which was the most potent
inhibitor of human IL 2 effects, was also tested on rodent IL 2 preparations.   Table 6 shows that this antibody also inhibited the effect of
rat IL 2 and even of mouse EL 4 thymoma derived IL 2 (3), indicating
that this antibody lacks species specificity.   The surprising finding
that a mouse anti-human monoclonal antibody reacts with mouse IL 2
suggests that the antibody is directed against a common preserved
determinant.

TABLE 6.   Inhibition of proliferation induced by heterologous IL 2

Source of IL 2[a]	^{3}H-TdR incorporation by CT6 cell line cells		
	−	+ antibody D-2[b]	
	cpm	cpm	% Inhibition
human	10,423	982	91.1
mouse	7,500	382	96.5
rat	8,589	641	92.5

[a] 10 units of IL 2 were used from human PBL supernatant, from mouse EL
4 thymoma supernatant or from rat spleen cell supernatant.

[b] 100 µg/ml of antibody D-2.

Production of Monoclonal Antibody Against IL 1

    A similar approach was used to produce monoclonal antibody to IL 1.
Human IL 1 was generated using LPS stimulation of ficoll hypaque separated
peripheral mononuclear cells.   The IL 1 activity was partially purified
by Sephacryl S-200 gel filtration yielding two peaks of IL 1 activity
with MW's of ∿ 50,000 and ∿ 15,000.   BALB/c mice were immunized 4 times
with the higher MW IL 1 activity in CFA.   Each immunization consisted of
1 ml of IL 1 activity with 50% of maximal activity at 1/250 dilution as
determined in the C3H/HeJ thymocyte assay.   On the day of adoptive
transfer, mice were injected I.P. with twice the previous dose of low MW

IL 1 activity. After hybridization 2/16 parental culture supernatants inhibited mouse thymocyte proliferation in response to human IL 1 and PHA. None of the supernatants inhibited the proliferation of the CT6 cells in response to IL 2. After cloning of the 2 active cultures, 6 clones were selected for in vivo ascitic antibody production. Table 7 shows that 4 different immunoglobulin classes were found. The inhibitory activity in the asatic fluid was increased by up to 1000 fold. This presumably reflects the increase in antibody concentration in ascites as compared to the hybridoma culture supernatants.

TABLE 7. Inhibition of human IL 1 enhanced thymocyte proliferation by monoclonal antibody

Clone	Antibody class	Antibody dilution that inhibits proliferation by 30%[a]	
		Hybridoma culture supernatant	Ammonium sulfate ppt.ascitic fluid
A-1	$\gamma1$,K	1/33	1/250
A-2	$\gamma3$,K	1/34	1/1900
A-3	$\gamma2a$,K	1/30	1/15000
B-1	$\gamma2a$,K	1/42	1/18000
B-2	μ,K	1/21	1/17000
B-3	$\gamma1$,K	1/8	1/240

[a]Titer that inhibited C3H/HeJ thymocyte proliferation induced by human IL 1 and PHA calculated by means of a linear regression analysis.

DISCUSSION

Although they are biologically very active, IL 1 and IL 2 are both obtained in only minute quantities in culture supernatants. Therefore, both have been partially purified in order to obtain material of increased specific activity for immunization purposes. Several preliminary attempts to obtain antigen reactive splenic B cells by the in vitro immunization method were unsuccessful (8). Additional polyclonal activation by lipopolysaccharide of the in vitro sensitized spleen cells failed to yield hybridomas that produced supernatants which inhibited lymphoproliferation in response to IL 1 or IL 2. Furthermore, we have not been able to demonstrate specific inhibitory activity in the serum of Interleukin immunized mice. Therefore, we used the method of adoptive transfer, which has been shown to greatly increase the frequency of antigen reactive B cells and successful hybridoma monoclonal antibody production (4). In the case of IL 2 we obtained clones secreting two immunoglobulin classes (IgG, or IgM), that not only inhibited the proliferation of mouse and human cells in response to homologous or heterologous IL 2 but reacted directly with the IL 2 molecule as shown by immunoaffinity absorption. However, the concentration of antibody needed to neutralize IL 2 is high. This observation suggests that these monoclonal antibodies are not directed against the active site of the IL 2 molecule, and that IL 2 antibody complexes may still be functional. The cross reaction of the monoclonal antihuman antibody (D-2) against rat and mouse IL 2 suggests that IL 2 is conserved similar structures on the IL 2 molecule which are essential for function. Interestingly, the crude anti IL 1 monoclonal antibodies did not inhibit the proliferation of IL 2 dependent cell lines which is compatible with the observations that IL 1 acts at an earlier stage in the immune response than IL 2 and also induces IL 2.

The monoclonal antibodies against the interleukins should provide an accurate tool for the study of the regulatory role of these mediators. The antibodies should also provide a powerful tool for the purification of IL 1 and IL 2 and for their use in other biochemical and biological assays.

REFERENCES

1. Andersson, J., and Melchers, F. (1978): Curr. Top. Micro. Immunol., 81:130–139.
2. Farrar, J. J., Mizel, S. B., Fuller-Farrar, J., Hilfiker, M. L. (1980): J. Immunol., 125:793–798.
3. Farrar, J. J., Fuller-Farrar, J., Simon, P. L., Hilfiker, M. L., Stadler, B. M., and Farrar, W. (1980): J. Immunol., 125:2555–2558.
4. Fox, P. C., Berenstein, E. H., Siraganian, R. P. (1981): Eur. J. Immunol. (in press).
5. Gefter, M. L., Margulies, D. H., and Scharff, M. D. (1977): Somatic Cell. Genet., 3:231–236.
6. Kearny, J. F., Radbruch, A., Liesegand, B., and Rajewsky, K. (1979): J. Immunol., 123:1548–1550.
7. Kennett, R. H., Denis, K. A., Tung, A. S., and Klinman, N. R. (1978): Curr. Top. Micro. Immunol., 81:77–91.
8. Luben, R. A., and Mohler, M. A. (1980): In The Biochemistry of Lymphokines, edited by A. L. deWeck, F. Kristensen and M. Landy pp. 55–65, Acad. Press, N.Y.
9. Smith, K. A., Lachman, L. B., Oppenheim, J. J. and Favata, M. F. (1980): J. Exp. Med., 151:1551–1556.
10. Stadler, B. M., Dougherty, S. F., Berenstein, E. H., Fox, P. C., Oppenheim, J. J., Siraganian, R. P. (1981): submitted.
11. Stadler, B. M., Dougherty, S. F., Farrar, J. J., and Oppenheim, J. J. (1981): submitted.
12. Stadler, B. M., Farrar, J. J. and Oppenheim, J. J. (1980): Behring Inst. Mitt., 67:245–248.
13. Togawa, A., Oppenheim, J. J., and Mizel, S. B. (1979): J. Immunol. 122:2112–2118.

*Lymphokines and Thymic Hormones: Their
Potential Utilization in Cancer Therapeutics,*
edited by A. L. Goldstein and M. A. Chirigos,
Raven Press, New York © 1981.

Purification and Biological Properties of Interleukin 3

James N. Ihle, Jonathan Keller, John C. Lee, William L. Farrar,
and Andrew J. Hapel

*Biological Carcinogenesis Program, Frederick Cancer Research Center,
Frederick, Maryland 21701*

INTRODUCTION

Lymphokines are known to play a central role in regulating immune responses. Factors such as migration inhibitory factor are important in macrophage localization at sites of inflamation. The macrophage derived factor interleukin 1 (IL-1), also termed LAF appears to play an essential role by facilitating the production of another lymphokine, interleukin 2 (IL-2), by helper T cells (14,25,26). IL-2 in turn appears to mediate the differentiation and amplification of cytotoxic T cells and has been particularly important in current research by virtue of its ability to maintain the growth in tissue culture of cytotoxic T cell lines (7,18,21, 27). In addition to these factors which have been characterized biochemically, a variety of additional factors are involved in diverse aspects of immune responses which have not been characterized. These factors include lymphokines which affect B cells either in allowing the differentiation of an antibody response in vitro or polyclonally activating immunoglobulin production, as well as factors promoting the differentiation and proliferation of myeloid cells or mast cells (8,20). From these observations, it appears reasonable to assume that the majority of the manifestations of humoral and cellular immune responses are regulated by lymphokines including not only the recruitment of nonantigen-specific components such as macrophages, but also the expansion of potentially antigen-specific components as well.

One of the central regulatory components of an immune response involves an antigen-specific helper T cell. Several lymphokines including MIF, T cell replacing factors in B cell responses, and IL-2 have been shown to be produced by helper T cells under appropriate conditions of antigen stimulation (6,11,12,23,24). More recently, cloned helper T cell lines have been established from immune mice by antigen stimulation in vitro and have been shown to produce several lymphokines (8,20). Interestingly, cloned helper T cells have also been shown to mediate a classical delayed type hypersensitivity reaction when put in vivo with the appropriate antigen, demonstrating the central regulatory role of this subpopulation of lymphocytes (3). In in vitro responses, antigen-specific helper T cells mediate classical blastogenic responses. Although this response had been previously considered to be simply the proliferation of antigen-specific lymphocytes, recent data has suggested that the response is more complex (15). In particular, proliferation appears to involve a variety of lymphocyte subpopulations responding to biochemically distinct lymphokines produced by an antigen-specific helper T cell. Although the blastogenic response has been related to a few lymphokines, the vast majority of the factors and subpopulations involved have not been characterized.

The factors produced by antigen-stimulated helper T cells clearly influence the functions of a variety of cell types. Perhaps one of the most potentially important class of factors, however, are those which directly influence T cell functions. From a speculative viewpoint it might be anticipated that antigen-activated T cells would produce factors which affect many stages of T cell differentiation which would allow the continued expansion of functional effector cell populations including helper and cytotoxic cells under conditions of antigen excess. The only factor to date which has this property is IL-2, and the available data suggest that this lymphokine only functions at a relatively terminal stage of cytotoxic T cell differentiation. In the results presented here, we demonstrate the existence of a second lymphokine which specifically influences T cell differentiation. This factor, however, promotes a very early stage of T cell differentiation and in vitro specifically promotes the differentiation of helper T cells.

MATERIALS AND METHODS

Mice.
Normal BALB/c mice were obtained from the Animal Production Facility of the Frederick Cancer Research Center. Mice were generally used at 4-6 weeks of age.
Preparation of Conditioned Media.
Unfractionated normal BALB/c splenic lymphocytes were seeded at a concentration of 5-10 x 10^6 viable cells/cm^2/ml. The cultures were incubated with 5 µg/ml of Con A for 48 hr at 37°C in RPMI 1640 containing 1% fetal calf serum (FCS). The cells were removed from culture fluids by centrifugation and the conditioned media filtered through a 0.45µ filter. Conditioned media were stored at 4°C.
Spleen Cell Preparations.
Spleens were removed aseptically and gently mashed. The suspension was passed through cotton gauze to remove large debris and the cells were pelleted by centrifugation. Erythrocytes were lysed by suspending cells in ACK buffer (0.155 M NH_4Cl, 0.1 mM Na_2 ethylene diaminotetraacetate, 0.01 M $KHCO_3$) and remaining cells were washed once in RPMI. T cells were further purified by a modification of the method of Julius et al. (11), as described by Lipsky and Rosenthal (16) with minor changes. Briefly, 50 ml syringes were packed with 5 g of washed nylon wool (Fenwal Laboratories) and were equilibrated just before use with RPMI 1640 medium with 20% FCS at 37°C. Spleen cells were incubated on the column for 1 hr then eluted with 80 ml of medium at a flow rate of 1 ml/min. Eluted cells were adjusted to appropriate concentrations as described in the text.
Purification of Interleukin 3 (IL-3).
Ammonium sulphate (560 g/L) was used to precipitate proteins from conditioned media. The precipitate, normally from 7-16 liters of medium, was

resuspended in a minimal volume of phosphate buffered saline (PBS) and dialyzed extensively against PBS. The dialysate was centrifuged at 15,000 rpm for 30 min and the soluble fraction filtered through a 0.45µ filter. The preparation was then applied to a G-100 Sephadex column equilibrated with PBS. Fractions were collected and assayed for lymphokine activity in the splenocyte proliferation assay and for induction of 20 alpha hydroxysteroid dehydrogenase (20αSDH). Active fractions were pooled and precipitated with ammonium sulphate (560 g/L). The precipitate was resuspended in a minimal volume of 0.01 M NaCl, 0.01 M sodium phosphate buffer (pH 7.0), and extensively dialyzed against the same buffer. The dialysate was clarified by centrifugation (15,000 rpm, 30 min) and the soluble fraction applied to a 1.5 x 30 cm DEAE cellulose column (Whatman DEAE 52) equilibrated with phosphate buffer. The column was then eluted with a 200-200 ml, 0.01-0.5 M NaCl linear gradient. Five ml fractions were collected and assayed for IL-2 and IL-3 activity. The fractions containing IL-3 activity were pooled, ammonium sulfated as above, dialyzed against 0.01 M sodium phosphate (pH 7.0) 0.01 M NaCL and applied to a CM cellulose column. Active fractions were pooled, lyophilized, resuspended, dialyzed against phosphate buffer as above, and used in the experiments described. Protein concentrations were determined by the method of Lowry et al. (17). Salt concentrations were determined by conductivity.

Induction and Assay of 20αSDH.

In order to follow the purification of IL-3, 10 ml of a suspension $(3 \times 10^6$ cells/ml) of splenic lymphocytes from nu/nu BALB/c mice were incubated at 37°C with samples taken from the column fractions and diluted with RPMI 1640 plus 10% FCS. After 24 hr at 37°C, the cells were harvested by centrifugation and assayed for 20αSDH. Cells were suspended in 0.01 M sodium phosphate buffer (pH 7.0) containing 1.0 mM $MgCl_2$ and sonicated for two cycles of 15 sec bursts at 50 watts in a Sonifer Cell Disruptor Sonicator (Heat Systems, Ultrasonics, Inc.). The sonicate was then centrifuged at 20,000 x g for 30 min. The supernatant was decanted and frozen in liquid nitrogen until enzyme analysis. The enzyme assay used was adapted from Weinstein et al. (29). Briefly, 0.1 ml of a cell extract was incubated for varying periods of time with 0.1 ml of ^{3}H-progesterone $(10^{-6}$ M) (New England Nuclear) and 0.2 ml of a NADPH regenerating system consisting of 0.1 mM NADPH, 1 mM glucose-6-phosphate, and 0.15 units of glucose-6-phosphate dehydrogenase (Sigma). Samples were assayed in duplicate at three time points; a zero time point was included in each assay to determine background conversion. The reaction was stopped by the addition of ether containing carrier progesterone and 20-alpha hydroxypregn4-en-3-one (20αOHP) (Sigma) with vigorous vortexing. The aqueous phase was frozen in liquid nitrogen and the ether phase was decanted into conical glass tubes and evaporated under a gentle stream of air. Methanol (0.02 ml) was added to each tube to dissolve the steroids and this solution was subjected to thin layer chromatography on silica gel thin layer chromatography plates (EM Laboratories) in an ether: chloroform system (3:10). The spots of progesterone and 20αOHP were identified under a shortwave UV lamp (Mineralight, UltraViolet Products, Inc.), scraped into scintillation fluid (16 g PPO and 0.4 g POPOP per gallon toluene), and counted in a Beckman liquid scintillation counter. The picomoles of 20αOHP formed were calculated from the percent conversion of ^{3}H-progesterone to ^{3}H-20αOHP minus background conversion and expressed as specific activity (pmoles/ h/10^8 viable cells). The reaction was linear with increasing extract concentration or time (data not shown) up to 40% conversion. Replicate analysis of the samples yielded a standard deviation of less than 2% conversion.

Treatment of Cells with Typing Antibodies.

The immunofluorescence assay for the detection of intracelluar terminal deoxynucleotidyl transferase was adapted from Gregoire et al. (9). Cell suspensions at 2×10^4/ 0.1 ml were spread onto glass microscope slides in a cytocentrifuge (Cytospin, Shandon Instruments). The cells were air dried and fixed in cold methanol for 30 min. The fixed cells were rehydrated in PBS. Rabbit anti-bovine TdT was purchased from Bethesda Research Laboratories and was used as the primary antibody. The primary antibody was allowed to incubate with the fixed cells for 30 min at room temperature. After extensive rinsing, fluorescein conjugated goat anti-rabbit IgG (Fab$_2$) was added as developing reagent for 30 min at room temperature. The slides were rinsed and examined for fluorescence using a Zeiss research microscope with an epi-illumination system. Appropriate positive and negative control cells and reagents were also included.

Cell Surface Phenotype Analysis by Indirect Immunofluorescence.

Monoclonal antibodies raised against Thy 1.2, Lyt 1 and Lyt 2 (obtained from New England Nuclear and Becton-Dickenson, respectively) were used except for conventional rabbit antisera to murine IgM and Ia^k (purchased from Litton Bionetics and Cederlane, respectively). Generally a 1:200 dilution of the monoclonal antibodies or 1:50 dilution of conventional reagents was used to treat 10^6 cells. FITC goat anti-rabbit IgG or FITC rabbit anti-mouse IgM was used as the developing reagent. The cells were lightly fixed with 1% phosphate buffered formalin for 10 min in the cold. After each treatment with the immunofluorescent reagents at 4°C for 30 min the cells were washed extensively with PBS. Immunofluorescence was determined by a Zeiss microscope equipped with epi-illumination system.

RESULTS

Distinct T cell subpopulations can be readily defined by the presence or absence of the enzymes terminal deoxynucleotidyl transferase or 20αSDH (22). TdT$^+$ lymphocytes are predominately thymic localized, hydrocortisone-sensitive, and are not active in various lymphocyte assays (2,13). In contrast, 20αSDH$^+$ lymphocytes comprise the majority of peripheral T cells, are hydrocortisone-resistant, and appear to constitute the mature functional subpopulation (22,28,29). The requirement for an intact thymus for the maturation of 20αSDH$^+$ lymphocytes is shown by the results illustrated in Fig. 1. In normal mice the levels of 20αSDH in splenic lymphocytes are high soon after birth and decrease to a relatively constant level at 4 weeks of age. In contrast, only low levels of 20αSDH are found in splenic lymphocytes from nu/nu athymic mice which, after approximately 4 weeks of age, increase slowly with time. These results suggested that nu/nu mice had precursor lymphocytes capable of becoming 20αSDH$^+$ although in young mice the factors required for the differentiation of such lymphocytes was limiting. For these reasons we began to explore various sources for the presence of a specific factor which could promote the differentiation, in vitro, of 20αSDH$^+$ lymphocytes from nu/nu splenic lymphocyte preparations.

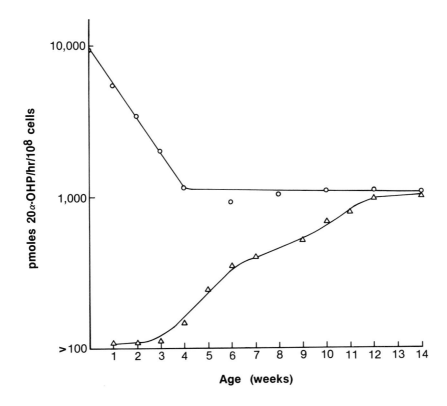

FIG. 1.   Age dependence for the expression of 20αSDH in normal and
athymic mice.   Either (C57BL/6 x C3H)F1 mice (o—o) or NIH Swiss nu/nu
mice (△—△) were sacrificed at the indicated ages.   Spleen lymphocyte
populations were obtained and assayed for the presence of 20αSDH
activity as described in Methods.

The ability of various factors to induce 20αSDH expression in vitro
is shown in Table 1.   In the presence of either Con A or LPS no 20αSDH
induction occurred.   Similarly, neither thymosin fraction V nor hydrocortisone or progesterone had any detectable activity.   In contrast, conditioned media from Con A or PHA stimulated normal lymphocytes had the
ability to induce the expression of 20αSDH.   The specificity of these
preparations is indicated by the inability of conditioned media from LPS
stimulated normal splenic lymphocytes to induce 20αSDH.   Last, conditioned media from mixed lymphocyte reactions had activity comparable to
Con A and PHA conditioned media.   These results suggested that associated
with T lymphocyte activation was the production of a factor capable of
inducing 20αSDH in nu/nu splenic lymphocytes.

TABLE 1. Ability of various factors to induce 20αSDH in nu/nu splenic
lymphocytes in vitro

Culture conditions	pmoles OHP/hr/10^8 lymphocytes	Fold stimulation
Media	220	1.00
Con A (5 µg/ml)	180	0.82
LPS (10 µg/ml)	170	0.77
Thymosin fraction V (10 µg/ml)	110	0.50
Hydrocortisone (10^{-7} M)	130	0.59
Progesterone (10^{-7} M)	140	0.64
LPS CM[a] (50%)	135	0.61
Con A CM (50%)	1320	6.00
PHA CM (50%)	1480	6.73
MLR CM (50%)	1370	6.23

[a]Conditioned media were prepared by incubating normal splenic lymphocytes (2 x 10^6/ml) with Con A (5 µg/ml), LPS (10 µg/ml), or PHA (25
µg/ml) for 48 hr and recovering the media after centrifugation to remove
the cells. MLR CM was prepared by incubating 2 x 10^6 lymphocytes/ml
each of BALB/c and C57BL/6 normal splenic lymphocytes. Conditioned media
was collected after 72 hr.

We next determined whether the production of this factor was associated with antigen-specific activation of T cells. In previous experiments we have demonstrated that during the regression of MoLV/MSV tumors
there is a T cell blastogenic response against the major envelope glycoprotein of the virus, gp70 (5). As shown in Table 2, conditioned media
from gp70 stimulated immune lymphocytes contained readily detectable
levels of a factor capable of inducing 20αSDH in nu/nu splenic lymphocytes. The specificity of the production of this factor is indicated by
the lack of comparable activity in conditioned media from gp70 treated
nonimmune lymphocytes or from immune lymphocytes incubated with the viral
core protein p30 which does not induce an immune response. The T cell
population required for the production of this factor is also shown in
Table 2. Treatment of immune lymphocytes with either antibodies against
Thy 1 or Lyt 1 abrogated production of the factor whereas treatment with
antibodies against Ig, Ia, or Lyt 2 had no effect. These results demonstrate that the production of the factor in immune reactions is dependent
upon an antigen-specific helper T cell.
Conditioned media from activated T cells are known to contain a variety of lymphokines which affect T cell differentiation and proliferation.
To determine whether the induction of 20αSDH was due to a known or
unique factor, we purified the activity. Similar to other lymphokines,
the activity could be precipitated from conditioned media at 75% ammonium
sulfate saturation. On G-100 columns the activity eluted at a position
corresponding to a molecular weight of 30,000-50,000 daltons (10). The
fractions from G-100 were subsequently chromatographed on DEAE cellulose. As shown in Fig. 2, the factor eluted from these columns in the

TABLE 2. Induction of 20αSDH in nu/nu splenic lymphocytes by factors in conditioned media from antigen stimulated immune lymphocytes

Culture conditions	pmoles OHP/hr/10^8 lymphocytes	Fold stimulation	% inhibition
Experiment 1[a]			
Media	80	1.0	-
Con A CM	980	12.25	-
gp70/immune CM	840	10.50	-
gp70/nonimmune CM	60	0.75	-
p30/immune CM	70	0.87	-
p30/nonimmune CM	70	0.87	-
Experiment 2[b]			
Media	180	1.0	-
gp70/immune CM +C'	1600	8.89	-
gp70/immune CM α Thy 1 + C'	250	1.39	84%
gp70/immune CM α Lyt 1 + C'	210	1.17	87%
gp70/immune CM α Lyt 2 + C'	1580	8.78	1.2%
gp70/immune CM α Ia + C'	1340	7.44	16.2%
gp70/immune CM α Ig + C'	1570	8.72	1.9%

[a]Nylon wool purified splenic lymphocytes from MoLV/MSV immune or normal C57BL/6 mice were stimulated for 48 hr with either MoLV gp70 (5 µg/ml) or p30 (5 µg/ml). The conditioned media from these cultures was then tested for their ability to induce 20αSDH at a concentration of 50%.

[b]Immune lymphocytes were used as above but were initially treated with the natibodies indicated and C' prior to incubation with gp70 (5 µg/ml). Conditioned media were subsequently assayed as above.

run through fractions and was clearly separated from another lymphokine, IL-2, which eluted from this column in the salt gradient at approximately 0.15 M NaCl. The active fractions from DEAE cellulose were subsequently applied to a CM-cellulose column and the activity was found to elute in the run through from this column. Last, the active fractions were applied to a blue sepharose column to which the activity bound and could be eluted in a salt gradient with the peak of activity eluting at approximately 0.1 M NaCl.

The results of these purification procedures are summarized in Table 3. The final preparation represents a 6,250-fold purification and generally results in a 20% recovery of activity. The purified factor generally has a specific activity (ED_{50}) of approximately 1 ng/ml. This value, assuming a molecular weight of 40,000 daltons, indicates an apparent affinity of about 2×10^{-11} M, a value close to known values for factors such as insulin and several growth factors. As shown in Fig. 3,

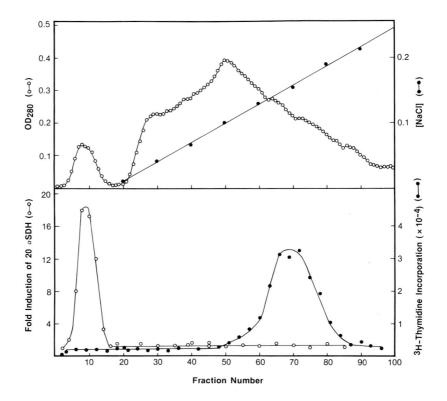

FIG. 2. DEAE cellulose fractionation of conditioned media. The active fractions from G-100 Sephadex fractionation of conditioned media were pooled, concentrated as described in Methods, and dialyzed against 0.01 M sodium phosphate buffer, pH 7.0, 0.01 M NaCL. The sample was then applied to a DEAE cellulose column (1.5 x 30 cm) equilibrated in the same buffer and eluted with a linear NaCl gradient. Fractions of 5 ml were collected, the optical density at 280 A (o—o), and the NaCL concentration were determined (●—●). The top panel fractions were subsequently assayed for their ability to induce 20αSDH (o—o) and for IL-2 activity (●—●); bottom panel as described in Methods.

the final preparations appeared homogenous by SDS-PAGE and gave a single major protein band with an apparent molecular weight of 40,000 daltons.

The activity of the purified factor in various lymphokine assays is shown in Table 4. This particular preparation had been purified through CM cellulose and was not completely pure. Nevertheless, no colony stimulating activity, interferon activity, or T cell replacing activity for B cell responses was detected. In addition, the factor did not support the growth of cloned cytotoxic T cells, an activity characteristic of IL-2. No thymocyte mitogenic activity was present either in the presence or absence of Con A, demonstrating the lack of IL-1-like activity.

TABLE 3. <u>Typical recoveries and purification of IL-3 from conditioned media (1% FCS)</u>

Purification Step	ED_{50}(ng/ml)[a]	Fold purification	Recovery
Conditioned media	5000	-	
$(NH_4)_2SO_4$ ppt	2200	2.3X	100%
G-100 fractions	320	15.6X	60%
DEAE	18	320X	50%
CM	3	1667X	45%
Blue Sepharose	0.8	6250X	20%

[a]ED_{50} effective dose in ng/ml giving 50% of maximal induction.

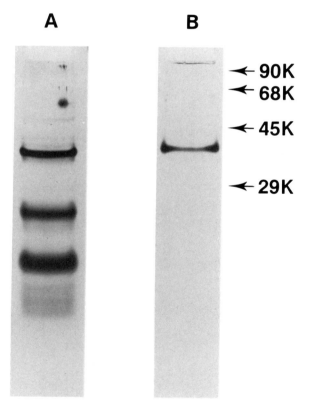

FIG. 3. SDS-PAGE analysis of purified IL-3. (A) Sample prior to blue sepharose column; (B) Peak of activity from blue sepharose.

TABLE 4. Relative activities of purified IL-3 in various lymphokine assays

Lymphokine assay	ED_{50} (ng/ml)
Induction of 20αSDH in nu/nu splenic lymphocytes	25
Induction of splenic lymphocyte proliferation	25
Growth of cloned cytotoxic T cells	>1000
Colony-stimulating activity	>1000
Interferon activity	>1000
T cell replacing activity in B cell responses	>1000
Thymocyte proliferation (-Con A)	>1000
Thymocyte prolfieration (+Con A)	>1000

In addition to the induction of 20αSDH, however, the purified factor induced proliferation of normal splenic lymphocytes with comparable ED_{50}s. Because this factor does not have a number of known lymphokine activities, is produced by antigen-specific helper T cells, and functions to promote the differentiation of early T cells, we have proposed the term interleukin 3 (IL-3).

Some of the properties from previous studies of the induction of 20αSDH in nu/nu splenic lymphocytes by purified IL-3 are summarized below (10). The induction of 20αSDH by IL-3 is rapid and after a lag of approximately 6 hr, linear increase in 20αSDH occurs over the next 24-36 hr resulting in increases in enzyme activity of 15- to 20-fold. The rapidity and the fold increases strongly suggest that IL-3 is inducing the enzyme rather than simply amplifying a population of 20αSDH positive lymphocytes. That IL-3 promotes differentiation is further suggested by the observation that the precursor lymphocyte is hydrocortisone-sensitive and unstable in tissue culture, whereas the induced population is hydrocortisone-resistant and stable in tissue culture. Similar to a number of differentiation events, the induction of 20αSDH requires cell division as demonstrated by the ability of mitomycin C to inhibit induction. The requirement for proliferation is interesting in view of the ability of IL-3 to induce proliferation of normal splenic lymphocytes. However, whether this proliferation is associated with induction of 20αSDH cannot be determined due to the normally high levels of 20αSDH in normal mice.

The characteristics of the lymphocyte population responding to IL-3 and the induced population have also been examined in previous studies (10). The precursor lymphocyte responding to IL-3 is not abrogated following treatment with antibodies against Thy 1, Lyt 1, Lyt 2, Ia or Ig and complement. Moreover, once induced to express 20αSDH, the lymphocytes are still insensitive to these treatments. These results and the above have demonstrated, therefore, that IL-3 promotes the differentiation of an early, hydrocortisone-sensitive Thy 1⁻ lymphocyte to become hydrocortisone resistant and Thy 1⁻. Presumably in the presence of additional factors this precursor gives rise to a mature Thy 1⁺ 20αSDH⁺ lymphocyte.

IL-2 has been shown to be capable of expanding the subpopulation of lymphocytes which responds to it. Therefore, it was conceivable that IL-3 in addition to promoting differentiation might cause the expansion of the resulting population in tissue culture. To explore this possibility we attempted to establish IL-3 dependent lymphocyte lines in vitro. The ability of IL-3 to support the growth of lymphocytes was initially determined by varying factor concentration, lymphocyte density and media. From these experiments, optimal conditions were found to involve plating 2-4 x 10^6 nylon wool purified normal splenic lymphocytes/cm^2 in RPMI 1640 containing 10% FCS with concentrations of IL-3 giving maximal induction of 20αSDH. The media is changed every 3 days and the cells transferred to fresh wells every 7 days to remove adherent cells. Under these conditions there is a transient period of growth during the first 2-3 days followed by a decrease in cell numbers over the next 10-20 days. After this the cultures increase in growth and after 4-6 weeks stable transferable cell lines are established. Such cell lines have been established 111 times in 117 attempts to date, whereas in the absence of IL-3 none have resulted. Therefore, IL-3 very reproducibly and efficiently is capable of establishing lymphocyte cell lines.

A number of the cell lines were examined for the various lymphocyte characteristics summarized in Table 5. For comparison, the characteristics of a cloned IL-2 dependent cytotoxic T cell line are also included. All of the IL-3 derived lines examined had comparable lymphocyte surface phenotypes of Thy 1$^+$, Lyt 1$^+$,2-, Ia- and Ig- and were clearly distinct from the IL-2 T cell line which was Thy 1$^+$, Lyt 1-,2$^+$. The results also demonstrate that with regard to the surface phenotype, IL-3 promotes the establishment of a very specific subpopulation of lymphocytes. Of the cell lines examined none expressed TdT, whereas all the lines examined had detectable 20αSDH. Consistent with these results all the cell lines examined were found to be resistant to hydrocortisone. The data, therefore, suggest that the IL-3 derived lines have the phenotypic properties of mature helper T cells.

During the course of examining the properties of the IL-3 derived lines, it became evident that none of the cell lines required exogenously added IL-3 for growth once they were established. Typical results indicating this independence are illustrated in Table 6, and come from cloning experiments in which the ability to form colonies in soft agar in the presence of various factors was examined. As shown, all of the

TABLE 5. Phenotypic characteristics of IL-3 derived T cell lines relative to an IL-2 dependent T cell line

Phenotype	IL-3 derived cell lines no. positive/total	CT6 Cell Line
Thy 1.2	41/41	+
Lyt 1	41/41	-
Lyt 2	0/41	+
Ia	0/41	-
Ig	0/41	-
TdT	0/6	-
20αSDH	4/4	+
Cortisone sensitivity	0/41	-

TABLE 6. Cloning efficiency of IL-3 derived T cell lines in soft agar in the presence or absence of lymphokines

Cell line	Cloning efficiency in agar supplemented with		
	IL-3	IL-2	Media alone
GN	67	68	72
HN	89	94	84
IN	100	100	100
JN	96	100	84
KN	100	100	100
A4A	92	74	84
CT$_6$	0	72	0

IL-3 derived lines have comparable cloning efficiencies in either media alone or IL-2 or IL-3 supplemented media. In contrast, the IL-2 derived cytotoxic T cell line was absolutely dependent on IL-2 for growth. Therefore, although IL-3 is absolutely required for the establishment of the cell lines, once established, growth is not dependent on exogenously added lymphokines.

The independence from lymphokines for growth and the obvious helper cell phenotype suggested that the IL-3 derived lines may be capable of producing their own lymphokines. We, therefore, examined conditioned media from several of the cell lines for the production of IL-3 and IL-2. As shown in Table 7, all of the lines examined produced readily detectable levels of IL-3, whereas no IL-3 was produced by the IL-2 dependent T cell lines. In contrast, none of the cell lines constitutively produced detectable IL-2, but in the presence of phorbol myristic acetate all the lines examined produced readily detectable IL-2. In addition, a number of the cell lines have been examined for the production of colony stimulating activity and all constitutively produced this factor (data not shown). Therefore, the IL-3 derived T cell lines appear to contain the functional characteristics of helper T cells.

DISCUSSION

Our results demonstrate the existence and properties of a previously unidentified lymphokine. Due to its source of production and the populations that it affects, we have proposed the term interleukin 3 to be consistent with the recently proposed standardized nomenclature for lymphokines (30). IL-3 has as its unique characteristic the capability of inducing 20αSDH activity in nu/nu splenic lymphocytes. As demonstrated here and previously, of a variety of lymphokines in conditioned media from activated T cells only a single factor appears to have this activity. In addition we have examined sources of IL-1 activity, such as P388D$_1$ conditioned media and have not detected IL-3 activity. Conversely, purified IL-3 does not have any activity in a variety of

TABLE 7. Production of IL-3 and IL-2 by IL-3 derived cloned T cell lines

Cell lines	Culture conditions	Lymphokine production no. positive/total	
		IL-3	IL-2
IL-3 derived cell lines	Media	41/41	0/8
	Media + PMA	8/8	8/8
CT6 (IL-2 line)	Media	0/1	ND
	Media + PMA	0/1	ND

other lymphokine assays, demonstrating its unique characteristics. The only additional activity we have detected is the ability to induce proliferation of normal splenic lymphocytes, but since the induction of 20αSDH requires proliferation, this is not unexpected.

Using conventional biochemical techniques, it has been possible to purify IL-3 to apparent homogeneity. In general, IL-3 is a relatively stable factor and retains its activity over long periods at 4°C in either crude preparations or in the purified form. The elution characteristics from ion exchange columns suggest that IL-3 is relatively uncharged at pH 7.0 and, therefore, unlike other murine lymphokines does not bind to DEAE cellulose. The purified IL-3 has an ED_{50} of approximately 1 ng/ml which is within the range of activity of such growth factors and suggests an apparent affinity of approximately 2×10^{-11} M. The purified factor has an apparent molecular weight of 40,000 daltons on SDS-PAGE analysis consistent with other data (not shown) from sizing columns under nondenaturing conditions. Experiments are currently in progress to establish the amino acid sequence of purified IL-3.

Our results demonstrate that with normal lymphocytes and with immune lymphocytes, IL-3 is a product of activated T cells. Similar to IL-2, IL-3 is produced by Con A, PHA or alloantigen-stimulated T cells. In addition, antigen-specific immune lymphocytes produce IL-3 in blastogenic reactions. In additional experiments we have demonstrated that in these reactions IL-3 represents one of the blastogenic factors which promotes proliferation. The phenotype of cells responding to antigen and producing IL-3 has a typical helper T cell phenotype of Thy 1+, Lyt 1+,2-. This subpopulation of lymphocytes has previously been shown to be responsible for the production of other lymphokines. These results as well as the results with cloned helper T cell lines as described below strongly suggest that a single class or subpopulation is responsible for lymphokine production. However, it is conceivable that the production of specific factors by this class of lymphocytes will require different physiological signals either as antigen or antigen plus mediators such as IL-1.

The physiological role that IL-3 plays in differentiation or regulation of the immune system is not yet entirely clear. Recent experiments (unpublished) have demonstrated that 20αSDH is a T cell marker enzyme found in both cloned functional cytotoxic T cells, as well as helper T cells. These results confirm previous experiments with more complex lymphocyte populations which suggested that 20αSDH is found in all mature T cells. Therefore, assuming that only IL-3 induces 20αSDH, the lymphocyte population responding to IL-3 would appear to represent a precursor for both helper and cytotoxic T cells. In addition, the lack of expression of Thy 1 on either the precursor or IL-3 induced populations would suggest that the induction of 20αSDH occurs in a relatively immature population of lymphocytes and that additional factors may be required for the continued differentiation to Thy 1+ functional T cells. Experiments are currently in progress to determine the properties of such factors. Nevertheless, the properties of hydrocortisone sensitivity and capability to respond to IL-3 appear to define an early pre-T cell subpopulation.

The data strongly suggest that in athymic mice one of the major factors limiting the differentiation of functional mature T cells is the conversion of 20αSDH- to 20αSDH+ lymphocytes, which in turn suggests that IL-3 may be a limiting factor. This is indicated by the ability of IL-3 to rapidly induce the expression of 20αSDH in vitro suggesting that the appropriate immediate precursors are present. Second, as previously noted (10), the specific activity of 20αSDH in maximally induced cells is comparable to that found for normal splenic lymphocytes, suggesting that only IL-3 is required to generate the normal frequency of 20αSDH+ lymphocytes. For these reasons it will be particularly interesting to examine the effects of purified IL-3 in vivo in nu/nu mice. Also of interest will be to determine why in the absence of a thymus early production of IL-3 does not occur and thus the differentiation of 20αSDH+ lymphocytes is blocked.

Perhaps the most unexpected result from our experiments was the ease with which IL-3 can be used to establish T cell lines. In a variety of experiments over the last 6 months, continuous T cell lines have been established with virtually 100% efficiency. Although not shown, this efficiency also applies to nu/nu splenic lymphocyte preparations. Equally striking has been the consistency of the cell type that is established with IL-3. This contrasts dramatically with recent results which have demonstrated that T cell clones isolated by growth in Con A depleted conditioned media have a variety of phenotypes (19). Taken together these results would suggest that conditioned media have a variety of factors capable of either allowing the differentiation or growth of distinct subpopulations of T cells. In addition it might be anticipated that multiple factors exist which could influence in vitro the pathways of differentiation resulting in unique subpopulations.

In the presence of IL-3, the predominant if not exclusive lymphocyte subpopulation isolated is of a helper T cell phenotype. This is exemplified by both the surface phenotype of the cell lines as well as their ability to produce lymphokines such as IL-3, IL-2, and CSF. The production of IL-3 is particularly interesting since although the establishment of the cell lines was dependent on IL-3, once established all the lines were independent of exogenously added IL-3 or other lymphokines for growth. Because of this we cannot at present determine whether the growth of the lines is independent of IL-3 or perhaps one of the other factors that the cell lines produce. These cell lines, however, are quite distinct from the IL-2 cytotoxic T cell lines, which require the continual addition of IL-2 for growth.

The ability of IL-3 to establish lymphocyte lines with characteristics of helper T cells was unexpected. As indicated above the precursor which responds to IL-3 and the resulting $20\alpha SDH^+$ lymphocyte are Thy 1^- suggesting that only an early T cell is involved. Therefore, during establishment of the cell lines the Thy 1^- $20\alpha SDH^+$ subpopulation must undergo additional differentiation to become a Thy 1^+, Lyt $1^+, 2^-$ lymphocyte. What these secondary events are is not known, but several preliminary observations suggest an interesting possibility. In particular, based on the observation that all the cell lines produce IL-3, we reasoned that they may be antigenically stimulated in tissue culture. The only source of "antigens" available would be fetal calf serum components. We, therefore, examined the growth of the cell lines in normal mouse serum and found that the cells failed to grow. Since the major serum component is bovine serum albumin, we examined the ability of pure BSA to "grow" uncloned lines and have observed that in the presence of NMS and BSA the cultures grow as well as in FCS. These results suggest, therefore, that the cell lines may represent helper T cells for FCS components and in turn suggest that IL-3 promotes the differentiation of a precursor helper T cell which in the presence of antigen can undergo differentiation to a functional helper T cell which then only requires antigen for continued growth. Experiments are currently in progress to determine the validity of this model.

Since the goal of these proceedings is to evaluate the possible use of various lymphokines in modifying host responses, it seems appropriate to consider the potentials of IL-3. Although considerable work needs to be done to better delineate precisely the physiological role of IL-3, the available data provide some interesting speculative possibilities. The fact that IL-3 promotes differentiation of early T cells suggests that with regard to amplifying the immune system in vivo, IL-3 may have more general effects than factors such as IL-2 which amplify terminal components of the system. Second, since IL-3 appears to be the initial limiting factor with regard to differentiation of T cells in nu/nu mice, replacement therapy in syndromes such as DiGeorge's disease and other T cell hypoplasias may be possible. From the in vitro experiments, it is clear that IL-3 can facilitate the differentiation of functional helper T cells and, therefore, may be useful as an immune adjuvant to facilitate the initial recruitment of helper T cells which in turn can then function to expand the response as determined by antigen presence or absence. Last, the available data also suggest that IL-3 can be used to efficiently generate in tissue culture antigen-specific helper T cells which will provide a unique opportunity to study the immune system in vitro as well as providing the potential for developing a protocol for an in vitro/in vivo establishment of immunity.

REFERENCES

1. Adelman, N.E., Ksiazek, J., Yoshida, T., and Cohen, S. (1980): J. Immunol., 124:825.

2. Barton, R., Goldschneider, I., and Bollum, F.J. (1976): J. Immunol., 116:462.

3. Bianchi, A.T.J., Hooijkaas, H., Benner, R., Tees, R., Nordin, A.A., and Schrier, M.H. (1981): Nature, 290:836.

4. David, J.R., and David, R.A. (1972): In: Progress in Allergy, edited by P. Kallos, B.H. Waksman, and A. deWeck, p. 300. S. Karger, Basel.

5. Enjuanes, L., Lee, J.C., and Ihle, J. N. (1979): J. Immunol., 112:665.

6. Farrar, J.J., Mizel, S.B., Fuller-Farrar, J.J., Farrar, W.L., and Hilfiker, M.L. (1980): J. Immunol., 125:793.

7. Gillis, S., and Smith, K.A. (1977): J. Exp. Med., 146:468.

8. Glasebrook, A.L., Quintans, J., Eisenberg, L., and Fitch, F.W. (1981): J. Immunol., 126:240.

9. Gregoire, K.E., Goldschneider, I., Barton, R.W., and Bollum, F.J. (1977). Proc. Natl. Acad. Sci. USA, 74:3993.

10. Ihle, J.N., Pepersack, L., and Rebar, L. (1981): J. Immunol., (in press).

11. Julius, M.H., Simpson, E., and Herzenberg, L.A. (1973): Eur. J. Immunol., 3:645.

12. Kuhner, A.L., Cantor, H., and David, J.R. (1980): J. Immunol., 125: 1117.

13. Kung, P.C., Silverstone, A.E., McCaffrey, R.P., and Baltimore, D. (1975): J. Exp. Med., 141:855.

14. Larsson, E.L., Iscove, N.N., and Coutinho, A. (1980): Nature, 283:664.

15. Lee, J.C., Enjuanes, L., Cicurel, L., and Ihle, J.N. (1981): J. Immunol., (in press).

16. Lipsky, P.E., and Rosenthal, A.S. (1976): J. Immunol. 117:1594.

17. Lowry, O.H., Rosebrough, N.J., Farr, A.L., and Randall, R.J. (1951): J. Biol. Chem., 193:265.

18. Morgan, D.A., Ruscetti, F.W., and Gallo, R. (1976): Science, 193: 1007.

19. Nabel, G., Fresno, M., Chessman, A., and Cantor, H. (1981): Cell, 23:19.

20. Nabel, G., Greenberger, J.S., Sakakeeny, M.A., and Cantor, H. (1981). Proc. Natl. Acad. Sci. USA, 78:1157.

21. Nabholz, M., Conselman, A., Acuto, O., North, M., Haas, W., Pohlit, H., von Boehmer, H., Hengartner, H., Mach, J.P., Engers, H., and Johnson, J.P. (1980): Immunol. Rev., 51:125.

22. Pepersack, L., Lee, J.C., McEwan, R., and Ihle, J.N. (1980): J. Immunol., 124:279.

23. Schimpl, A., and Wecker, E. (1972): Nature (New Biol.), 237:15.

24. Shaw, J., Caplan, B., Paefkau, V., Pilarski, L.M., Delovitch, T., and McKenzie, I.F.C. (1980): J. Immunol. 124:2231.

25. Smith, K.A., Gilbride, K.J., Favata, M.F. (1980): Nature, 287:836.

26. Smith, K.A., Lachman, L.B., Oppenheim, J.J., and Favata, M.F. (1980): J. Exp. Med., 151:1551.

27. Watson, J., Gillis, S., Marbrook, J., Mochizuki, D., and Smith, K.A. (1979). J. Exp. Med., 150:849.

28. Weinstein, Y. (1977): J. Immunol., 119:1223.

29. Weinstein, Y., Linder, H.R., and Eckstein, B. (1977). Nature, 266:632.

30. Letter to the Editor. (1979): J. Immunol., 123:2928.

*Lymphokines and Thymic Hormones: Their
Potential Utilization in Cancer Therapeutics,*
edited by A. L. Goldstein and M. A. Chirigos,
Raven Press, New York © 1981.

Lymphotoxins: Purification and Biological Parameters

Jim Klostergaard, Robert S. Yamamoto, and G. A. Granger

*Department of Molecular Biology and Biochemistry, University of California, Irvine,
Irvine, California 92717*

It is in part the purpose of this symposium to review the state-of-the-art of the field of lymphokines. These nonimmunoglobulin lymphocyte factors have been the focus of a great deal of effort from many laboratories since they were first termed lymphokines by Dumonde and colleagues (6) about twelve years ago. These studies were, with some notable exceptions, largely descriptive in nature. It is probably not a coincidence that both the fields of cellular immunology and lymphokines pale in comparison to humoral immunology with regard to a sophisticated understanding of basic molecular mechanisms. Our group will present in this treatise its progress in the purification of a complex system of interrelated cell-toxins elaborated by actvated lymphocytes. Some of their biochemical and biological parameters will be considered within the context of their possible role in cell-mediated immune responses, including cell lysis.

I. Chemical characterization of lymphotoxins

A. Quantitation of bioassay

The ability to quantitate a particular biological effect is one of the principal factors underlying the difference in sophistication between humoral immunology and the lymphokine field. It should be noted that this is at least in part a result of the limited quantity of lymphokines usually available in lymphocyte supernatants. A bioassay which can be quantitated is indispensable in attempts to purify a particular mediator, for without it, determination of yields in isolation steps is impossible. Since most lymphokine assays depend on the determination of an effect on an indicator cell, the development of sensitive targets for the lymphokine activity clearly contributes to the sensitivity with which the factor can be detected.

In our work, a valuable lymphotoxin-sensitive strain of the murine α-L-929 cell has been developed and is currently being utilized. By plating a defined number of mitomycin C-treated L-cell targets (1×10^5), a titer of a particular lymphotoxin preparation is defined as the reciprocal of the dilution causing 50% lysis of the targets, i.e., one unit. This sensitive bioassay has permitted detection of

---

J.K. is a Senior Postdoctoral Fellow of the American Cancer Society, California Division.

lymphotoxins in the low femtomole range.

B. Purification of lymphotoxins

1. Preparations of supernatants

The other major impediment to biochemical research in the lymphokine field is that in general only very limited amounts of these
factors are elaborated by activated lymphocytes. This has necessi-
tated, in some cases, starting a purification scheme with very large
volumes of supernatant. Some investigators have attempted to surmount
these difficulties by superinduction techniques or by employing continuous lymphoblastoid lines which produce high titers of lymphokines.
Although the latter can only be maintained in the presence of serum,
release of the mediator may occur spontaneously in serum-free media.
The concern for reducing the load of exogenous protein in supernatants
of primary activated lymphocyte culture and for eliminating particular
contaminants secreted by the cells has led to the use of serum-
substitutes and to the exacting timing of collection of supernatants.
For example, Jegasothy and Battles (23) found that inhibitor of DNA
synthesis (IDS) could be harvested optimally between 48 and 72 hours
after activation of rat lymphocytes; hence, the cells were removed from
culture after two days, and then recultured in fresh serum-free media.
This manipulation greatly reduced the complexity of the supernatant,
and they were able to achieve a homogeneous product with a purification
scheme which increased the specific activity only about 300-fold.

This approach is not invariably successful, however. Russel and
coworkers (42) have reported a purification scheme for human alpha-
light class lymphotoxin (α_L-LT) in which lectin-activated lymphocytes
are cultured first in the presence of serum, and then allowed to
release LT after resuspension in serum-free media. The release in
serum-free media somewhat compromises the total potency of the supernatant compared to release in serum; however the specific activity of
the serum-free supernatant is much higher because no exogenous protein
(other than PHA) is added. Nevertheless, after three consecutive
separation procedures, i.e., molecular sieving, ion-exchange chromatography, and preparative electrophoresis, their LT preparation was
still heterogeneous by gel analysis. In contrast, Klostergaard and
coworkers (25,27) employed starting supernatants from PHA-activated
lymphocytes cultured with a small amount of a heat stable fraction of
calf serum, termed boiled serum (30). We have been able to demonstrate
an electrophoretically homogeneous preparation of α_L-LT after a purification scheme similar to that of Russel, et al. (42). This suggests
that in their case a considerable burden of contaminating proteins was
released by the lymphocytes during lymphotoxin release in serum-free
media (perhaps reflecting compromised cell viablilty) and that by
adding the proper exogenous protein (e.g., boiled serum), a higher
specific activity supernatant may be obtained. We have employed a
similar approach to the purification of alpha-heavy lymphotoxin (α_H-LT)
(26; and Klostergaard, et al., in preparation). Despite these low
protein conditions, the specific activities of both α_L and α_H rose
about four orders of magnitude before homogeneity could be achieved.

2. Biochemical separations

The choice of the first separation technique employed in a purification scheme should be as considered as the effort to increase the specific activity of the starting supernatant. Because of the zonal mixing observed in conventional liquid chromatography, the success of a purification scheme will be enhanced if the largest burden of contaminants may be disposed of early in the scheme. For example, in the purification of α_L-LT from boiled serum-containing supernatants, an initial molecular sieving step is fruitful because most of the exogenous protein is found in the void volume (25,30). In other cases, an affinity-chromatographic step might be employed to the same end and eliminate the need for a separate concentration step as well.

It should be evident from the successful schemes reported for the purification of lymphokines that multiple tandemized purification steps are generally required to obtain a homogeneous product. By employing distinct separation techniques, molecular polymorphism of a particular lymphokine may become apparent. For example, in the case of lymphotoxins, six different molecular weight classes have been described: Complex; Cx, Precursor alpha-heavy, $P\alpha_H$; alpha-heavy, α_H; alpha-light, α_L; beta, β; and gamma, γ; (10,12,15,39,47,50). These can in turn be shown to be polymorphic on the basis of behavior on ion-exchange, lectin-affinity, and hydrophobic-affinity columns, and in electrophoretic systems (10,11,13,14,25,26,39,45,47). Therefore, a resolution of this complex system requires the refinement of many components. Some other lymphokines appear also to be quite polymorphic (4,51); the reason for this is not at all apparent. However, precedent for this is becoming well documented in the interferon systems (46).

Since the purpose of a purification scheme for any protein is to increase the specific activity of the preparation, it is imperative that an accounting of the distribution of proteins following an isolation procedure be performed. Unfortunately, many protocols reported for lymphokine purification do not do so, and are therefore of doubtful value. Again, since these mediators are present in low amounts, highly sensitive protein assays must be applied. Our laboratory has found that based on the criteria of sensitivity and economy, external trace radiolabeling with ^{125}I has distinct advantages over most internal radiolabeling procedures. We have introduced the isotope using the Iodogen procedure, which we have found to be much milder than other oxidative methods, to a specific activity approaching 10^7 cpm/µg into many proteins (25; and Klostergaard, et al., unpublished observations), and this has allowed us to verify the effectiveness of our purification protocols and document purity in gel systems for both α_L and α_H lymphotoxins (25-27) (Table I). It is our experience that crude preparations of proteins (or supernatants) may be successfully radioiodinated to allow determinations of increases in purity early in a purification scheme. However, in order to obtain a pure component of suitable specific activity (radioactivity) for radioautographic procedures, it is more satisfactory to label a more refined preparation from later in the scheme.

We obtain α_L class (70-90,000 d) human lymphotoxin from PHA-activated tonsil and adenoid lymphocytes, cultured in RPMI-1640

TABLE 1. Radioiodination of human α_{L2} lymphotoxin by the Iodogen
          procedure: Effect of chloramide dose and time on efficiency
          and residual lytic activity

Iodogen (µg)	Time (min)	Efficiency (Percent)	Lytic Activity (Percent)
10	10	≈30	≈85
3	10	≈25	≈95
1	5	≈25	≈100
0.5	5	≈25	≈100

supplemented with boiled serum. This yields culture supernatants with
lymphotoxin titers comparable to that for lymphocyte cultures employing
serum, and therefore with far higher starting specific activities (30).
The α_L class can be resolved into charge subclasses by ion-exchange
chromatography on DEAE-Sepharose. The predominant subclass, α_{L2},
is enriched about fivefold over the activity in the molecular sieving
fractions, and about 75-fold over the supernatant. Polyacrylamide
gel electrophoretic (PAGE) analysis, where both biological activity
and protein is monitored, reveals this preparation is only 1% pure.
The resident contaminating proteins are removed by preparative
electrophoresis (27) or preparative isoelectricfocusing (Klostergaard,
et al., unpublished observations) yielding a homogeneous product
(Table 2).

TABLE 2: Steps involved in the purification of ^{125}I-labeled human α_{L2}
          LT subclass

	Specific Activity LT units/µg protein[a]	Increase compared to whole supernatant
A. Whole supernatant	<1	--
B. Molecular sieving (AcA 44) (α class obtained)	≈5	≈12-15
C. DEAE chromatography (α_2 subclass obtained)	≈25	≈75
D. Preparative PAGE	≈2,500	≈7,500
E. Analytical tube PAGE	≈5,000	≈15,000

[a] Protein determined by fluorescamine assay using BSA as a standard.

The other α_L subclasses, α_{L1} and α_{L3} are present in very minute
quantities and their purification has not yet been attempted. The
relationship between these charge subclasses has been shown to be
only partly due to carbohydrate, on the basis of reactions with
exoglycosidases (45). However, these subclasses are interrelated
because they express common antigenic determinants (31,56).

Supernatants containing a stable form of α_H-LT are generated from
Con A-activated tonsil and adenoid lymphocytes in RPMI-1640 supplemented with lactalbumin hydrolysate (LAH). This form is of the same
size (120-150,000 d) and reacts with anti-F(ab')$_2$ reagents as does the
α_H from lectin-stimulated T-enriched peripheral blood lymphocytes or MLC

lymphoblasts. Residual exogenous LAH peptides are removed by molecular sieving which entails a purification factor of about five- to tenfold. The α_H preparation shows very significant reversible binding to Con A-Sepharose, and a 50-fold increase in specific activity is realized. A final purification step on preparative isoelectric- focusing yields a homogeneous product (26). Polymorphism is apparent in the lectin affinity chromatographic step, as 10-15% of the α_H lytic activity appears in the breakthrough and 85-90% binds the sorbent; microheterogeneity is also apparent from electrofocusing, as the α_H pI's range from 6-7 (Table 3).

TABLE 3:   Steps in the purification of human α_H LT

		Estimated Percent Yield	Estimated Specific Activity	
			LT units/μg protein[a]	Increase compared to whole supernatant
A.	Whole Supernatant	--	<1	--
B.	Molecular Sieving Ultrogel AcA 44	⌄70	⌄2	⌄5-10
C.	Lectin-Affinity Chromatography Con A-Sepharose	⌄50	⌄100	⌄250-500
D.	Preparative Isoelectricfocusing	⌄30	⌄2,000	⌄5-10,000

3. Documentation of purity

An essential prerequisite for the analysis of the peptide sub- structure and primary structure of lymphokines, as for any proteins, is a rigorous documentation of homogeneity. The underlying rationale for such documentation, which is frequently ignored, is that a component is homogeneous only if it resists an increase in specific activity when subjected to any isolation procedure.

Electrophoretic analysis in polyacrylamide gel (PAGE) systems has proven to be a very valuable aid in such documentation, when properly employed. When performed under native conditions (no SDS), PAGE has excellent resolving power, capable of discriminating even between molecules of very similar size and charge characteristics. Most bio- logical activities tolerate the relatively mild conditions, and thereby PAGE analysis allows the assignment of a particular protein component to the active molecule. In contrast, analysis of the same preparation by PAGE in the presence of SDS frequently abrogates the biological activity, and may not be able to resolve multiple components in a prep- aration which has already been subjected to molecular sieving, and is therefore comprised on components of similar size. However, some reports indicate that some lymphokines survive SDS treatment; this is probably the exception, rather than the rule, especially for lymphokines of high molecular weight or for those comprised of multiple peptide chains.

We have documented the purity of human α_L-LT obtained by the scheme detailed in the previous section by the following criteria: 1) the lytic activity migrates with a single radioiodinated component in native PAGE (Figure 1);

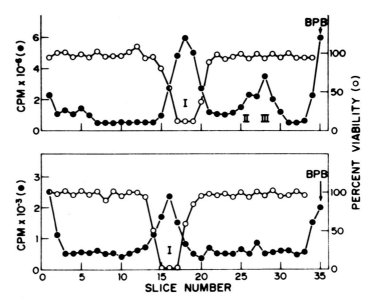

FIG. 1. (Top Panel) Electrophoretogram in a 7% acrylamide gel of ^{125}I-α_{L2} which had been purified by molecular sieving, ion-exchange chromatography, and preparativve electrophoresis (Table 2). Lytic activity (O——O) and radioactivity (●——●) in each gel slice is indicated -- (Bottom Panel) Electrophoretogram in a 7% acrylamide gel of Peak I from top panel. Lytic activity (O——O) and radioactivity (●——●) is indicated. (Reproduced from Molecular Immunology by written permission of the Editor).

2) this labeled component is a single peak on analytical isoelectric-focusing (Figure 2); 3) the labeled component and lytic activity are totally immunoprecipitated with identical amounts of a specific rabbit anti-α_L antiserum (Figure 3) (27). The pure molecule has been analyzed by SDS-PAGE, and two distinct polypeptide chains of about 27,000 and 68,000 are detected (Johnson, et al., unpublished observations).

To date, our evidence for purity of the human α_H-LT preparation obtained by the scheme described in the previous section is based on the fact that the radioiodinated component migrates in coincidence with the lytic activity (Figure 4) (26). We are currently attempting to further substantiate its homogeneity by analysis in native PAGE at different acrylamide concentrations, and by specific immunoprecipitations with reagents recognizing determinants on the molecule.

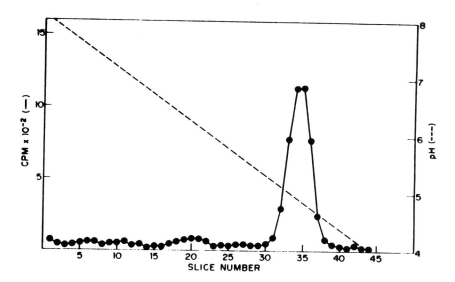

FIG. 2. Analytical isoelectricfocusing in polyacrylamide of Peak I from Figure 1, Top Panel. Radioactivity (●——●) in each slice is indicated, as is the range of the pH gradient (———). Reproduced from <u>Molecular Immunology</u> by written permission of the Editor).

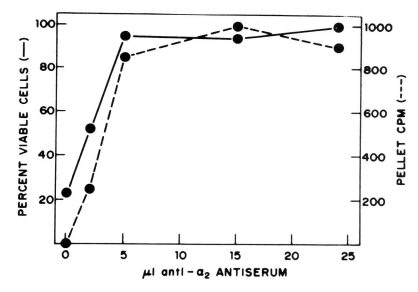

FIG. 3. Immunoprecipitation by specific anti-α_{12} antiserum of ^{125}I-α_{L2} from Peak I of Figure 1, Top Panel. Aliquots of Peak I were reacted with the rabbit antiserum, and these complexes precipitated with a goat antiserum to rabbit serum. Lytic activity (●——●) remaining in the supernatant, and radioactivity (●--●) in the pellet is indicated. (Reproduced from <u>Molecular Immunology</u> by written permission of the Editor).

II. Mechanism of action of lymphotoxins

   A. Growth-inhibitory and cell-lytic effects

     Lymphotoxins were originally described as weakly cell-lytic or
growth inhibitory molecules, acting only on a protracted time scale
($\approx$24 hr), and only effective on certain cell types (28,40). As
biochemical studies advanced and revealed the multicomponent nature
of lymphotoxins, it became apparent that certain lymphocyte populations were responsible for the biosynthesis and secretion of particular molecular weight classes (Figure 5). Activated B-cells and
B-cell lymphoblastoid lines appear to only produce the α_L molecular
weight forms (70-90,000 d) (8). In contrast, activated T-enriched
human peripheral blood lymphocytes and lymphoblasts from mixed lymphocyte culture (MLC) release the higher molecular weight forms: Complex
- >200,000 d, and α_H - 120-160,000 d (12,50).

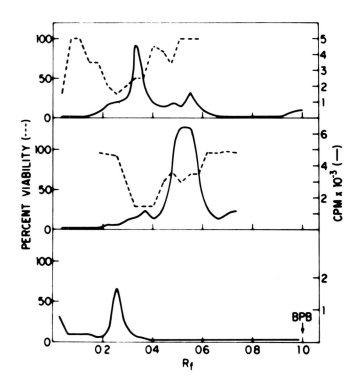

FIG. 4. (Top Panel) Electrophoretogram in a 7% acrylamide gel of
^{125}I-α_H which had been purified by molecular sieving and lectin-
affinity chromatography (Table 3). Lytic activity ($- - -$) and radioactivity ($\underline{\quad\quad}$) in each slice is indicated -- (Middle Panel) Electrophoretogram in a 5% acrylamdie gel of the same separation -- (Bottom
Panel) Electrophoretogram in a 7% acrylamide gel of ^{125}I-α_H which had
been purified by molecular sieving, lectin-affinity chromatography,
and preparative isoelectricfocusing (Table 3). (Reproduced from
Molecular Immunology by written permission of the Editor).

The smaller forms (α_L, β, γ) are the more stable, and are probably the components the first investigators examined. Indeed, we have observed that only uniquely sensitive cells are susceptible to their effects. Cell lysis is protracted, although the kinetics observed appear to depend on the concentration of toxin employed. The larger forms (Cx, α_H) are distinctly less stable, and unless they are rapidly handled properly, they are degraded into the smaller LT molecules. These larger forms are cell-lytic and growth inhibitory for a much wider spectrum of cells, although lysis is <u>still</u> relatively protracted (8-16 hr) (57).

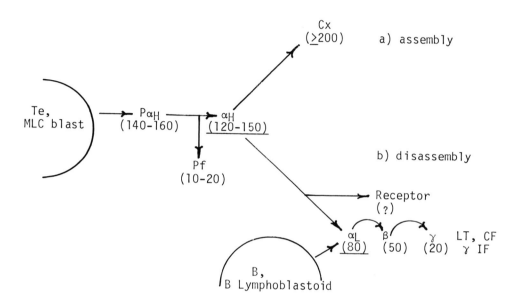

FIG. 5. Cellular origin and processing of lymphotoxins in the fluid phase. T-enriched cells and MLC-blasts yield receptor-directed $P\alpha_H$ form (see text). B cells and B lymphoblastoid lines release α_L form, which is not receptor-associated. $P\alpha_H$ is either processed to highly lytic receptor-associated Cx, or degraded to weakly lytic, non-receptor-associated, α_L, β or γ (molecular weight X 1,000).

Of particular interest and relevance to a molecular model of lymphocyte mediated killing is that the Cx and α_H appear to be associated with nonimmunoglobulin antigen-binding receptor(s). The serological evidence for this in the human system is that heterologous anti-F(ab')$_2$ (IgG) reagents can block their cell-lytic capacity, and anti-heavy and anti-light chain reagents react poorly or not at all (12,17,20,50). Functional evidence for a "selective" receptor is obtained from studies in two species. Murine Cx and α_H from allo-immune splenocytes demonstrate enhanced lysis of the immunizing allogeneic target, compared to other allogeneic targets (18,19,21). In the human, two lines of functional evidence exist. Human MLC blasts can be triggered to release cell-lytic molecules, principally

Cx and α_H, into the supernatant. These supernatants lose lytic activity if they are adsorbed on fixed monolayers of the stimulator cell employed in the MLC, and not on monolayers of unrelated targets (20). These supernatants show enhanced lysis of the specific target as well (20,56). When peripheral blood lymphocytes from donors immune to a particular antigen are stimulated with that antigen in vitro, they release cell-lytic molecules. These can be specifically adsorbed to antigen-affinity columns, and their nonspecific cell-lytic activity for α-L-929 cells can be blocked by the specific antigen, but not unrelated antigens (20).

In attempting to establish the specificity of killing in both the murine alloimmune system and in the human peripheral blood lymphocyte (PBL) MLC system, it must be considered that these lymphoid tissues contain very heterogeneous effector cell populations. These include anomalous killer (AK) and natural killer (NK) populations in addition to the desired cytotoxic T-lymphocytes (CTL). Since all three populations are activated to some degree with the protocols employed, the lytic molecules found in the supernatant may be derived from diverse sources. In fact, it is now established that NK rich cell populations do release cell-lytic molecules in response to lectin stimulation, which bind to and lyse target cells which are susceptible to lysis by the intact NK cell (55). While the response of AK cells is not as well characterized, it is apparent that the lytic activity found in the supernatants from lectin-activated murine spleen cells and human PBLs will reflect the cellular heterogeneity of these lymphoid tissues. These considerations currently preclude the definitive statement that cell-lytic supernatant forms kill specifically. The challenge then will be to obtain cell-lytic molecules from cloned cytotoxic T-lymphocyte lines.

B. Delivery to the target cell

Serological evidence from several laboratories suggests that the family of lymphotoxin molecules is involved in the lytic mechanism(s) of several types of in vitro cell-mediated cytotoxicity (CMC). These CMC reactions include human and guinea pig lectin-induced cellular cytotoxicity (16,44), human natural killing (54), human antibody-dependent cellular cytotoxicity (29), and human and guinea pig cytotoxic T-lymphocyte mediated cytotoxicity (9,48,49). The cell-lytic reactions may be blocked at some point in their lytic phase(s) by reagents reactive with components of the lymphotoxin system. These findings must now be extended to the isolation and characterization of the structure expressed by the different effector cell populations which react with the immunological blocking reagents.

Evidence from our own laboratory indicates that lectin-stimulated T-enriched human PBLs and MLC blasts, which include NK, AK, and CTL populations, release cytotoxins in a carefully controlled temporal sequence (12,20). The first form released into the supernatant is termed precursor alpha-heavy ($P\alpha_H$) (Figure 5). This component is highly unstable, expresses $F(ab')_2$ determinants and functional receptor activity, has strong cell-lytic capacity, and does not react with an anti-α_L antiserum (12,50). Under mildly perturbing forces, the $P\alpha_H$ degrades to the α_H form. This form has all the functional features of the $P\alpha_H$, but also reacts with the anti-α_L antiserum. This change in immunological reactivity occurs upon the reversible release of a 10-20,000 d component from the $P\alpha_H$ (12). The α_H may then apparently be processed along one of two routes: either aggregation to form highly cell-lytic Complexes (Cx), or breakdown to weakly lytic α_L, β, and γ LT components. Some evidence suggests that at least some aspects of the release and processing of these toxins is controlled and modulated by cellular proteases.

An important distinction and comparison with the complement system can be drawn. In that system, all the subunits are available in the blood vascular system of the host. As subunits, their biological effects are minimal; only upon appropriate triggering in a very complex mechanism do these subunits assemble to precipitate a cascade into the membrane attack complex with extremely potent cell-lytic capacity. The lymphotoxin system appears to operate with opposite polarity: the effector cell delivers to the target cell high molecular weight forms (Cx, $P\alpha_H$, α_H) with potent and receptor-directed cell-lytic capacity. These high molecular weight forms may be disarmed, if they do not rapidly interact with antigen by breakdown, possibly by proteolytic action, into the lower molecular weight forms (α_L, β, γ) which have weak anti-cellular effects.

Since the effector cell is able to deliver these potent toxins in the absence of deleterious effects to itself (polarity of lysis), a mechanism involving initial production of zymogen-like, non-lytic high molecular weight form, or involving unique processing of the toxins by the target cell might be invoked. Although no evidence for the former exists yet, some studies support the latter possibility. Weitzen and Granger (53) have reported the α_L-LT mediated lysis of α-L-929 cells requires an active target cell protease(s). Their results are consistent with many of the features of murine CTL-mediated lysis reported by Redelman and Hudig (37), who found that lysis required active proteases and intact thiol groups. However, the relevance of a mechanism for lysis of a uniquely sensitive target cell (α-L-929) by a weakly lytic toxin (α_L) to that for specific or selective killing of a variety of targets by the highly potent cell-lytic forms (Cx, $P\alpha_H$, α_H) is not clear. It will be of great importance to conduct similar inhibition studies employing cloned effector populations with defined specificities, as well as on the Cx and α_H forms themselves, in lysis of a wide variety of targets.

C. Relationship to other lymphokine activities

In drawing analogies between the lymphotoxin and complement cell-lytic systems, the question arises whether, as with the latter system, the weakly cell-lytic subunits of the lymphotoxin system may participate in other types of cellular responses, currently perceived as other lymphokine functions. This is an extension of the concept of "mother factors" (5) in lymphokines, whereby other mediators are derived from a common precursor(s), and it is the mode of processing this precursor which dictates the types of activities which are found in a given supernatant. Preliminary experimental evidence supporting this hypothesis has become evident. For example, in the human, serological evidence indicates that a specific anti-α_L lymphotoxin antiserum blocks monocyte chemotactic factor activity (Granger and Yoshida, unpublished results). It will be of interest to test the homogeneous human α_L and α_H lymphotoxin molecules for activity in other lymphokine assays in collaboration with other investigators. We may also employ monospecific antisera against the α_L and α_H molecules to test for blocking of activities in these systems. In view of the similar anticellular effects of proliferation inhibitory factor (PIF), γ-interferon (γ-IFN) and lymphotoxin, it will be especially rewarding to examine the possible relationships between these mediators.

III. Prospects for therapeutic utilization

Reports from many laboratories have lent support to the concept that lymphotoxins may be selectively cytotoxic or cytostatic for transformed cells compared to normal cells in vitro (7,32,33,38,41). There is also evidence that these molecules are tumoricidal in vivo in both animals and humans (1-3,22,24,34-36,43,52,58,59). While these are very exciting and potentially fundamental observations, they are severely limited by the fact that many of the studies employed very crude lymphocyte supernatants as their "lymphotoxin" preparations. Since these supernatants contain multiple lymphokine activities with anticellular effects, it is not clear that lymphotoxin is the only causative agent. Even those investigators who have attempted to control for resident interferon cannot readily discount the possiblity of synergy between different anticellular mediators (as has been observed for different interferons). Clearly, these studies must be verified with the pure molecules now available in our laboratory. In order to establish a justification for the possible use of these agents in human patients, a thorough investigation of their effects in vitro on transformed cells and in vivo in animal tumor systems must be conducted.

REFERENCES

1. Bast, R. C., Jr., Zbar, B., Machaness, G. B., and Rapp, K. J. (1975): J. Natl. Cancer Inst., 54:749-756.
2. Berstein, I. D., Thord, D. E., Zbar, B., and Rapp, K. J. (1971): Science, 172:729-731.
3. Biozzi, G., Stiffel, C., Halpern, B. N., and Mouton, D. (1958): Amer. Inst. Pasteur, 94:681-689.
4. Brown, A. P., and Rocklin, R. C. (1979): J. Immunol., 122:1059.
5. Cohen, S. (1980): In: Biochemical Characterization of Lymphokines, edited by A. L. DeWeck, F. Kristensen and M. Landy, pp. 607-609, Academic Press, New York.
6. Dumonde, D. C., Wolstencroft, R. A., Panayi, G. S., Matthew, M., Morley, J., and Houson, W. T. (1969): Nature, 224:34-42.
7. Evans, C. K., Rabin, E. S., DiPaolo, J. A. (1977): J. Cancer Res., 37:898-903.
8. Fair, D. S., Jeffes, E. W. B., and Granger, G. A. (1979): Molec. Immunol., 16:186-192.
9. Gately, M. K., Mayer, M. M., and Henney, C. S. (1976): Cell. Immunol., 27:82-93.
10. Granger, G. A., Yamamoto, R. S., Fair, D. S., and Hiserodt, J. C. (1978): Cell. Immunol., 38:388-402.

11. Granger, G. A., Klostergaard, J., Weitzen, M. L., Yamamoto, R. S., and Johnson, D. L. (1981): In: Thirteenth Midwinter Miami Symposia, edited by W. A. Scott, R. Werner, and J. Schultz, V. 18, Academic Press, New York.

12. Harris, P. C., Yamamoto, R. S. Crane, J., and Granger, G. A. (1981): J. Immunol. (in press).

13. Hiserodt, J. C., Fair, D. S., and Granger, G. A. (1976): J. Immunol., 117:1503-1506.

14. Hiserodt, J. C., and Granger, G. A. (1976): Cell. Immunol., 26: 211-216.

15. Hiserodt, J. C., Prieur, A.-M., and Granger, G. A. (1976): Cell. Immunol., 24:277-288.

16. Hiserodt, J. C., and Granger, G. A. (1977): J. Immunol., 119: 374-380.

17. Hiserodt, J. C., Yamamoto, R. S., and Granger, G. A. (1978): Cell. Immunol., 38:417-433.

18. Hiserodt, J. C., Tiangco, G. J., and Granger, G. A. (1979a): J. Immunol., 123:317-324.

19. Hiserodt, J. C., Tiangco, G. J., and Granger, G. A. (1979b): J. Immunol., 123:332-341.

20. Hiserodt, J. C., Yamamoto, R. S., and Granger, G. A. (1979): Cell. Immunol., 41:380-396.

21. Hiserodt, J. C., Granger, G. A., and Bonavida, B. (1981): In: T and B Lymphocytes, Recognition and Function, Academic Press, New York (in press).

22. Holtermann, O. A., Klein, E., Djerassi, I., Bernhard, J. D., and Parmett, S. R. (1976): In: Immunobiology of the Macrophage, edited by D. S. Nelson, pp. 577-591. Academic Press, New York.

23. Jegasothy, B. V., and Battles, D. R. (1979): J. Exp. Med., 150: 622-632.

24. Klein, E. (1969): Cancer Res., 29:2351-2362.

25. Klostergaard, J., Yamamoto, R. S., and Granger, G. A. (1980): Molec. Immunol. 17:613-623.

26. Klostergaard, J., and Granger, G. A. (1981): Molec. Immunol. (in press).

27. Klostergaard, J., Long, S., and Granger, G. A. (1981): Molec. Immunol. (in press).

28. Kolb, W. P., and Granger, G. A. (1968): Proc. Natl. Acad. Sci., 61:1250-1255.

29. Kondo, L. L., Rosenau, W., and Wara, D. W. (1981): J. Immunol., 126:1131-1133.

30. Lewis, J. E., Yamamoto, R. S., Carmack, C., Lundak, R. L., and Granger, G. A. (1976): J. Immunol. Meth., 11:371-383.

31. Lewis, J. E., Carmack, C. E., Yamamoto, R. S., and Granger, G. A. (1977): J. Immunol. Meth., 14:163-176.

32. Lisafeld, B. A., Minowada, J., Klein, E., and Holtermann, O. A. (1980): Int. Arch. Allergy Appl. Immunol., 62:59-66.

33. Meltzer, M. S., and Bartlett, G. L. (1972): J. Natl. Cancer Inst., 49:1439-1443.

34. Old, L. J., Benacerraf, B., Clarke, D. A. Carswell, E. A., and Stockert, E. (1961): Cancer Res., 21:1281-1301.

35. Papermaster, B. W., Holtermann, O. A., Klein, E., Djerassi, J., Rosner, D., Dao, T., and Costanzi, J. (1976): Clin. Immunol. and Immunopathol., 5:31-47.

36. Papermaster, B. W., Holtermann, O. A., Klein, E., Parnett, S.,
     Dobkin, D., Laudio, R., and Djerassi, J. (1976): Clin. Immunol.
     and Immunopathol., 5:48-59.
37. Redelman, D., and Hudig, D. (1980): J. Immunol., 124:870-878.
38. Rosenberg, S. A. Henrichon, M., Coyne, J. A., and David, J. R.
     (1973): J. Immunol., 110:1623-1629.
39. Ross, M. W., Tiangco, G. J., Horn, P., Hiserodt, J. C., and
     Granger, G. A. (1979): J. Immunol., 123:325-331.
40. Ruddle, N. H., and Waksman, B. H. (1968): J. Ex. Med., 128:
     1267-1279.
41. Rundell, J. O., and Evans, C. H. (1981): Immunopharmacology,
     3:9-18.
42. Russell, S. W., Rosenau, W., Goldbeg, M. L., and Kumitomi, G.
     (1972): J. Immunol., 109:784-790.
43. Salvin, S. B., Younger, J. S., Nishio, J., and Neta, R. (1975):
     J. Natl. Cancer Inst., 55:1233-1236.
44. Sawada, J.-I., and Osawa, T. (1978): Transplant., 26:319-324.
45. Toth, M. K., and Granger, G. A. (1979): Molec. Immunol., 16:
     67-75.
46. Vilcek, J. T., Yip, J. K., Pang, R. H. L., Thayer, K.,
     Henriksen, D., Urban, C., and Taniguchi, T. (1981): In:
     Thirteenth Midwinter Miami Symposia, edited by W. A. Scott,
     R. Werner, and J. Schultz, V. 18, Academic Press, New York
     (in press).
47. Walker, S. M., Lee, S. C., and Lucas, Z. J. (1976): J. Immunol.,
     116:807-815.
48. Ware, C. F., and Granger, G. A. (1981a): J. Immunol. (in press).
49. Ware, C. F., and Granger, G. A. (1981b): J. Immunol. (in press).
50. Ware, C. F., and Granger, G. A. (1981): J. Immunol. (in press).
51. Weiser, W. Y., Greineder, D. K., Demold, H. G., David, J. R.
     (1980): Biochemical Characterization of Lymphokines, edited by
     A. L. DeWeck, F. Kristensen, and M. Landy, pp. 1-5. Academic
     Press, New York.
52. Weiss, D. W., Bonhag, R. S., and DeOme, K. B. (1961): Nature,
     (London), 190:889-891.
53. Weitzen, M., and Granger, G. A. (1980): J. Immunol., 125:719-724.
54. Weitzen, M. L., and Granger, G. A. (1981): Cell. Immunol.
     (submitted).
55. Weitzen, M. L., Yamamoto, R. S., Granger, G. A. (1981): Cell.
     Immunol. (submitted).
56. Yamamoto, R. S., Hiserodt, J. C., Lewis, J. E., Carmack, C. E.,
     and Granger, G. A. (1978): Cell. Immunol., 38:403-416.
57. Yamamoto, R. S., Hiserodt, J. C., and Granger, G. A. (1979):
     Cell. Immunol., 45:261-275.
58. Youdim, S. (1977): Cancer Res., 37:572-577.
59. Youdim, S., Moser, M., and Stutzman, O. (1974): J. Natl. Cancer
     Inst., 52:193-198.

*Lymphokines and Thymic Hormones: Their
Potential Utilization in Cancer Therapeutics,*
edited by A. L. Goldstein and M. A. Chirigos,
Raven Press, New York © 1981.

Isolation and Purification of an Acid-Soluble Polypeptide with Lymphokine Properties from a Human Lymphoblastoid Cell Line

John E. McEntire, Pamela A. Dunn, *Charles W. Gehrke,
and Ben W. Papermaster

*Cancer Research Center, Columbia, Missouri 65201; *University of Missouri,
Columbia, Missouri 65211*

INTRODUCTION

Lymphokines refer to cell-free soluble factors produced by lympho-cytes which are non-specific in their action (7). More recently, they have become established as soluble secretory products of activated lymphocytes that stimulate motility, proliferation, phagocytosis, chemotaxis and cell lysis in target cells (5). Targets include both T and B lymphocytes, monocytes, neutrophils, endothelial cells and fibro-blasts (32). The list of predominantly in vitro, biologic activities ascribed to lymphokines has included over 90 functions and the molecular basis for most of these has remained undefined (6). Lymphokines com-prise a subgroup of a more generic term, cytokines, which have come to include a large family of polypeptide growth factors controlling cell division, differentiation, function, and interaction (32).

The inflammatogenic potential of crude supernatant culture fluids from antigen- or mitogen-stimulated lymphocyte cultures and lymphokine production by long-term lymphoblastoid cells in culture has been pre-viously described by others (1-4,20,25,27,30,31,34,35). Our initial experiments were performed with concentrated supernatant preparations of the lymphoblastoid cell line, RPMI 1788, grown in human serum-containing medium (22,24). Our previously published studies reported that often complete regression of dermal metastatic tumor lesions could be initiated by local injections of crude lymphokine preparations (23). Similar studies have been reported with RPMI 1788 lymphokines by Hamblin et al (12).

Purification and characterization of human and murine lymphokines are of current interest for their potential value in diagnostics and therapeutics (21). Partial purification of lymphotoxins (11), inter-leukins (9,14), and MIF (29) have been reported. However, purification to homogeneity and complete characterization as established for Type 1 interferons (36) and α_1-thymosin (18) have not been achieved as yet with lymphokines. We now report partial purification and characteriza-tion of an acid-soluble polypeptide which demonstrates properties of macrophage phagocytic promotion and activation.

Supported by NCI grants CA-26224, CA-29145, and CA-25740, DHHS; Frater-nal Order of the Eagles, Order of the Eastern Star, and the A.P. Green Foundation.

METHODOLOGY AND RESULTS

The cell line RPMI 1788 was established in 1968 (13). Immunoglobulin and HL-A typing of the lymphoblastoid cell line RPMI 1788 were published in 1970 (26), and at later intervals in 1972 and 1978 by Drs. S. Ferroni and R. Reisfeld (Scripps Clinic and Research Foundation, La Jolla, California) (personal communication). A recent test for surface antigens by Dr. J. Minowada, Roswell Park Memorial Institute, in June, 1979, gave the following results: E(-), EA-, EAC+, SmIg-IgM CyIg-Igm, low TDT, low ADA and normal karyotype. Recent HLA-typing by Ferroni and Reisfeld gave a profile of HLA-H2, B , 14 1a-DW 4,14. The cell line does not produce the third component of complement and fails to phagocytize C. albicans when treated with donor opsonins and peripheral blood. The evidence from present marker studies would suggest that the RPMI cell line 1788 has remained genetically stable for over 10 years in continuous culture and continues to retain the characteristics of B-lymphoblastoid cell lines. The cell line grows with a generation time of approximately 24 to 30 hours in RPMI 1640 medium in 10% fetal bovine serum at a density of 1 to 1.5 x 10^6 cells per ml. The cell line is maintained at the American Type Culture Collection, Rockville, MD.

Stock RPMI 1788 cells at a concentration of 1-5 x 10^7/ml are frozen in medium consisting of 67% RPMI 1640 (Flow), 30% fetal calf serum (FCS) (Gibco), and 3% dimethylsulfoxide (DMSO) (Sigma), pH 7.2. Cell suspensions are equilibrated at room temperature for 30 to 60 minutes in one milliliter freezing vials (Nunc). Temperature is subsequently lowered to -90°C at a rate of 1°C per minute in a Revco ultra low freezer. Stocks are routinely rotated every 3 to 6 months to preserve viability of the cells.

Frozen stocks for initiation of seed cultures are rapidly thawed at 37 to 42°C and transferred to fresh, prewarmed (37°C) RPMI 1640 containing 20% FCS and a mixture of penicillin-streptomycin (Gibco) at a final concentration of 100 i.u. and 100 mcg per milliliter (complete medium), respectively. DMSO is removed by gentle centrifugation and washing twice at 100 x g in the above medium. After washing, cells are resuspended to a concentration of 1-2 x 10^6 viable cells/ml in complete medium and incubated at 37°C. Cells are maintained at this concentration for 3 to 4 days or until vigorously growing at which time FCS is diminished to 10%. Cell numbers and viability determinations are accomplished by hemocytometer counting and trypan blue exclusion.

Preparation of Lymphokine-containing Supernatants

Human plasma was obtained from the Red Cross Mid-Missouri Blood Center. Pooled plasma was brought to 0.02 M in calcium by the addition of appropriate volumes of 40% $CaCl_2$. Plasma was allowed to clot for 3 hours at 37°C in a circulating water bath, then rapidly frozen at -70°C to initiate clot retraction. Serum was harvested after thawing by centrifugation at 200 x g for 3 hours. Lipids were removed by centrifugation at 125,000 x g for 3 hours in a swinging bucket rotor. Sterilization was performed by filtration through 0.2 micron Nalge filters. All serum was stored at -70°C until used. Prior to use, serum was heat-inactivated at 56°C for 30 minutes.

Cells growing vigorously in culture medium supplemented with FCS were transferred to spinner flasks and stirred at the rate of approximately 50 to 60 rpm. After adaption to spinner culture (1 to 3 days), cells were stepped to human serum-containing medium by alternating centrifugations and washing twice in excess volumes of RPMI 1640 containing 2% pooled human serum and antibiotics. Cells were suspended after the final wash at a concentration of 1-2 x 10^6 viable cells/ml in RPMI 1640 plus 2% human serum and no antibiotics for generation of lymphokine-containing supernatants.

Cells were cultured for 24 hours in a medium consisting of 98% RPMI 1640 and 2% pooled human serum in spinner flasks with stirring at 50 to 60 rpm. Cells and supernatants were separated by centrifugation at 200 x g. Supernatants were further clarified by centrifugation at 18,000 x g and stored at -20°C until further processed. Sterility of cultures was tested daily by incubation of culture fluids in thioglycollate broth.

The clarified supernatant was concentrated over PM-10 membranes in a TCE-5 ultrafiltration device (Amicon Corp.) from 20 L to about 1 L (20:1). The concentrate was layered onto a 10 x 100 cm column of Sephadex G-25 (Pharmacia), which had been equilibrated with a volatile buffer, 0.05 M ammonium bicarbonate. The column was eluted with the same buffer and the void volume was collected. The desalted protein was frozen and lyophilized in trays on an FTS20-54VP freeze dryer. The powdered protein was resuspended in pyrogen-free sterile saline at 20 mg dry weight/ml with slow stirring and the solution was centrifuged at 37,000 x g for 30 minutes. After this initial clarification, the solution was ultracentrifuged at 144,000 x g for 3 hours. After centrifugation, the material was tested for sterility, endotoxin and mycoplasma. Sterile material was dispensed into 5 ml vials, lyophilized and stoppered under vacuum.

Bioassays

Assays for skin inflammatory activity were carried out *in vivo* in guinea pigs as described previously (22). Specific activity was measured by intradermal injection of groups of three guinea pigs with appropriate dilutions of lymphokine fractions into three different sites on each animal and a dose reponse curve was determined by linear regression (22). Lymphotoxin activity *in vitro* was measured as described by Smith et al, with the exception that target cells were prelabeled with tritiated amino acids and washed with RPMI 1640 medium containing 10% FCS (28).

Phagocytic uptake was used to detect subnanogram amounts of active lymphokine fractions obtained during purification procedures as described by Dunn et al (8,17). Fluorescent intracellular beads in macrophages were counted manually by fluorescence microscopy. Uninduced, adherent mouse macrophages responded sensitively and reproducibly to added lymphokine in the micro-phagocytosis assay. This technique was used to generate linear dose response curves to log dilutions of lymphokine fractions with significantly increased uptake as low as 0.2 nanograms of protein. Lineweaver-Burke plots on phagocytic rates for bead uptake under variable concentrations of beads per cell were used to calculate rate constants of lymphokine-stimulated and control cells (17).

Acid Extraction of Biologically Active Peptides

A simple procedure for rapid, large-scale preparative extraction was carried out with 75 liters of supernatant. Cell culture supernatant was prepared as above. The lyophilized powder was resuspended in 0.15 molar NaCl to 40 mg/ml, stirred for 1 hour at 4°C, and centrifuged at 19,000 x g for 30 minutes. Trichloroacetic acid (TCA) was added slowly while stirring to a final concentration of 10% (w/v). After an additional 10 minutes of stirring at 4°C, the resulting slurry was centrifuged at 19,000 x g. The supernatant was neutralized with 5N NaOH to pH 7.0, filtered over a 0.45 micron Nalge filter, desalted on Sephadex G-25 equilibrated with 0.05 M ammonium bicarbonate buffer, and lyophilized. The powder was resuspended in distilled water, dispensed into vials, and lyophilized.

Samples of this preparation were tested for endotoxin, as described by J. H. Jorgensen et al (16), and biologic activity, and were shown to satisfy the safety standards for clinical investigation according to Federal Register, 38 (223): 610.11-610.12 (1973).

Biological activity of the TCA soluble extract was evaluated using assays for MAF, NK cell activity, lymphotoxin, guinea pig skin reactivity, phagocytosis and suppression of mouse L1210 tumor growth (Table 1) (10,12, 21,22).

TABLE 1. Biological Properties of LK 1788 and Fraction AE

Assay	Protein Required For Unit Activity		Activity Increase
	Crude	Fraction	
In Vivo NK	1500 MCG	9 MCG	167X
In Vitro MAF	328 MCG	7 MCG	47X
Guinea Pig Skin RX	510 MCG	11 MCG	47X
Antitumor Activity			
Human Basal Cell	(NT)	+	
Mouse L1210	+	+	

Assays are defined in references 10, 12, 21, 22.

Purification of the Acid Extract

The lymphokine prepared as above and extracted in trichloroacetic acid was further purified by high performance liquid chromatography (HPLC) on molecular sieving columns (Water's I-125, I-250) and reverse phase columns (Water's C18). Chromatography was carried out on a Water's system consisting of two Model 6000 pumps, a Model 440 absorbance monitor equipped with both 254 nM and 280 nM channels, a Model 660 gradient programmer, Model R401 refractive index detector and a Model U6K injector. Samples in various buffer systems as described below were chromatographed, monitored for absorbance, and assayed for biological activity. Active, biosynthetically-labeled protein fractions were rechromatographed and single peaks were dissociated with 6M guanidine hydrochloride and further purified. The Water's I-125 protein sieving column has an 80,000 dalton nominal exclusion limit, and the separation of fractions consisted of several peaks eluting in a size range comparable to the markers used to calibrate the column. The markers consisted of blue dextran (2,000,000 daltons), human albumin (68,000 daltons), and myoglobin (17,500 daltons). The material applied to the column was biosynthetically-labeled with tritiated amino acids as described elsewhere. Figure 1 demonstrates the elution profile with the I-125 molecular sieving column in 0.05 M phosphate buffer, 0.15M NaCl at pH 7.2, at a rate of 2.0 ml per minute. Phagocytic activity was found in the second major peak.

Peak 2 eluted from the column in Fig. 1 was applied to a Water's I-250 column equilibrated in 6M guanidine HCl, also previously calibrated with protein markers as above. These results (Fig. 2) suggest that the peak eluting after albumin, which contains a predominance of the tritiated amino acid incorporated counts, is in the size range of 8400 daltons and often is found in association with albumin in the absence of dissociating agents. A comparable picture can be shown when aggregated fraction, which voids a G-100 Sephadex column, is chromatographed on BioGel A-1.5M agarose in 6M guanidine hydrochloride (Fig. 3). The predominance of the tritium-labeled material eluted at a volume corresponding to 8400 daltons. This same fraction was subjected to additional resolution on a reverse phase C18 column. The tritiated fraction was added to the column which was equilibrated in water and eluted with a gradient of 0-100% CH_3CN at the rate of 5% per minute (Fig. 4). A single labeled peak eluted with the water phase of the column prior to CH_3CN, reflecting the polar nature of the molecule. Amino acid composition studies were performed on the eluted peak, and the predominant amino acids were shown to be aspartic and glutamic, each comprising about 15% of the peptide content. Upon assay of this peak for phagocytic enhancement (Table 2), an increase of 78,290-fold is shown with a yield of less than 1 μg/L of culture supernatant.

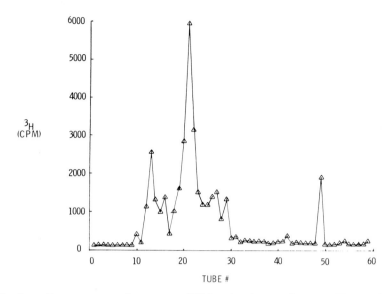

FIG. 1. Chromatography on an HPLC sieving column. The acid-extracted lymphokine was chromatographed on a Water's I-125 column in 0.05 M phosphate, 0.15 M NaCl, pH 7.2. Under these conditions, the tritium label cochromatographs with albumin as well as in the lower molecular weight range.

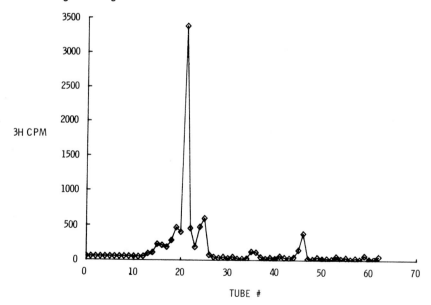

FIG. 2. HPLC in 6M guanidine HCl. Samples in 6M guanidine HCl were chromatographed over a Water's I-125 column. The major peak, which eluted at a volume corresponding to 8400 daltons, was purified by repeated chromatography.

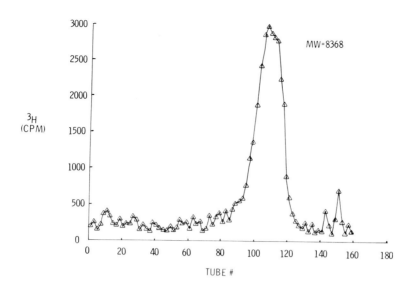

FIG. 3. Chromatography of labeled lymphokine in the presence of
6M guanidine HCl. The acid extract of lymphokine 1788, which had been
biosynthetically-labeled with tritiated amino acids, was chromatographed
on BioGel A1.5M in 6M guanidine HCl. Fractions were collected and
aliquots counted in a liquid scintillation counter. The major radio-
labeled peak has dissociated from carrier proteins and corresponds to
approximately 8400 daltons by comparison to calibration standards, blue
dextran, ovalbumin, and myoglobin.

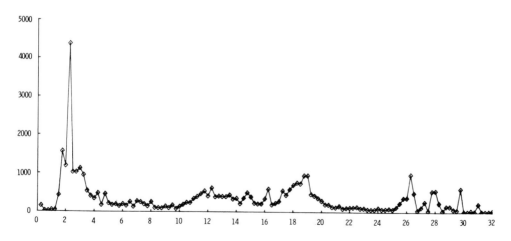

FIG. 4. Reverse phase C18 HPLC of ^{3}H-lymphokine acid extract fraction. The column, equilibrated in water, was loaded and eluted with
water for 5 minutes, then a gradient of 0 - 100% CH_3CN was applied.
Fractions were monitored for A_{280} and radioactivity.

TABLE 2. Purification of Activity in Fractions of RPMI 1788 Culture
          Supernatant in Amounts Per 100 L Starting Supernatant Fluid

Fraction	Protein (mg)	(%)	[a]Activity (Units)	(%)	Specific Activity (Units/mg)	Relative Specific Activity
Crude	104,000	(100%)	1,008,800	(100%)	9.7	1.0
Acid Extract	100	(0.1%)	165,000	(16.3%)	1,650	170
HPLC Peak	0.019	(0.0002%)	14,429	(1.4%)	759,440	78,290

[a]Activity is expressed as phagocytic index as defined by Lopatin, et al
(17) and Dunn and Tyrer (18). Recoveries are normalized to 100 L lots
as if the entire starting material were taken through all purification
steps.

DISCUSSION

Our approach to purification of biologically active lymphokines has
been guided by the principles of simplicity and large scale preparation.
Solubilization in trichloroacetic acid provides preferential solubility
to highly polar compounds. From the complex mixture of proteins and
other substances in the crude concentrate obtained by filtration and
lyophilization, only small amounts of albumin and several peptides are
identifiable in the TCA soluble extract. Moreover, the soluble TCA
extract clearly contains entities synthesized by the cell line identifiable as biosynthetically-labeled fractions which have incorporated
tritiated amino acids. At least one of these has been identified as a
polar, acidic peptide of 8400 daltons, which promotes phagocytosis and
macrophage activation. Preliminary characterization by amino acid
composition yields a high percentage of asp and glu, comprising 30% of
the relative percent composition.

Since the overall yield of this peptide is less than 0.001% of the
starting material, not enough of the purified fraction has been accumulated for amino acid sequence determination or other chemical characterization at this time. We intend to pursue large-scale preparation for
structural analysis and biologic characterization in macrophage test
systems, particularly macrophage-mediated tumor cell cytotoxicity.
Beyond the immediate goals of characterization, the calculated concentration of purified peptide (less than 1 μg per liter) precludes production with other than recombinant DNA techniques (15,33) or direct
chemical synthesis (19).

SUMMARY

Supernatants from the long-term cultured human lymphoblastoid cell line, RPMI 1788, contain lymphokine activities and promote tumor regression. Lymphokine activities in 1788 supernatants include lymphotoxin, MIF, enhancement of phagocytosis, and macrophage activation. They promote human and guinea pig inflammatory reactions, and mouse and human tumor regression. Concentrates of 1788 cell culture supernatants were prepared for purification by diafiltration, desalting, and lyophilization and further subjected to ultracentrifugation, acid extraction, dissociation in guanidine HCl, and high performance liquid chromatography (HPLC) to yield a product free of detectable serum proteins. Bioassays on an acid-soluble fraction prior to chromatography indicated total recovery in the range of 0.05 to 0.1% of total protein. Specific activities were increased by acid extraction as follows: skin test response, 50 to 250x; spleen cell-mediated cytotoxicity, 170x; phagocytic uptake, 170x. A peptide isolated by HPLC gel filtration demonstrated an approximate additional 450-fold increase in phagocytic stimulation over the acid-soluble starting material. The active peptides are acidic, and one with an apparent molecular weight of 8400 daltons could be detected by both biologic and isotopic (^{3}H) activity following biosynthetic incorporation of ^{3}H amino acids. Amino acid composition analysis of this peptide demonstrates approximately 15% relative content each of aspartic and glutamic acids.

ACKNOWLEDGMENT

The authors would like to acknowledge Academic Press, New York, and the journal <u>Cellular Immunology</u> for permission to reproduce Figures 1-4.

REFERENCES

1. Bennett, B., and Bloom, B.R. (1968): <u>Proc. Nat. Acad. Sci.</u>, 59: 756.
2. Bernstein, I.D., Thor, D.E., Zbar, B., and Rapp, H.J., (1971): <u>Science</u>, 172:729-731.
3. Bloom, B.R., and Glade, P.R., editors (1971): <u>In Vitro Methods in Cell-Mediated Immunity</u>. Academic Press, New York.
4. Cohen, S. (1981): <u>Fed. Proc.</u>, 40:51-53.
5. Cohen, S., Pick, E., and Oppenheim, J.J., editors (1979): <u>Biology of the Lymphokines</u>. Academic Press, New York.
6. de Weck, A.L., Kristensen, F., and Landy, M., editors (1980): <u>Biochemical Characterization of Lymphokines</u>. Academic Press, New York.
7. Dumonde, D.C., Wolstencroft, R.A., Panayi, G.S., Matthew, M., Morley, J., and Howson, W.T. (1969): <u>Nature</u>, 224:38-42.
8. Dunn, P.A., and Tyrer, H.W. (1981): <u>J. Lab. Clin. Med.</u> (in press).
9. Gallo, R. (1981): In: <u>Proceedings of the International</u> Workshop on Lymphokines and Thymic Factors. Raven Press, New York. (Article included in this publication.)

10. Gilliland, C.D., McEntire, J.E., Woods, W.L., Tyrer, H.W., and Papermaster, B.W. (1981): In: Cellular Responses to Molecular Modulators, edited by W.A. Scott, R. Werner, J. Schultz, and L.W. Mozes. Academic Press, New York (in press).

11. Granger, G.A. (1981): In: Cellular Responses to Molecular Modulators, edited by W.A. Scott, R. Werner, J. Schultz, and L.W. Mozes. Academic Press, New York (in press).

12. Hamblin, A.S., Wolstencroft, R.A., Dumonde, D.C., Den Hollander, F., Schuurs, A.H.W.M., Backhouse, B.M., O'Connell, D., and Paradinas, F. (1978): In: Developments in Biological Standardization, edited by International Association of Biological Standardization Council, pp. 335-341. S. Karger, Basel.

13. Hatt, H.D., and Gantt, M.J., editors (1979): The American Type Culture Collection. American Type Culture Collection, Rockville, MD.

14. Ihle, J. (1981): In: Proceedings of the International Workshop on Lymphokines and Thymic Factors. Raven Press, New York. (Article included in this publication.)

15. Itakura, K., Hirose, T., Crea, R., Riggs, A.D., Heyneker, H.L., Bolivar, F., and Boyer, H.W. (1977): Science, 198:1056-1063.

16. Jorgensen, J.H., and Smith, R.F. (1973): Appl. Microbiol., 26:43-48.

17. Lopatin, E., Dunn, P.A., McEntire, J.E., Eaton, W., and Papermaster, B.W. (1981): J. Immunol. Meth. (in press).

18. Low, T.L.K., Thurman, G.B., McAdoo, M., McClure, J., Rossio, J.L., Naylor, P.H. and Goldstein, A.L. (1979): J. Biol. Chem., 254:981-986.

19. Meienhofer, J.N. (1973): In: Hormonal Proteins and Peptides, edited by C.H. Li, pp. 46-267. Academic Press, New York.

20. Papageorgiou, P.S., Henley, W.H., and Glade, P.R. (1972): J. Immunol., 108:494-504.

21. Papermaster, B.W., and Dumonde, D.C. (1981): In: Proceedings of the First International Congress on Immunopharmacology. Pergamon Press, London (in press).

22. Papermaster, B.W., Holtermann, O.A., Klein, E., Parmett, S., Dobkin, D., Laudico, R., and Djerassi, I. (1976): Clin. Immunol. Immunopathol., 5:48-59.

23. Papermaster, B.W., Holtermann, O.A., Klein, E., Rosner, D., Dao, T., and Costanzi, J.J. (1976): Clin. Immunol. Immunopathol., 5:31-47.

24. Papermaster, B.W., Holtermann, O.A., Klein, E., Rosner, D., Dao, T., and Djerassi, I. (1974): Res. Comm. Chem. Pathol. Pharmacol., 8:413-416.

25. Pick, E., Krejci, J., Cech, K., and Turk, J.L. (1969): Immunology, 17:741-767.

26. Reisfeld, R.A., Pellegrino, M., Papermaster, B.W., and Kahan, D.B. (1970): J. Immunol., 104:560-565.

27. Salvin, S.B., Youngner, J.S., Nishio, J., and Neta, R. (1975): J. Nat. Cancer Inst., 55:1233-1236.

28. Smith, M.E., Laudico, R., and Papermaster, B.W. (1977): J. Immunol. Meth., 14:243-251.

29. Sorg, C. (1981): In: Proceedings of the International Workshop on Lymphokines and Thymic Factors. Raven Press, New York. (Article included in this publication.)

30. Tubergen, D.G., Feldman, J.D., Pollock, E.M., and Lerner, R.A. (1972): J. Exp. Meth., 135:255-266.

31. Valdimarsson, H., and Gross, N.J. (1973): J. Immunol., 111:485-491.
32. Waksman, B.H., and Namba, Y. (1976): Cell. Immunol., 21:161-179.
33. Wetzel, R., Heyneker, H.L., Goeddel, D.V., Jhurani, P., Shapiro, J., Crea, R., Low, T.S.K., McClure, J.E., Thurman, G.B., and Goldstein, A.L. (1981): In: Cellular Responses to Molecular Modulators, edited by W.A. Scott, R. Werner, J. Schultz, L.W. Mozes. Academic Press, New York (in press).
34. Yoshida, T., and Cohen, S. (1974): J. Immunol., 112:1540-1547.
35. Yoshida, T., and Cohen, S. (1977): In: Mechanisms of Tumor Immunity, edited by I. Green, S. Cohen, and R.T. McCluskey, pp. 87-108. John Wiley & Sons, New York.
36. Zoon, K.C., Smith, M.E., Bridgen, P.J., Zur Nedden, D., and Anfinsen, C.B. (1979): Proc. Nat. Acad. Sci., 76:5601-5605.

*Lymphokines and Thymic Hormones: Their
Potential Utilization in Cancer Therapeutics,*
edited by A. L. Goldstein and M. A. Chirigos,
Raven Press, New York © 1981.

Human Transfer Factor: Specificity and Structural Models

*†§Denis R. Burger, *†Arthur A. Vandenbark, **Terry Lee, **G. Doyle
Daves, ‡Phillip Klesius, and *§R. Mark Vetto

*Surgical Research Laboratory, Veterans Administration Medical Center and Departments of
†Microbiology and Immunology and of §Surgery, University of Oregon Health Sciences Center,
Portland, Oregon 97201; ‡U.S. Department of Agriculture, SEA-AR-SR, Regional Parasite Research
Laboratory, Auburn, Alabama 36830; and **The Oregon Graduate Center, Beaverton, Oregon 97005*

INTRODUCTION

Components in dialyzates of leukocyte extracts (DLE) have been
defined by the effects they exert in various immunologic assays.
Lymphocyte proliferation in vitro has detected mitogenic and
suppressive activity as well as antigen-dependent activities in
leukocyte extracts (9). Similarly, other immunologic assays
(leukocyte migration inhibition, chemotaxis, etc.) have implicated
additional properties or activities in DLE. We use the term
transfer factor (TF) to denote the ability of DLE to transfer dermal
reactivity in man. None of the other in vitro or in vivo phenomena
attributed to DLE have been directly shown to detect or assess the
dermal transfer component. Since this activity is still evaluated
in a transfer system in man, the nature, specificity, and mode of
action of the responsible component(s) have remained controversial.

The strategy that we employed to investigate the nature of the
dermal transfer component was (a) to develop a reproducible system
to assess passive transfer in man; (b) to fractionate DLE by
exclusion chromatography, electrofocusing, and HPRP chromatography
in order to purify the active component for structural analysis; and
(c) to assess the enzymatic sensitivities and behavior of TF on
immunoadsorbents in order to characterize structural features before
purification. This presentation describes (a) recent experiments
designed to evaluate the specificity of the dermal transfer
component and (b) constraints placed on structural models for TF by
experiments on affinity adsorption characteristics and enzymatic
susceptibilities of TF.

PREPARATION AND ASSAY OF TRANSFER FACTOR

Classically microbial antigens have been used to evaluate responsiveness in both donors and recipients in order to assess passive transfer (21). The drawbacks to the use of common microbial antigens as markers of biologic activity are many and have been previously summarized (9, 22). The approach employed here was to use large batches of TF from leukapheresed human donors or TF from calves who were immunized to non-microbial antigens. This has enabled us to relate the dermal reactivity in the recipient to the immunization of the donor (12). In this way our data argue for the concept of specific TF raised through immunization and support the specificity of TF reported in the literature.

Donors of Transfer Factor

Donors of TF were normal, healthy adults with well-documented delayed dermal hypersensitivity to Keyhole limpet hemocyanin (KLH), Horseshoe crab hemocyanin (HCH) and/or Tularemia (Tul). We selected these antigens since the frequency of reactivity in the unimmunized population of our geographic region (Northwest USA) was extremely low (less than 1%). After donors were selected, they were leukapheresed and TF prepared. These donors were then immunized with one of the three antigens and leukapheresed a second time two months later. Some of the donors were then immunized to a second antigen to provide TF with two defined reactivites.

We have reported (11, 12, 26) the detailed methodology for preparation and testing of TF from KLH-immunized donors. Briefly, leukocytes harvested by pheresis were lysed by five freeze-thaw cycles and subjected to vacuum dialysis (11). The vacuum dialyzates were stored at -20 C. In general, 10 to 20 units (systemic transfer doses) were prepared from a single leukapheresis procedure. Individual batches were reproducibly active (i.e. 18/20 positive transfers with a mean skin test diameter of 16.5 mm). Since no adverse effects from the leukapheresis were noted, TF could be prepared before and after immunization to these antigen.

Recipients of Transfer Factor

Recipients of TF were selected from patients hospitalized for care for other than immunologic, malignant or infectious diseases. None of the patients were anergic and all responded to common microbial antigens and mitogens in vivo and in vitro.

Recipients were tested in vitro by lymphocyte proliferation but were not tested intradermally with KLH, HCH, or Tul prior to TF administration. One TF unit (5×10^8 lymphocyte equivalents) was injected subcutaneously into the abdominal area. Two to five days later the recipients were skin tested intraderamlly with 100 ug KLH, 50 ug HCH, and 1/1000 Tul (Foshay vaccine 5-56). The skin tests were read blind at 24 and 48 hours for erythema and induration.

A crucial feature of the KLH transfer system was the naive status of the recipients before receiving TF from KLH-immunized donors. We presumed that this antigen would rarely be encountered by the recipient population. This presumption allowed us to avoid subjecting recipients to a "priming" exposure in the form of a skin test which would have been required to select non-reactive individuals to microbial antigens. Although the extent to which the recipient pool was naive to KLH was unknown in absolute terms, considerable evidence was obtained which support this contention (10).

ANALYSIS OF SPECIFICITY OF TRANSFER FACTOR

The specificity of the skin test conversion has been in question since the first description of TF. To test specificity one would like to employ donors immune to antigen A, but not B, and donors immune to antigen B, but not A. In addition, donors immune to both A and B, and others immune to neither should be selected. For TF to produce an immunologically specific skin test conversion, the recipients must strictly reflect donor immunities. This sort of protocol has not been previously carried out in man; most studies have included only one phase of this experiment (i.e., administration of TF from donor A and testing recipients with both antigens A and B). A summary of published studies that tested specificity in this manner is found in reference 8. In this analysis the frequency with which TF produced skin test conversions consistent with specificity was 157/200, whereas only 12/151 conversions were observed with TF from nonimmune donors. A serious criticism of these pooled data is that only a few of the studies were conducted as blind protocols. Positive transfers depend upon skin test conversions that are often subtle (5 to 15 mm induration in most cases) and the reliability of the assay would benefit by objective evaluation which is best accomplished by blind or double-blind protocols.

The specificity of TF has also been questioned by reports of altered responsiveness to dinitrochlorobenzene (DNCB) (19) and in mixed lymphocyte culture (15) following administration of TF. Several patients with immunodeficiencies, after repeated failures to become immunized to DNCB, have reacted to this agent following administration of TF from donors not known to been DNCB immune. The interpretation of these results has been that TF acts nonspecifically to boost cellular immunity. The interpretation is probably correct, since TF may improve the condition of a patient and raise the patient's ability to respond immunologically to DNCB. Since results in immunodeficient patients cannot differentiate between the relevant alternatives (i.e., specific, nonspecific or both specific and nonspecific components in TF) these data were not taken in account in evaluating specificity from the published literature on TF. Similar arguments apply to improved reactivity in mixed lymphocyte cultures following TF injection.

Our previous data (5, 6, 7, 9, and unpublished observations) are consistent with specificity but could not offer formal proof. Keyhole limpet hemocyanin (KLH)-immunized donors transfer KLH reactivity but not tuberculin sensitivity, whereas tuberculin donors transfer PPD reactivity but not KLH reactivity. Moreover, we (11) showed that donors can not transfer KLH reactivity (0/6 recipients positive) until after KLH immunization (24/26 recipients positive).

A double blind protocol was recently designed to evaluate critically the specificity of human and bovine TF. Human TF was prepared from four donor groups: (a) KLH+, (b) HCH-, (c) KLH and HCH+, and (d) KLH and HCH- donors. Bovine TF was prepared prior to and at specified intervals after immunization of calves with either or both of these hemocyanins. We have previously shown that bovine TF effectively transfers KLH reactivity to human recipients (4). In the protocol using calves, the visceral trunk was cannulated prior to immunization and lymphocytes collected by chronic drainage procedures during a 28 day period. Bovine TF was prepared from the visceral trunk lymphocytes as we described for human transfer factor. Human recipients received a single coded TF preparation 48-96 hours before skin testing with all three antigen preparations (100 ug KLH, 50 ug HCH and 1/1000 Tul). The skin tests were read at 24 and 48 hours by a third party and subsequently the codes broken and results compiled. In this experiment human TF converted human recipients directly proportional to the immune status of the donors. (Table 1)

TABLE 1.   Specificity of human transfer factor

Immunization of donors	Dermal Reactivity in Recipients to the following antigens		
	KLH	HCH	Tul
Preimmunization	2.1 ± 1.2(4)[a]	1.6 ± 1.0(3)	1.8 ± 1.2(4)
KLH+, HCH-	12.1 ± 3.2(4)	2.2 ± 1.1(4)	2.2 ± 1.0(3)
HCH+, KLH-	2.5 ± 1.0(4)	8.6 ± 2.3(4)	1.9 ± 0.8(4)
KLH+, HCH+	13.3 ± 4.1(3)	7.9 ± 2.1(3)	2.3 ± 1.1(4)

[a]mean ± standard deviation (N) of the diameter of induration at 24 hours

The reactions to the KLH skin tests were strong (10 mm) in recipients of KLH+TF and clearly negative in recipients of KLH-TF. Although the positive responses to HCH in HCH+TF recipients were weak (5-10mm range) there was a clear distinction between the HCH+ and HCH- TF recipients. Double positive or negative TF converted recipients as would be predicted from a specificity model.

In a separate specificity trial using bovine TF, human recipients only responded to a dermal challenge with antigen if they received TF from calves that were immune to that antigen. Before immunization, bovine TF was ineffective whereas after immunization only reactivity to the immunizing hemocyanin was observed in the recipients (Tables 2 & 3). Consistent with the responses in recipients of human TF, recipients of HCH+ bovine TF developed only weak reactions to HCH.

TABLE 2.   Specificity of calf transfer factor in human recipients

Days after immunization with antigen		Dermal Reactivity in Human Recipients		
HCH	KLH	KLH	HCH	Tul
0	0	2.1 ± 1.2(3)[a]	2.0 ± 1.1(4)	2.1 ± 1/0(4)
7	0	3.1 ± 1.1(4)	7.4 ± 2.1(4)	1.2 ± 0.7(3)
14	7	10.1 ± 2.5(3)	8.2 ± 2.1(4)	2.0 ± 1.0(4)
28	21	19.5 ± 4.1(4)	10.3 ± 3.1(3)	1.1 ± 1.2(3)

[a]mean ± standard deviation (N) of the diameter of induration at 24 hours.

TABLE 3.   Specificity of calf transfer factor in human recipients

Days after immunization with antigen		Dermal Reactivity in Human Recipients		
KLH	HCH	KLH	HCH	Tul
0	0	2.2 ± 1.0(4)[a]	2.1 ± 0.9(3)	1.1 ± 1.0(5)
7	0	9.5 ± 1.5(4)	1.7 ± 1.4(4)	2.3 ± 0.7(4)
14	7	20.7 ± 4.5(4)	6.1 ± 1.2(4)	2.1 ± 1.0(4)
28	21	22.3 ± 5.0(4)	9.2 ± 1.7(4)	3.2 ± 1.3(4)

[a]mean ± standard deviation (N) of the diameter of induration at 24 hours.

Although these protocols were not as ideal as we would have liked (low HCH reactivity, small number of recipients/group), the results obtained (stated conservatively) make it very difficult to exclude specificity for TF or (stated optimistically) argue in favor of a specificity model for TF. Further confirmation of the specificity model for TF will come from structural and immunochemical analysis of the active components. It should be noted that recent experiments from Borkowski and Lawrence (1) and Peterson and Kirkpatrick (personal communication) offer additional evidence for the specificity of TF assessed in vitro or in mice.

Augmentation of dermal reactivity by factors in DLE has been reported to be unrelated to the immune status of the donor (17, 26). Since no background level of antigen reactivity was detected in potential recipients before TF, we doubt that augmentation of a low level of reactivity played a significant role in these

experiments. Two other considerations that add to this argument
are: (a) the augmentation activity would have to be found
exclusively in DLE from KLH-immunized donors even three years after
sensitization since "transfer" of KLH reactivity was exclusively
restricted to DLE from immunized donors, and (b) no dermal
augmenting activity was detected in Sephadex Fraction IIIa (26) from
which all other preparations were made.

ENZYMATIC SENSITIVITIES OF HUMAN TRANSFER FACTOR

It has been possible to place constraints on structural models of
TF by determining the enzymatic susceptibilities of active
preparations. The general experimental design for the experiments
involving enzymatic treatment of TF consisted of (a) demonstrating
enzyme activity using known substrates (b) treatment of TF
containing fractions under optimal enzymatic conditions; (c) removal
of residual enzyme components by rechromatography on Sephadex G-25;
(d) analysis of the resulting preparations for residual enzyme
contamination and (e) systemic transfer of dermal reactivity. Sham
controls (identical conditions but without enzymes) were done in
parallel to assure that loss in TF activity was enzyme related.
The resistance of TF to pancreatic deoxyribonuclease, pancreatic
ribonuclease and trypsin reported in the earlier literature (22)
suggested that the active moiety was not a conventional nucleic acid
or protein. A polypeptide composition for TF has been an attractive
hypothesis, since it is feasible to generate the multiple
combinations required to account for specificity with a dictionary
of amino acids. A diversity of 10^7 to 10^8 combinations can be
generated from a polypeptide chain with eight residues available for
substitution even with seven residue substitutions required to
derive a new specificity (20). More recently some evidence arguing
for a polypeptide moiety in TF has come from both animal (24) and
human (25) transfer systems. Our approach (13) to determine if a
polypeptide component was essential for TF activity was to select
two nonspecific peptidases (pronase and proteinase K) for
degradation experiments. Treatment of TF with high doses of
peptidases completely destroyed passive transfer (from a mean of
11.8 mm induration sham treated to 3.8 mm with pronase and 3.0 mm
with proteinase K. As a control traysylol (a synthetic polypeptide)
was used to selectively inhibit peptidase activity of the pronase
during exposure to TF. If the destruction of TF was due to the
peptidase action of the enzyme rather than a contaminating enzymatic
activity, one would expect the traysylol to inhibit pronase
destruction of TF. This proved to be the case in subsequent
bioassays (Table 4).

Table 4. Enzymatic treatment of transfer factor containing fractions.

DLE fraction[a]	Enzymatic treatment	Dermal response x ± s.d. (N)
DLE	None	13.9 + 5.3 (8)
IIIa	None	14.6 + 4.1 (16)
IIIa	Sham, no enzyme	11.8 + 1.9 (9)
IIIa	Pronase, 2 mg/TFU	17, 20 (2)
IIIa	Pronase, 30 mg/TFU	3.8 + 0.5 (4)
IIIa	Pronase, 30 mg/TFU + Traysylol	11, 18 (2)
IIIa	Proteinase K, 1 mg/TFU	10.0 + 1.0 (4)
IIIa	Proteinase K, 25 mg/TFU	3.0 + 1.0 (3)
IIIa	Leucine aminopeptidase	14.0 + 2.0 (3)
IIIa	Carboxypeptidase A	2.0 + 1.0 (4)
IIIa	Alkaline phosphatase	13.4 + 1.9 (10)
IIIa, APT	Phosphodiesterase I	4.8 + 0.5 (4)
IIIa, APT	Phosphodiesterase II	11.3 + 1.0 (5)
IIIa	NADase	11.0 + 2.0 (4)
IIIa	NADase + pyrophosphatase	12.0 + 2.0 (4)
IIIa	Ribosyl transferase A	14.1 + 2.1 (4)
IIIa	Ribosyl transferase B	6.1 + 5.2 (4)

[a]DLE = vacuum dialyzed extract; IIIa = Sephadex fractions IIIa;; IIIa, APT = alkaline phosphatase treated fraction IIIa. The enzyme treatments were carried out according to Burger et al. (13). Ribosyl transferase A is the favored reaction (ADP-ribosylation of peptides) whereas ribosyl transferase B is the reverse.

In additional experiments, we employed terminal-specific peptidases to characterize further the polypeptide portion of the TF structure. Carboxypeptidase A which is specific for the carboxy-terminus of a peptide destroyed TF activity (mean skin test size was 2.1 mm after treatment). Leucine aminopeptidase which is specific for the amino-terminus did not destroy activity (Table 4).

To investigate the possibility of a phosphodiester linkage in the TF structure, we compared the sensitivity of TF to two exonucleases, snake venom phosphodiesterase I (3' exonuclease) and bovine spleen phosphodiesterase II (5' exonuclease). Phosphodiesterase I destroyed TF activity (mean = 4.8 mm after treatment), whereas phosphodiesterase II did not (mean = 11.3 after treatment, Table 4).

The sensitivity of TF to somewhat more specialized enzymatic treatments was also investigated. Pyrophosphatase was used to investigate the possibility of a pyrophosphate linkage in the TF structure. Since nicotinamide adenine dinucleotide (NAD) blocks the action of pyrophosphatase, NADase was used as a pretreatment to remove contaminating levels of NAD from TF preparations. NADase treatment itself had no effect on biologic activity but was judged by high pressure liquid chromatography to remove the available NAD in the preparations. However, even after treatment of the TF

preparation with NADase, pyrophosphatase did not destroy biologic
activity (Table 4). These observations would seem to restrict the
type of phospholinkages that could be in TF model structures.
However, these observations must be interpreted cautiously since
when pyrophophatase was tested on model structures consisting of
adenine dinucleotide phosphoribosylated (ADPR-)-peptides,
destruction of this type of pyrophosphate linkage was not observed.

Ribosyl transferase (chlora toxin) is known to be a potent
inhibitor of delayed type hypersensitivity (3) and displays
specificity for ADPR-peptides. The favored reaction of this enzyme
is to add ADP-ribose to proteins or peptides. This activity can
also be reversed to remove the ADPR from peptides ( ). In
examining the effects of ribosyl transferase on TF bioactivity, we
observed that the favored reaction, that is to add an ADP-ribose to
proteins, did not influence biologic activity of TF. When the
reaction was reversed, that is to remove ADPR from proteins,
biologic activity seemed to be destroyed. However we observed
considerable variability in these transfers. Moreover, additional
experiments are required to demonstrate that it was ribosyl
transferase activity in the cholera toxin preparation that led to
the destruction of biological activity.

There are some important pitfalls to consider when structural
constraints are based on enzymatic susceptibilities. Some of these
considerations include (a) contaminating enzymes in the preparations
employed; (b) enzymatic activation of an inhibitor of activity
rather than direct destruction of bioactivity; and (c) adsorption of
bioactivity to the enzymes and therefore, non-specific loss of
bioactivity. One approaches these concerns by using enzyme
preparations with different substrate specificities and by employing
as many alternative approaches as possible. This is often not
sufficient and necessitates that enzyme sensitivities must be
interpreted cautiously and backed up by independent analysis.
However, even taking these concerns into account the general
approach has proved useful and we envisage it to be useful in the
future.

AFFINITY ADSORPTION OF TRANSFER FACTOR

The general experimental design to assess the ability of various
affinity adsorbents to bind TF activity was as follows. (A) Each
adsorbent was demonstrated to have binding capacity for the
appropriate structure. (B) TF or sham preparations were incubated
with the adsorbents for 24-48 hours with mixing at 4°C. (C) The
supernatant fluid was harvested and tested for biologic activity by
systemic transfer of KLH dermal reactivity. (D) The binding
capacity of the adsorbents were re-evaluated where possible. It
should be noted that it has not as yet been possible to evaluate
bioactivity of materials eluted from these adsorbents.

Immunoadsorbents discussed in this section have been prepared by
the method of Cuatrecasas (14) using cyanogen bromide activated
Sepharose 4B or N-hydroxysuccinimide-activated Sepharose 4B-CK beads
as described by Gottlieb et al. (18). Specific purified antibody or
antigen was prepared using these immunoadsorbents as follows:
samples were applied directly to the immunoadsorbents which were
then washed until the effluent absorption was negligible. The

adsorbents were then eluted with 3 M sodium thiocyanate (a chaotropic agent which disrupts the hyrophobic and electrostatic association between antigen and antibody) until the absorption was again negligible.

KLH and Anti-KLH Immunoadsorbents

One hypothesis to account for the transfer of KLH reactivity to naive recipients suggests that TF behaves as an antigen receptor (has avidity for KLH). An additional hypothesis is that the structure contains a "super antigen" activity (possibly contains a KLH determinant). Use of a KLH adsorbent and anti-KLH antibody adsorbent could provide a plausible approach for the isolation of structures with these characteristics. KLH was conjugated to Sepharose 4B and this adsorbent was demonstrated to specifically isolate anti-KLH antibody. Rabbit anti-KLH antibody from a hyperimmune animal and human anti-KLH antibody were specifically purified using this adsorbent and conjugated to succinimide activated sepharose containing a 6 carbon atom spacer group from the agarose bead. This minimizes possible steric interactions between the bead and the antibody molecule. The conjugated beads were then shown to be active by specifically binding radiolabeled KLH. Tubes containing KLH or anti-KLH immunoadsorbent beads were incubated with and without TF for 24-36 hours. The tubes were centrifuged and the supernatant fluid collected and assayed for biological activity. The anti-KLH adsorbents did not remove TF activity from the preparations (Table 5).

TABLE 5. Does transfer factor contain antigen?

Immunoadsorbent	Specificity of TF	Dermal Reactivity of Recipients x $\pm$ sd(N)
none	KLH	14.1 $\pm$ 3.3(6)
Sepharose-anti KLH(Rb)	KLH	15.3 $\pm$ 2.6(4)
Sepharose-anti KLH(Hu)	KLH	12.6 $\pm$ 4.5(4)

(Rb) = rabbit antibody, (Hu)=human antibody from KLH+TF donor.

A decrease, however, in the size of the KLH skin tests (about 60% reduction, Table 6) was observed when TF was incubated with the KLH-adsorbent.

TABLE 6.   Does transfer factor have avidity for antigen?

Immunoadsorbent	Specificity of TF	Dermal Reactivity of Recipients x ± sd(N)
none	KLH	12.1 ± 3.0(9)
	HCH	8.0 ± 3.1(3)
Sepharose-KLH	KLH	4.1 ± 2.6(6)
	HCH	7.2 ± 2.8(3)
Sepharose-KLH+anti-KLH	KLH	9.6 ± 3.1(3)

Whether this apparent decrease in activity was specifically related to the affinity approach was investigated further by incubating HCH (+) TF with this adsorbent. The KLH adsorbent did not remove HCH reactivity from the HCH (+) TF preparation. Moreover, saturation of the KLH adsorbent with anti-KLH antibody blocked the ability of this adsorbent to remove most of the KLH transfer activity. The results presented in Tables 5 and 6 must be cautiously interpreted. The KLH (+) TF could have strong avidity for KLH when associated with a complementary framework on T cells but may only have weak avidity for this adsorbent as we present it on the beads. Although TF does not bind to the anti-KLH adsorbent (Table 4) one cannot rule out the possibility that TF contains a KLH determinant that is not recognized by the rabbit or human antibody, i.e., a T-cell recognized determinant.

If these data are substantiated they could support the possibility that the specificity in TF may be due to a V_H region in the structure. Attempt to demonstrate this with anti-KLH idiotype sera have had mixed success and additional experiments along these lines are in progress. These data support the recent findings of Borkowski and Lawrence (2) who have shown that TF has avidity for antigen coated polystyrene.

Anti-Ia Immunoadsorbents
Because of the association of Ia with several lymphocyte/macrophage factors the question of an Ia determinant on TF has been raised. This question can be addressed in the human TF system. We have selected TF from KLH-immune donors with different DR haplotypes (DR-2, w-6 and DR-w6). The gamma globulin portion of monospecific polymorphic and monoclonal supertypic antisera was prepared and conjugated to succinimide activated sepharose. The activity and specificity of the conjugated beads was assessed by incubation of the beads with DR-2 and DR-w6 positive human B cells. Loss of dermal transfer activity from TF by incubation with the appropriate adsorbent would implicate the presence of this Ia determinant in the biologically active TF molecule. No loss of

biological activity was observed with TF from either donor when the preparations were incubated with anti-DR immunoadsorbents. It would have been surprising to find DR (Ia) determinants on TF since the polypeptide portion appears to have a relatively small molecular size. This experiment showing no loss of activity after incubation of the TF with the anti-DR adsorbent does not prove that Ia is absent from the TF molecule but does at least say that if Ia is present it is not available for complexing with the adsorbent.

Table 7.   Does transfer factor express Ia determinants?

HLA-Dr Specificity of Donor	Immunoadsorbent	Dermal Reactivity or Recipients $x \pm sd(N)$
DR-2,w6	none	9.6 ± 2.3(14)
	Sepharose-anti DR-2	8.7 ± 3.1(3)
	-anti DR-w6	10.2 ± 3.4(3)
	Sepharose-anti MT-1(1,2,4,7)	9.8 ± 2.8(3)
	-anti MT-2(3,5,6,8)	8.1 ± 2.6(3)
	-anti MT-4(4,5,7)	nd
DR-w6	none	13.5 ± 3.1(18)
	Sepharose-anti DR-w6	15.2 ± 3.2(3)
	-anti DR-2	12.8 ± 4.6(3)
	Sepharose-anti MT-1(1,2,4,7)	11.6 ± 3.7(3)
	-anti MT-2(3,5,6,8)	15.8 ± 3.9(3)
	-anti MT-4(4,5,7)	13.1 ± 3.3(3)

Lectin and Cis-diol Binding Adsorbents

Lectins possess binding affinities for specific carbohydrate residues which are attached to proteins or lipid structures (23). Lectin adsorbents therefore can be prepared which will bind sugar-containing compounds. Table 8 presents the results of incubating TF with a combination lectin adsorbent. Each lectin was shown to be active after conjugation to sepharose beads by removing specific agglutination effects of various sugars on treated type A red cells. A mixture of these lectin adsorbents did not adsorb biological activity from any of five TF preparations tested. These findings indicate that TF does not contain any of these sugar moieties which are accessible to the adsorbent.

Boronate derivatives on various solid supports display a high capacity for binding and separating low molecular weight compounds with coplaner cis-diol groups (ribonucleotides, -sides, sugars, catecholamines, and co-enzymes). The adsorbent used here was n-aminophenyl boronic acid immobilized on Bio-Gel P (polyacrylamide gel). Of particular interest is that ribose and ribose-containing compounds will bind to this adsorbent. Since our preliminary data suggested that TF contained a ribose moiety we expected binding. Binding of TF activity to this adsorbent in six experiments confirmed the presence of a cis-diol (ribose) functionality but could not provide more specific data (i.e. ribonucleotide versus ribonucleoside, Table 8).

In future experiments this technique may provide a preparative tool for separating cis-diol containing compounds from other constituents in the preparations if biological activity can be eluted from the adsorbent.

TABLE 8. Does transfer factor contain carbohydrate or sugar residues?

Adsorbent	Sugar Specificity	Dermal Reactivity of Recipients $x \pm sd(N)$
none	none	$14.6 \pm 3.8(11)$
Combination lectin	galactose glucose mannose fucose sialic acid N-acetylglucosamine D-glucopyranoside	$13.1 \pm 4.2(5)$
n-aminophenyl boronic acid	ribose (coplaner cis-diol groups)	$3.8 \pm 1.2(6)$

CONSTRAINTS ON STRUCTURAL MODELS FOR TRANSFER FACTOR

The experiments done in our laboratory over the past three years regarding the specificity, purification, and structure of TF are summarized in Table 9. These experiments suggest that the TF structure possesses a polypeptide component with a free carboxy terminus and a phosphodiester linkage to a moiety with a free 3' hydroxyl. Retention characteristics on high pressure, reverse phase chromatography and behavior to alkaline phosphatase treatment are consistent with an additional phosphate residue in the TF molecule. We have previously presented a model structure based on these characteristics (13). The additional constraints presented by experiments presented here suggest the inclusion of V_H region in the structure.

Table 9: Summary of properties of human transfer factor to KLH.

1. Non-immune donors do not transfer KLH reactivity.
2. TF activity is only observed after immunization of donors to the antigen.
3. TF activity elutes at 2-3 V_o on Sephadex G-25 compared to all other fractions.
4. TF has an isoelectric point below 2.
5. TF activity is found in two chromatographic regions by high pressure reverse phase chromatography.
6. TF activity to KLH could not be adsorbed by anti-KLH immunoadsorbents but was bound to KLH-adsorbents.
7. TF does not contain an Ia specificity that could be adsorbed by anti-DR antisera.
8. A combination lectin immunoadsorbent would not adsorb KLH TF activity.
9. An adsorbent with a coplaner cis-diol binding capacity (ribose) adsorbed TF acitivity.
10. TF is inactivated by pronase, proteinase K, and carboxypeptidase A.
11. TF is not inactivated by leucine aminopeptidase.
12. TF is inactivated by phosphodiesterase I but not phosphodiesterase II, alkaline phosphatase, NADase, or pyrophosphatase.

*This work was supported by the Veterans Administration, Department of Agriculture, and NIH grant AI 14699-01. The skillful technical assistance of Douglas Dawson and manuscript preparation by Mary Hagen is sincerely acknowledged.

REFERENCES

1. Borkowsky, W., and Lawrence, H. S. (1979): J. Immunol. 123:1741.
2. Borkowsky, W., and Lawrence, H. S. (1981): J. Immunol. 126, 486.
3. Bourne, H. R., Lichtenstein, L. M., Melmon, K. L., Henney, C. S., Weinstein, Y., and Shearer, G. M. (1973). Science 184, 19.
4. Burger, D. R., Klesius, P., Vandenbark, A. A., Vetto, R. M. and Swann, I. (1979). Cell. Immunol. 43, 192.
5. Burger, D. R., Nolte, J. E., Vandenbark, A. A., and Vetto, R. M. (1976): In Transfer Factor: Basic Properties and Clinical Applications (M. S. Ascher, A. A. Gottlieb and C. H. Kirkpatrick, eds). p. 323. Academic Press, New York.
6. Burger, D. R., Vandenbark, A. A., Daves, D., Anderson, W. A., Jr., Vetto, R. M. and Finke, P. (1976): J. Immunol. 117, 789.
7. Burger, D. R., Vandenbark, A. A., Daves, G. D., Anderson, W. A., Vetto, R. M. and Finke, P. (1976): Journal of Immunology 177,797.
8. Burger, D. R., Vandenbark, A. A., Dunnick, W., Kraybill, W. G., Vetto, R. M. (1978): J. Reticuloendothel. Soc. 24(4), 389.
9. Burger, D. R., Vandenbark, A. A., Finke, P., Nolte, J. E. and Vetto, R. M. (1976). Journal of Immunology 117, 782.

10. Burger, D. R., Vandenbark, A.A., and Vetto, R. M. (1980): In Thymus, Thymic Hormones, and T-Lymphocytes. Proc. Serono Symposia, Vol. 38. Edited by F. Aluti and H. Wigzell. Academic Press, New York. Pp. 431-439.

11. Burger, D. R., Vandenbark, A. A., Finke, P. and Vetto, R. M (1977): Cellular Immunology 29, 410.

12. Burger, D. R., Vetto, R. M. and Vandenbark, A. A. (1974). Cellular Immunology 14, 332.

13. Burger, D. R., Wampler, P., Vandenbark, A. A., and Vetto, R. M. (1979): In Immune Regulators in Transfer Factor (A Khan, C. H. Kirkpatrick, and N. O. Hill, eds) 377-388. Academic Press, London and New York.

14. Cuatrecasas, P. (1970): Journal of Biological Chemistry 245, 3059.

15. Dupont, B., Ballow, M., Hansen, J., Quick, C., Yunis, E. and Good, R. (1974): Proc. Natl. Acad. Sci. USA 71, 867.

16. Gill et al (1978): Proceedings of the National Academy of Sciences 75, 3050.

17. Gottlieb, A. A., Foster, L. G., Saito, K., Sutcliffe, S., Wrigley, P., Oliver, T., Cullen, M. and Fairley, G. H. (1976): In Transfer Factor: Basic Properties and Clinical Applications (M. S. Ascher, A. A. Gottlieb, and C. H. Kirkpatrick eds) 263-282. Academic Press, London and New York.

18. Gottlieb, A. B., Seide, R. K. and Kindt, T. J. (1975) Journal of Immunology 114, 51.

19. Griscelli, C., Revillard, J., Betuel, H., Herzog, C. and Touraine, J. (1973): Biomedicine 18, 220.

20. Kirkpatrick, C. H. and Smith, T. K. (1977): In Regulatory Mechanism in Lymphocyte Activation (D. O. Lucas, ed.) 174-188. Academic Press, London and New York.

21. Lawrence, H. S. (1969): In Advances in Immunology, 239. Academic Press, London and New York.

22. Lawrence, H. S. (1974): In Harvey Lectures, series 68. Academic Press, London and New York.

23. Lis, H. and Sharon, N. (1973). Annual Reviews of Biochemistry 42, 541.

24. Rifkind, D., Frey, J. A., Peterson, E. and Dinowitz, M. (1977): Infection and Immunity 16, 258.

25. Spitler, L. E., Webb, D., von Muller, C. and Fudenberg, H. H. (1973): Journal of Clinical Investigation 52, 802.

26. Vandenbark, A. A., Burger, D. R., Dreyer, D., Daves, G. D. and Vetto, R. M. (1977): Journal of Immunology 118, 636.

Lymphokines and Thymic Hormones: Their Potential Utilization in Cancer Therapeutics, edited by A. L. Goldstein and M. A. Chirigos, Raven Press, New York © 1981.

The Response of Macrophages to Migration Inhibitory Factors and Other Signals

Clemens Sorg

Department of Experimental Dermatology, Universitäts-Hautklinik, 4400 Münster, West Germany

I. INTRODUCTION

Monocytes and macrophages are characteristic components of cellular infiltrates associated with acute or chronic inflammatory reactions. It is well established that antigen activated lymphocytes represent one possibility out of several others to cause an inflammatory reaction. Activated lymphocytes release a number of factors called lymphokines, which are believed to initiate and promote cellular infiltration. The lymphokine described first was the macrophage migration inhibitory factor (MIF) (2,4) which is thought to play an important role in the early events of cellular immune reactions by its action on macrophages. In the following I am going to describe our work on the chemical and functional characterization of MIF in three different species (guinea pig, mouse, man). In the second part I will report on our work on the analysis of the mononuclear phagocyte system in its response to MIF and other signals.

II. CHEMICAL AND FUNCTIONAL CHARACTERIZATION OF MIF

a) Guinea Pig

Guinea pig lymph node cells were stimulated with Concanavalin A (Con A) and simultaneously labeled with radioactive leucine (24,25,26,28). The 24 h culture supernatants were fractioned, using repeated Sephadex chromatography and various electrophoretic techniques (14,31). Using an anti-lymphokine antibody raised against purified migration inhibitory factor containing fractions which had been characterized extensively before (5,6,7,9,29), three lymphocyte activation products were identified initially with molecular weight 60.000 (a), 45.000 (b), and 30.000 (c), which all had an isoelectric point of around 5.2. With these materials the following characterizations have been performed: a, b and c were inhibitory in the macrophage migration assay. The buoyant density in a CsCl gradient was g = 1.278 for all three molecules. Treatment with neuraminidase did not cause a shift to pI greater than 5.2 and did not destroy biological activity. Reduction and alkylation or treatment with EDTA did not change the molecular weight of a, b or c. No proteolytic activity could be detected in any of the preparation, nor did any of the MIF activities contain Ia determinants. Because of the similarities in their chemical and biological properties, it was assumed that the three molecules are oligomers of a common subunit of a molecular weight of 15.000 and a pI of 5.2. A molecule of this size was detected in low amounts in stimulated culture supernatants which also exhibited marked migration inhibitory activity. It is concluded that MIF activity is not associated with a single molecule but rather with a group of structurally related molecules.

In another study we investigated the cellular sources of migration inhibitory factor (30), since it had been reported earlier that MIF was also produced by nonlymphoid cells (1, 21, 34). Using the anti-lymphokine serum and radiolabeled supernatants from various cells, migration inhibitory activity reacting with the anti-lymphokine serum and properties identical to those determined on MIF from lymphocytes was found in the following cell types: purified B cells, activated with staphylococcus aureus, L_2C leukemia (strain 2), growing embryonic fibroblasts. No activity was found in supernatants of peritoneal macrophages. Furthermore, no cross-reactivity of the antiserum with human or murine MIF was found. The results indicate that MIF with similar molecular properties may be produced by a variety of cells under appropriate stimulation. This situation is reminiscent of the production of interferons by a diversity of cell types.

b) Mouse

Con A stimulated and nonstimulated supernatants from spleen cells of BALB/c mice were fractionated on Sephadex G-100 and each fraction was tested in the macrophage migration assay, using medium containing 15% fetal calf serum as control (27). In the stimulated supernatants several distinct peaks of inhibitory activity were found, eluting at the molecular weight range of about 56.000 (a), 42.000 (b), 28.000 (c) and 14.000 (d). Activity was also found at higher molecular weight ranges and in the void volume, even though this was less consistent. In nonstimulated control cultures only a minor amount of inhibitory activity at the molecular weight 56.000 was observed. Similar results were obtained with stimulated and unstimulated thymocytes. Major activities were found here at molecular weight 56.000 and 28.000, while no or only minor activity was found at the molecular weight 42.000 and 14.000. When the materials of peak activity were pooled and subjected to isoelectric focussing, inhibitory activity was found for all molecular weight ranges (a-d) at pH 4.5 - 5.5. Neuraminidase treatment of all activities did not destroy activity and did not cause a significant shift to a higher pI. These data are very similar to the ones described above for the guinea pig, suggesting that inhibitory activity is associated with a group of structurally similar molecules rather than with a single molecule.

In order to determine further effects of MIF on macrophages, stimulated supernatants were fractionated by Sephadex chromatography and isoelectric focussing. Preparations (a-d) were tested for MIF activity. Figure 1 shows typical dose response curves for such preparations. Note, that at high concentrations there is no migration inhibition but rather a tendency to enhanced migration as compared to the controls. Further, there is always an indication for a biphasic course of the dose response for which we have no explanation ready.

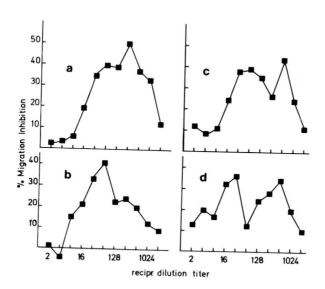

FIG. 1. Dose response of oil induced peritoneal macrophages to
purified migration inhibitory factors a, b, c, d.

Aliquots of these preparations were sent to a number of laboratories, each performing a particular test on macrophages. The results are summarized in table 1. The functional profile of MIF preparations show that they are contaminated to a certain degree with other lymphokine activities, e.g. as expected TRF is a contaminant in preparation (c) (11). Induction of Leishmania enrietti killing was only observed with (a) and not with (b), (c) and (d). Tumor cytotoxicity could be induced with all four preparations, however, we would not conclude that MIF is identical with the macrophage cytotoxic factor (11), since our preparations were not endotoxin-free and the observed effect could be a cooperative phenomenon between MIF and endotoxin (22). Yet, the experiment quite clearly shows that MIF has no chemotactic activity and is unrelated to interferon. It is also not an inducer of interferon. Furthermore, it shows that tumor cytostasis and tumor cell kill may be regulated through different pathways. From these experiments we would conclude that MIF is not identical with most macrophage activating activities which was the widely accepted assumption of the past years (for review see Sorg, 1979 (26).

c) Human

Chemical characterization of human MIF is currently at a less advanced state. Human lymphocytes are gained from peripheral blood of volunteer donors by leukapheresis. Lymphocytes are stimulated with mitogen and the superna-

TABLE 1.   Biological properties of murine MIFs

	a	b	c	d
Mol.wt.	56.000	42.000	28.000	14.000
pI	5.2	5.2	5.2	5.2
Activities				
- Interferon	-	-	-	-
- TRF[1]	±	±	+	-
Chemotactic for				
- PMN	±	±	±	±
- Monocytes	-	-	-	-
Induction in macrophages of:				
- Tumor cytotoxicity[2]	+	+	++	+++
- Tumor cytostosis[3]	-	-	-	-
- Killing of Leishmania enrietti[4]	+++	-	-	-
- Prostaglandin $E_1 + E_2$ release	±	++	+	+
- Interferon	-	-	-	-

tested by [1]Dr. A.Schimpl, Würzburg,   [2]Dr. E.Kniep, Freiburg,
[3]Dr. D.Gemsa, Heidelberg,   [4]Dr. J.Mauel, Lausanne.

tants are assayed on human monocytes/macrophages which are also obtained by
leukapheresis in high yields. From the current data a similar picture on the
molecular characteristics emerges as described already for MIF of mouse and
guinea pig, that is, several molecular weight species from below 10.000 up to
greater 60.000 can be identified. The isoelectric point of the various molecular
weight species is at 5.2, yet activity is also found at lower pH (unpublished
observations).

III. FUNCTIONAL HETEROGENEITY OF MACROPHAGES IN RESPONSE
TO LYMPHOKINES AND OTHER SIGNALS

In the course of our studies on the interaction of lymphokines with macrophages we noticed a great heterogeneity of macrophages in response to lymphokines. Our studies were dealing with the induction of plasminogen activator (12)
and interferon by lymphokines (17, 18). Functional heterogeneity of macrophages
has been documented before in many cases (for review see Sorg and Neumann,
1981 (32). The question on the biological basis of macrophage heterogeneity at
present cannot be answered with certainty. One assumption is that we are dealing with true subpopulations as it is known for the T cell B cell lineages.
Another possibility would be that macrophages which are bone marrow derived
pass through different maturation stages or intermediate relatively stable
phenotypes on their way to maturity and senescence, thus expressing charac-

teristic functions in each maturation stage. In order to approach this problem we adopted the bone marrow liquid culture system which had been introduced by Sumner et al., 1972 (33), and Goud et al., 1975 (8), several years ago.

Bone marrow cells from mice were cultured on teflon membranes in the presence of a colony stimulating factor produced by L cells (20). Parallel cultures were harvested daily and a series of functions was recorded over 12 days. The growth curve was declining rapidly after onset of culture until day 2 - 3 due to death of granulocytes and erythrocyte precursors. At day 4 - 5 the yield of cells increased, reaching a maximum at day 6 - 8 and then declined again. When the cells were stained (Pappenheim stain) and the macrophage content was determined according to the criteria of Cline and Sumner (3), the first appearance of macrophages could be seen at day 2 which increased linearly and reached a plateau at day 6. When the cells were stained for unspecific esterase (alpha-naphthyl-acetate) weakly stained cells peaked at day 2 and 3 and again at day 5 and 6 whereas heavily stained cells appeared for the first time at day 3 and then again at day 6 and on, reaching a maximum of nearly 90% at day 9. The phagocytosis of latex beads was observed very early in culture, reaching a plateau at day 7 - 8. Phagocytosis of immunoglobulin-coated sheep red blood cells was also performed with adherent cells. Phagocytic activity was apparent at day 2, decreasing by day 3 and reaching again a maximum at day 5 and 6. From day 7 on only few cells phagocytosed 3 or more red blood cells.

In another series of experiments the response to three different stimuli was investigated. Mouse serum was rendered chemotactic by zymosan as described by Snyderman and Pike, 1976 (23). The chemotactic response was measured in Boyden chambers using cellulose nitrate filters. Results showed a sharp maximum at day 3 - 4 for the chemotactic response of mononuclear cells (Figure 2). No chemotactic response was observed after day 5. When the response to MIF containing supernatants of Concanavalin A-stimulated spleen cells was measured, again a sharp maximum at day 4 and 5 was found, whereas no response could be detected before and after this period, even though the cells were vigorously migrating in the earlier days. Since interferon production by lymphokine induced macrophages requires an incubation time of 24 - 48 h and since this time would be too long in order to draw any conclusion on the momentous differentiation state of a cell culture, it was decided to use the LPS-induced production of interferon which - like migration inhibition and chemotaxis - requires only 3 - 4 h incubation. When tested daily, interferon induction by LPS was successful only at day 5 and 6.

As a further function the plasminogen activator production was recorded. Plasminogen activator was detected with a fibrinolysis assay which allows the simultaneous detection of fibrinolysis inhibitors (13). No plasminogen activator or significant amounts of fibrinolysis inhibitors were found during the first three days of culture. Beginning at day 4, plasminogen activator was readily produced reaching a maximum at day 6 and 7 and then decreased rapidly. At day 8 the cells had ceased the produced plasminogen activator and at day 9 they began to produce inhibitors of fibrinolysis for the rest of the culture period.

When we surveyed our data we noticed that those macrophages either derived from bone marrow liquid cultures or from peritoneal exudates, which did not produce plasminogen activator could also not be induced to release interferon

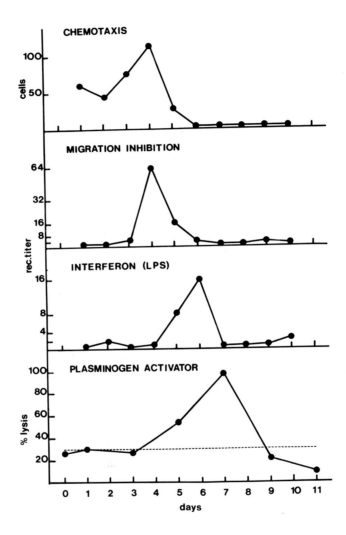

FIG. 2. Sequential expression of functions during maturation of
macrophages in bone marrow liquid culture system.

neither by LPS nor by lymphokines. Further, it was observed that those macrophages that responded best to LPS in terms of interferon production were close to or at the plasminogen activator producing state (20). We therefore asked the question whether plasminogen activator production might be a constitutive trait of those macrophages which can be induced to interferon production. In a series of experiments we found an almost perfect correlation between these two parameters, i.e. macrophage populations which produced plasminogen activator within 25 h of culture could be induced to release interferon. From these observations we would have to conclude that certain macrophages have the ability to produce plasminogen activator and are inducible to interferon production at the same time. Whether we are dealing with subpopulations or phenotypes of different maturation stages we still can't decide.

It has been described by Vassalli et al. (35) that macrophages may be induced to plasminogen activator production by the tumor promotor phorbol myristate acetate (PMA), which is also mitogenic to macrophages. The following question was then asked: are macrophages pushed by PMA and similar signals such as lymphokines into a certain phase of the cell cycle in which plasminogen activator production is expressed. And further, what role plays the cell cycle in macrophage heterogeneity.

In a series of experiments it was found that macrophages produce substantial amounts of plasminogen activator 2 - 22 h after exposure to PMA (32). The production of plasminogen activator then steadily decreases. In contrast, the number of cells in S-phase peaks later at 26 - 46 h. This indicates that macrophages after exposure to PMA are pushed towards the S-phase of the cell cycle. On their way to S, probably in late G_1, macrophages express plasminogen activator as a constitutive trait and also become sensitive to activation by lipopolysaccharides.

IV. HYPOTHESIS

Based on our summarized data and those from different laboratories we are able to describe the following picture (Figure 3): first, what is likely to happen in the bone marrow liquid culture system? Macrophages differentiate from precursors in the presence of colony-stimulating factor. After a phase of intensive proliferation of precursors and differentiation into macrophages, the young macrophages still keep on cycling, thus accumulating cells in late G_1, which are characterized by plasminogen activator production, inducibility of interferon, and their response to MIF and certain chemotactic factors. When proliferation is fading away, the cells differentiate gradually in G_1, loosing a series of constitutive functions and pass on to a G_0-like state characterized by production of fibrinolysis inhibitors. In this model the functional state of normal resident macrophages should be compatible with G_0, that of proteose peptone elicited macrophages with "early" and thioglycollate induced macrophages with "late" G_1. In kinetic studies with PMA, the time needed to induce normal resident macrophages to plasminogen activator production was considerably longer than that needed for proteose peptone elicited macrophages. The model proposes further that macrophage differentiation in G_1 is reversible and that macrophages of various functional states have to go through the bottle neck of "late" G_1 before entering S.

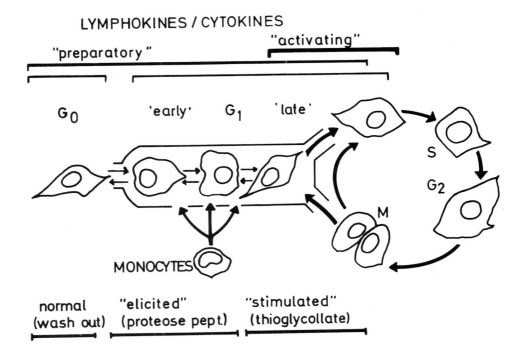

FIG. 3.   Hypothesis on the biological basis of macrophage heterogeneity.

What then is an activated macrophage and how can the action of lympho-kines be fitted in? As shown first by Mackaness (15) and subsequently by many others, activated macrophages express special functions, in particular bacteri-cidal and tumoricidal properties. Several collegues (10, 22) have demonstrated that macrophages can be rapidly activated by lipopolysaccharides to kill tumor cells. However, not all macrophages respond the same. Nonresponding macro-phages can be made responsive, however, by preincubation with lymphokines which serve as preparatory signals. In our model this would mean that macro-phages are pushed first from G_0 or "early" G_1 into "late" G_1, where macro-phages become inducible to kill tumor cells. These findings are paralleled by ours on the induction of interferon by LPS.

According to the proposed model one now could divide lymphokines and also cytokines into differentiogenic, mitogenic and activating signals. Until present only cumulative effects on macrophages of a cocktail of lymphokines have been studied. Using purified lymphokines in macrophage populations which are functionally characterized according to our model, we should be able to define the precise nature of a lymphokine signal and the nature of the cellular response to it. While it is still a widespread believe that MIF and macrophage activating factor are different manifestations of the same molecule, evidence has come out recently that they are not identical (16,11; see also this article). On the basis of our model we would predict that differentiation, activation and homeostasis of the mononuclear phagocytic system is regulated by a complex network of lymphokines and other factors.

REFERENCES

1. Bigazzi, P.E., Yoshida, T., Ward, P.H., and Cohen, S. (1975): Am.J.Pathol., 80:69-77.

2. Bloom, B.R., and Bennett, B. (1966): Science, 153:80-82.

3. Cline, M.J., and Sumner, M.A. (1972): Blood, 40:62-69.

4. David, J.R. (1966): Proc.Natl.Acad.Sci.USA, 56:72-77.

5. Geczy, C.L., Friedrich, W., and de Weck, A.L. (1975): Cell.Immunol., 19:65-77.

6. Geczy, C.L., Geczy, A.F., and de Weck, A.L. (1976): J.Immunol., 117:66-72.

7. Geczy, C.L., Geczy, A.F., and de Weck, A.L. (1976): J.Immunol., 117:1824-1881.

8. Goud, T.J.L.M., Schotte, C., and van Furth, R. (1975): J.Exp.Med., 142:1180-1199.

9. Hentges, F., Geczy, C.L., Geczy, A.F., and de Weck, A.L. (1977): Immunology, 32:905-913.

10. Hibbs, Jr., J.B., Taintor, R.R., Chapman, Jr., H.A., and Weinberg, J.B. (1977): Science, 197:279-282.

11. Hübner, L., Kniep, E.M., Laukel, H., Sorg, C., Fischer, H., Gassel. W.D., Havemann, K., Kickhöfen, B., Lohmann-Matthes, M.-L., Schimpl, A., and Wecker, E. (1980): Immunobiology, 157:169-178.

12. Klimetzek, V., and Sorg, C. (1977): Eur.J.Immunol., 7:185-189.

13. Klimetzek, V., and Sorg, C. (1979): Eur.J.Immunol., 9:613-619.

14. Klinkert, W., and Sorg, C. (1980): Molec.Immunol., 17:555-564.

15. Mackaness, G.B. (1969): J.Exp.Med., 129:973-992.

16. Meltzer, M.S., Wahl, L.M., and Leonard, E.J. (1980): In: Biochemical Characterization of Lymphokines, edited by A. de Weck, F. Kristensen, and M. Landy, pp. 161-167. Academic Press, New York.

17. Neumann, Ch., and Sorg, C. (1977): Eur.J.Immunol., 7:719-725.

18. Neumann, Ch., and Sorg, C. (1978): Eur.J.Immunol., 8:582-589.

19. Neumann, Ch., and Sorg, C. (1980): Eur.J.Immunol., 10:834–840.

20. Neumann, Ch., and Sorg, C. (1981): J.Reticuloendothel.Soc., in press.

21. Papageorgiou, P.A., Henley, W.L., and Glade, P.R. (1972): J.Immunol., 110:449–504.

22. Ruco, L.P., and Meltzer, M.S. (1978): Cell.Immunol., 41:35–51.

23. Snyderman, R., and Pike, M. (1976): In: In Vitro Methods in Cell Mediated and Tumor Immunity, edited by B.R.Bloom, and J.R.David, pp. 651–661. Academic Press, New York.

24. Sorg, C. (1976): Eur.J.Biochem., 55:423–430.

25. Sorg, C. (1978): J.Immunol.Meth., 19:173–179.

26. Sorg, C. (1979): Mol.Cell.Biochem., 28:149–167.

27. Sorg, C. (1980): Molec.Immunol., 17:565–569.

28. Sorg, C., and Bloom, B.R. (1973): J.Exp.Med., 137:148–170.

29. Sorg, C., and Geczy, C.L. (1976): Eur.J.Immunol., 6:688–693.

30. Sorg, C., and Geczy, C.L. (1978): J.Immunol., 121:1199–1205.

31. Sorg, C., and Klinkert, W. (1978): Fed.Proc., 37:2748–2753.

32. Sorg, C., and Neumann, Ch. (1981): In: Lymphokines, Vol. 3, edited by E. Pick, pp. 85–118. Academic Press, New York.

33. Sumner, M.A., Bradley, T.R., Hodgson, G.S., Cline, M.J., Fry, P.A., and Sutherland, L. (1972): Br.J.Haematol., 23:221–234.

34. Tubergen, D.B., Feldman, J.D., Pollock, E.N., and Lerner, R.A. (1972): J.Exp.Med., 135:255–261.

35. Vassalli, J.-D., Hamilton, J., and Reich, E. (1976): Cell, 8:271–281.

*Lymphokines and Thymic Hormones: Their
Potential Utilization in Cancer Therapeutics,*
edited by A. L. Goldstein and M. A. Chirigos,
Raven Press, New York © 1981.

Specific and Nonspecific Macrophage Migration Inhibition

Gary B. Thurman, Teresa L. K. Low, *Jeffrey L. Rossio,
and Allan L. Goldstein

*Department of Biochemistry, The George Washington University School of Medicine and Health
Services, Washington, D.C. 20037; *Department of Microbiology and Immunology,
Wright State University School of Medicine, Dayton, Ohio 45431*

The central role of the thymus gland in the development and maturation of lymphocytes responsible for cell-mediated immune reactions is
well-documented [1]. During fetal or neonatal development (depending
on the species), the thymus gland "seeds" the peripheral lymphoid
tissue with its armamentarium of post-thymic cells [23]. These cells
initiate and participate in cell-mediated immune responses upon appropriate antigenic stimulus. Once this "seeding" has taken place, the
thymus gland has accomplished one of its major purposes, and its presence in the body is no longer an absolute requirement for expression
of cell-mediated immune responsivity [22]. Removal of the thymus
gland after this "seeding" phenomenon has taken place does not greatly
interfere with immune responses or place the thymectomized host in immediate jeopardy. That is not to say that thymectomy is not eventual-
ly deleterious to health and longevity or is without adverse effects.
It simply indicates that most of the effects of thymectomy are subtle
and take relatively long periods of time to develop. This is in contrast to the effects seen with the removal of other endocrine glands
such as the pancreas or adrenals. In those cases the effects are almost immediate and are far from subtle.

Because the effects of adult thymectomy are subtle and not immediately obvious, the thymus gland was long neglected by scientists. The
thymus gland was classified in the vestigial organ category along with
the tonsils and the appendix. Pioneering studies in the early 1960's
demonstrated the dramatic effects of neonatal thymectomy and established the primary importance of the thymus in immunological development [for example, REFERENCE 17]. Since those basic observations
were made, a great deal of interest has focused on the thymus gland,

Present address of G.B.T.: Biological Response Modifiers Program, NCI –
Frederick Cancer Research Center, Frederick, Maryland 21701.

its cellular products, its polypeptide hormones and its interactive
role with other organs [see reviews REFERENCES 24 and 26]. Most of the
research on the thymus gland has revolved around its central role in
immunological maturation and cell production. The interactive role of
the thymus gland in systemic responses to antigens was largely ignored
and felt to be of little consequence. There have been relatively few
studies that have seriously investigated the effects that antigenic
stimuli have on the thymus gland, and even fewer studies on the effects
the thymus gland itself has on an adult animal responding to antigens.

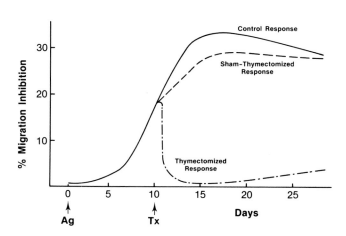

FIGURE 1 – Schematic representation of the time dependent development
of the cell-mediated immune response to antigen (Ag) of peripheral
blood lymphocytes as measured by their capability to inhibit the migration of macrophages. The effects of thymectomy (Tx) and sham-thymec-
tomy on this response are shown.

Our interest in this area was further stimulated by a report by
Field and Shenton in 1975 [4]. They found that removal of the thymus
gland 10 days after immunization of guinea pigs with purified protein
derivative (PPD) in complete Freund's adjuvant, led to the rapid decline of the PPD responsivity of the guinea pigs' peripheral blood
lymphocytes (PBL) as measured by macrophage migration (schematically
shown on Figure 1). They speculated that the unreactivity was due to
the loss of circulating thymosin due to thymectomy. They showed that
serum from a thymus-bearing animal could restore the in vitro response
to PPD and that serum from a thymectomized animal could not (see Figure
2).

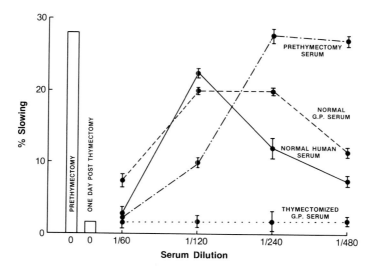

FIGURE 2 — Effects of sera from various sources on the response of peripheral blood lymphocytes to PPD as measured by % slowing in the macrophage electrophoretic mobility test [data compiled from REFERENCE 4].

We reported in 1976 [25], that the loss of reactivity to PPD following thymectomy in guinea pigs could be demonstrated using the capillary
tube macrophage migration inhibition (MMI) technique. We showed the
responsivity of the PBL to PPD could be restored in this assay by adding extracts from bovine thymus glands with hormonal-like activity
called thymosin [7]. We showed activity with a partially purified
preparation called thymosin fraction 5 and showed that one polypeptide
component, thymosin α1 was very active in this assay, while another,
polypeptide α3 was not (see Table 1).

TABLE 1

EFFECT OF THYMOSIN ON THE MMI RESPONSE
TO PPD OF PBL FROM THYMECTOMIZED GUINEA PIGS

CHAMBER CONTENTS	CONCENTRATION	SPECIFIC INHIBITION
Thymosin Fr. 5	10 μg/ml	−24.5%
	50 μg/ml	20.8%
	100 μg/ml	34.6%
Thymosin α1	1 ng/ml	12.6%
	10 ng/ml	26.5%
	100 ng/ml	54.5%
Polypeptide α3	1 ng/ml	−29.9%
	10 ng/ml	−47.8%
	100 ng/ml	−36.7%

This report expands those initial observations and reports the finding that two thymosin polypeptides, β3 and β4, have MMI capabilities themselves, independent of antigen.

MATERIALS AND METHODS

Thymosin and Control Polypeptides

Thymosin fraction 5 was prepared as reported by Hooper et al. [10]. Thymosin α1 was prepared from thymosin fraction 5 as reported [6] and synthetic thymosin α1 and tyrosine-thymosin α1 was obtained from Hoffmann-La Roche (Nutley, NJ). Thymosin α1, made by recombinant DNA Technology (N^α-desacetyl thymosin α1) [27], was obtained from Genentech (San Francisco, CA). Thymosin β3 (Low and Goldstein, unpublished and β4 [15] were prepared in our laboratories and synthetic thymosin β4 was obtained from Hoffmann-La Roche. Spleen fr. 5, kidney fr. 5 and angiotensin II were also supplied by Hoffmann-La Roche. Polypeptide β1 (also known as ubiquitin) was prepared in our laboratory as previously described [16]. Bovine serum albumin (BSA) was obtained from Sigma Chemical Co. (St. Louis, MO) and endotoxin (lipopolysaccharide) was obtained from Difco (Detroit, MI). Prealbumin and Facteur Thymique Serique (FTS) was supplied by Syntex (Palo Alto, CA).

Macrophage Migration Inhibition Assay

PBL Preparation. Hartley-strain outbred guinea pigs (Camm Labs, Wayne, NJ) were immunized with PPD (Connaught Labs, Toronto, Canada) in complete Freund's adjuvant (Difco), receiving 10 μg PPD in 0.1 ml adjuvant i.d. on a shaved flank. Ten days following the adjuvant, the guinea pigs were anesthetized and thymectomized using sterile precautions. Two days later the animals were exsanguinated while under light anesthesia. Autopsies were performed to insure that complete thymectomies had been accomplished. Animals with thymic remnants were not used in the study.

The blood was diluted with an equal volume of Hanks' balanced salts solution (GIBCO, Grand Island, NY) and gently layered on a Ficoll-Hypaque gradient (Lymphoprep, Nyegaard and Co., Oslo, Norway). Following centrifugation at 400 x g for 40 min, the PBL were recovered from the interface and washed in HEPES buffered RPMI 1640 (GIBCO), by centrifugation at 200 x g. The PBL were adjusted to 5 x 10^6/ml in 20% fetal calf serum and 9% DMSO, rate-frozen at -1°/min and stored at -70° until used.

Guinea Pig PEC Preparation. Peritoneal exudate cells (PEC) were prepared in Hartley strain guinea pigs by injecting 20-30 ml of sterile mineral oil (Elkins-Sinn, Inc., Cherry Hill, NJ) 3-5 days prior to the assay. On the day of the assay, the guinea pigs were anesthetized and injected i.p. with 50 ml of RPMI-1640. Following abdominal massage, the peritoneum was opened with a one inch incision in the umbilical region and the peritoneal fluids withdrawn. The peritoneal fluids were centrifuged at 200 x g for 10 min and the pelleted cells resuspended in a small volume of RPMI for transfer to clean tubes. Following three more washes, the cells were resuspended, counted and adjusted to 45 x 106/ml for use.

Mouse PEC Preparation. In some experiments mouse PEC were used in place of guinea pig PEC. The mouse PEC were induced in BALB/c normal or nude mice by injecting 1 ml of mineral oil i.p. 3 days prior obtaining the cells by washing the peritoneum with 5 ml of RPMI 1640.

Macrophage-like Cell Lines as Indicator Cells. In some experiments macrophage-like cell lines, WEHI-3 and FC-1, were used in place of PEC. The WEHI-3 cells migrate and have been reported to respond to migration inhibitory factor (MIF)(14). Likewise, the FC-1 cells are also migratory and respond to MIF(18).

Specific MMI Assay. The agarose droplet MMI technique of Harrington (9) was used, as briefly described below. The PBL were rapidly thawed, slowly diluted and washed 2 times in RPMI 1640. They were counted and resuspended at 5×10^6 viable cells per ml. Equal volumes of PBL and PEC were added together in a conical centrifuge tube and centrifuged at 200 x g for 10 min. Following removal of the supernatant, the cell button was warmed to 37° in a water bath.

An aliquot of a stock solution of 0.4% SeaPlaque agarose in water (Marine Colloids, Rockland, ME) was melted in a boiling water bath and cooled to 37°. An equal volume of 2X RPMI at 37° was added to the agarose. The agarose - RPMI solution was added to the cell button, using the total cell number to determine the amount added (1 ml per 10^9 cells). The cells were resuspended gently in the agarose at 37° using a Hamilton Repeating Dispenser with a 0.05 ml gas-tight syringe (Hamilton Company, Reno, NV) and 0.001 ml droplets were centrally placed in flat-bottomed microtiter plates (Falcon, Oxnard, CA). The droplets were solidified at 4° for 5 minutes and 0.05 ml of RPMI was added to each well. Various polypeptides were prepared in RPMI with or without PPD and 0.05 ml of the peptide, peptide plus PPD, or PPD alone were added to the appropriate wells. Control wells received medium alone. Samples were tested in triplicate or quadruplicate. The microtiter plates were incubated for 24 hours in a humid, 5% CO_2-in-air atmosphere on a perfectly level shelf of an incubator. The areas of migration were computed on a TI-59 programmable calculator from the dimensions measured by projecting the image of the droplet and cells on a grid using a Bausch and Lomb Trisimplex Microprojector (Fisher Scientific, Silver Spring, MD). The shape of the migration was assumed to be eliptical and the major and minor axes of the agarose droplet and the cell migration pattern were measured. The area of migration was calculated as the area of the cell migration pattern minus the area of the agarose droplet. Means and standard errors of the replicate samples were also calculated by the TI-59. The percent specific inhibition (PSI) was calculated as:

$$PSI \leqslant = 100 - \left| \frac{Area (thymosin \& PPD)}{Area (PPD)} \times \frac{Area (RPMI)}{Area (thymosin)} \times 100 \right|$$

If the area of the thymosin & PPD replicates was not statistically less (p $\leqslant$ 0.05 by Student's t-Test) than the area with PPD alone, the inhibition was considered insignificant. PSI's of less than 20% were also considered insignificant.

Nonspecific MMI Assay. The nonspecific MMI assay did not involve antigen and measured the direct effect various polypeptides had on macrophage inhibition. The percent nonspecific inhibition (PNSI) was calculated as:

$$PNSI = 100 - \left| \frac{Area\ (thymosin)}{Area\ (RPMI)} \times 100 \right|$$

If the means of the replicates for various polypeptides were not significantly different from the mean of the RPMI control by Student's t-Test (p ◁0.05), the inhibition was considered insignificant. Percent nonspecific inhibition of migration of less than 20% was also considered insignificant.

RESULTS

A variety of polypeptides isolated from thymosin fr. 5 were tested in both the specific and the nonspecific MMI assays and only 3 polypeptides showed significant activity, thymosin α1, β3 and β4 (Table 2). Thymosin α1 was active in specifically restoring the MIF production capability of the PBL of thymectomized guinea pigs, whereas thymosin β3 and β4 were not. However, thymosin β3 and β4 inhibited the migration of the PEC themselves in a nonspecific manner without antigen. Even at a concentration of .005 nM (25 pg/ml), both β3 and β4 significantly inhibited the migration of the PEC.

TABLE 2

EFFECT OF THYMOSIN POLYPEPTIDES ON THE MIF RESPONSE
TO PPD OF PBL FROM THYMECTOMIZED GUINEA PIGS

CHAMBER CONTENTS	CONCENTRATION	SPECIFIC INHIBITION	NON-SPECIFIC INHIBITION
Thymosin α1	.5nM	36%	NONE
Thymosin β3	.5nM	NONE	47%
	.05nM	NONE	44%
	.005nM	NONE	35%
Thymosin β4	.5nM	NONE	33%
	.05nM	NONE	37%
	.005nM	NONE	24%

Further evaluation of other polypeptides and of other thymic hormone preparations are presented in Table 3. With one exception, the only polypeptide preparations active in the specific MIF assay were thymosin α1 and its parent fraction, thymosin fr. 5. The one exception was angiotensin II, which repeatedly showed activity in this assay at concentrations in the same range as thymosin α1. Other controls, BSA, endotoxin, spleen fr. 5 and kidney fr. 5 were all negative. Three other polypeptides with reported effects on T-cell maturation, polypeptide β1 (ubiquitin), prealbumin and FTS were also negative in this assay system. Synthetic thymosin α1 was as active as the natural molecule, and tyrosine-thymosin α1, made for use in the development of a radioimmunoassay for thymosin α1 was also active. Of great interest was the observation that thymosin α1 made by recombinant DNA technology (N^α-desacetyl thymosin α1, REFERENCE 27) was also very active in this system. Neither thymosin β3 nor thymosin β4 (synthetic or natural) were active in the antigen-dependent MMI assay.

TABLE 3

ACTIVITY OF THYMOSIN AND CONTROL PEPTIDES IN THE MMI ASSAY

PREPARATION TESTED	SPECIFIC MMI RESPONSE TO PPD	NON-SPECIFIC MIGRATION INHIBITION
Thymosin Fr. 5	++	−
Thymosin α1	+++	−
Thymosin β3	−	+++
Thymosin β4	−	+++
Peptide β1	−	−
Prealbumin	−	−
Facteur Thymique Serique	−	−
BSA	−	−
Endotoxin	−	−
Spleen Fr. 5	−	−
Kidney Fr. 5	−	−
Angiotensin II	+++	−
Synthetic thymosin α1	+++	−
N^α-desacetyl thymosin α1	+++	−
Tyrosine-thymosin α1	+++	−
Synthetic thymosin β4	−	+++

−(<15%), + (15-20%), ++ (20-25%), +++ (>25%)

Repetitive experiments summarized in Table 3 indicated that the only components of thymosin fraction 5 tested to date that have shown non-specific macrophage migration inhibitory activity have been thymosin β3 and β4. Even the parent compound (thymosin fr. 5) did not inhibit migration. Thymosin α1 and polypeptide β1 did not show any migration inhibitory activity. The testing of other thymic factors and control substances (See Table 3) did not reveal any evidence of their capability to inhibit macrophage migration.

To investigate whether or not thymosin β3 and β4 were acting directly on macrophages or were stimulating lymphocytes to release MIF, the polypeptides were tested against PEC from various sources and against macrophage-like cell lines that had been reported to migrate and respond to MIF.

TABLE 4

TARGET CELLS FOR THYMOSIN POLYPEPTIDES' MIGRATION INHIBITORY EFFECT

PERCENT MIGRATION INHIBITION

THYMOSIN POLY-PEPTIDE	CONC. nM	PERITONEAL EXUDATE CELLS			MACROPHAGE LINES	
		G.P.	MOUSE	NUDE	WEHI-3	FC-1
$\beta 3$	5×10^{-1}	31.7	35.0	33.1	17.9	0
	5×10^{-2}	23.4	25.0	26.7	4.8	4.2
	5×10^{-3}	21.6	21.7	12.7	ND	ND
$\beta 4$	5×10^{-1}	40.9	37.6	18.8	29.7	11.6
	5×10^{-2}	39.4	29.2	20.7	18.1	0
	5×10^{-3}	37.8	8.4	23.1	ND	ND
$\alpha 1$	5×10^{-1}	6.5	5.7	3.7	2.2*	ND
	5×10^{-2}	7.5	6.3	0	8.1*	ND
	5×10^{-3}	0	25.1	0.5	11.6*	ND

* Done with 2.5% FCS

The data in Table 4 indicate that thymosin $\beta 3$ and $\beta 4$ inhibit macrophage migration of PEC without added PBL. Even PEC from T-cell deficient nude mice were inhibited by these 2 polypeptides. Thymosin $\beta 4$ significantly and repeatedly inhibited the migration of the WEHI-3 cells whereas thymosin $\beta 3$ only marginally inhibited the migration of WEHI-3 cells. Neither polypeptide inhibited the migration of the FC-1 cells. However, the FC-1 cells migrated poorly in the serum-free conditions used in this assay system and further experimentation is necessary before definitive conclusions are deduced from these negative results.

Thymosin $\alpha 1$ was used as a control polypeptide and did not significantly inhibit the migration of any of the cell types, except at one concentration for normal mouse PEC. This has not proven to be reproducible and may have been due to an unusual population of cells in the PEC obtained in this particular experiment.

The amino acid sequence of thymosin $\alpha 1$ and thymosin $\beta 4$ are shown in Fig. 3.

Thymosin $\alpha 1$ was the first polypeptide isolated and sequenced from thymosin fr. 5. It was isolated by ion-exchange chromatography on CM-cellulose and DEAE-cellulose, and gel filtration on Sephadex G-75. The yield of thymosin $\alpha 1$ from fr. 5 is about 0.6%. Thymosin $\alpha 1$ is an acidic polypeptide consisting of 28 amino acid residues with an acetyl group blocking the amino terminus. It has a molecular weight of 3108 daltons and an isoelectric point of 4.2. Computer analysis has established that the sequence of thymosin $\alpha 1$ bears very little homology to any of the protein sequences published, and shows no homology to thymopoietin II(20), FTS(2) or angiotensin II (5).

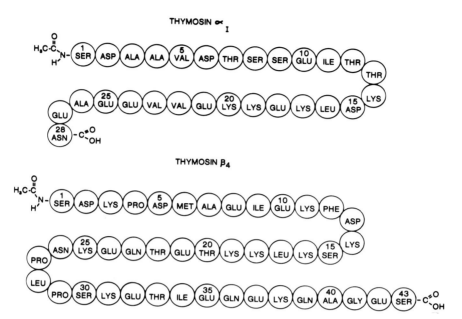

Fig. 3. The amino acid sequence of thymosin α1 and thymosin β4.

Thymosin β4 has now been sequenced (15) and synthesized. It was pre-pared from thymosin fr. 5 by chromatography on CM-cellulose and by gel filtration on Sephadex G-50. Thymosin β4 has an isoelectric point of 5.1 and a molecular weight of 4982 daltons. A computer search has indicated that the sequence of thymosin β4 does not have any significant homology with the sequences of other reported proteins.

The complete sequence for thymosin β3 has not yet been established. Preliminary studies (Low and Goldstein, unpublished) indicate that thy-mosin β3 has a sequence similar to that of thymosin β4 for most of its amino-terminal portion, with thymosin β3 being several amino acids longer than thymosin β4 at the carboxy-terminal end. Thymosin β3 has a molecular weight of approximately 5500 and an isoelectric point of 5.2.

DISCUSSION

At 10 days post-sensitization to PPD, guinea pigs are involved in a reaction which sensitizes circulating uncommitted lymphocytes to the in-jected antigen. These cells evidently undergo maturation to become anti-gen reactive cells under the influence of circulating thymosin polypep-tides and home to either the spleen or lymph nodes. A number of studies (reviewed in ref. 3) have established the concept that lymphocytes in the early stages of reaction to antigen are selectively removed from the circulation by the spleen and lymph nodes. Thoracic duct cells from mice, which had received allogeneic or xenogeneic cells in an intravenous challenge 1-2 days before, demonstrate a deficiency of specific reactivity to the cellular antigens which were injected (19,21).

Our studies indicate that when the thymus gland is removed during the sensitization period, some lymphocytes which have begun to react to the antigen are unable to undergo further maturation or home to the spleen or lymph nodes. Instead they remain in the circulation, and when challenged in vitro with the sensitizing antigen, are unable to react by MIF production unless thymosin is present.

We have found that thymosin α1 is the only polypeptide tested to date capable of restoring the reactivity of PBL from thymectomized guinea pigs. We have also shown that synthetic, tyrosine-modified and E.coli produced thymosin α1 are all active in this system.

The exact reasons why thymectomy following immunization causes a build-up of antigen-committed immature cells in the circulation are not known. When lymphocytes are taken from the spleen or the lymph nodes, they respond to antigen by MIF production without thymosin polypeptides being present (data not shown). Similarly, immunized, thymectomized guinea pigs give skin test responses to PPD of a similar magnitude to those given by non-thymectomized guinea pigs. This would seem to indicate that the immunologically defective site is the blood and that thymectomy may play an adverse and almost immediate role on the antigen reactivity of circulating lymphocytes. This model provides an excellent tool to further investigate the effects of thymectomy on immune reactivity. It may be of benefit in unraveling the complexities of thymus-dependent lymphocyte maturation into antigen reactive cells which can produce lymphokines upon stimulation.

The observation that angiotensin II can mimic thymosin α1 in this system has yet to be fully explained. Goetzl et al. (5) recently reported that the amino – and carboxy – terminal substituent tetrapeptides of angiotensin II, Asp-Arg-Val-Tyr and Ile-His-Pro-Phe, elicit substantial human mononuclear leukocyte chemotactic responses in vitro. They also noted that the amino-terminal tetrapeptide exhibits significant amino acid homology with the pentapeptide Arg-Lys-Asp-Val-Tyr, that has been reported to be the functionally critical constituent of the thymic polypeptide, thymopoietin II (8). We have not evaluated thymopoietin II or its active pentapeptide component in this assay.

An unexpected dividend of testing the various thymosin component polypeptides was the observation that thymosin β3 and β4 were nonspecifically (without antigen) capable of inhibiting the migration of macrophages. These two polypeptides inhibit migration in the pg/ml range and do not display any evidence of toxicity for the cells (data not shown). Preliminary data indicate that thymosin β3 and β4 act directly on the macrophages to inhibit their migration. However, the possibility that they act on lymphocytes and induce them to release a macrophage migration inhibitory factor (MIF) has not been completely ruled out.

One intriguing interpretation for this data is that thymosin β4 is an active component of the lymphocyte-produced MIF molecule itself. Several observation would support this possibility. Klinkert and Sorg (13) reported that MIF activity is not associated with a single molecule, but with a group of structurally related molecules. Using anti-lymphokine antibody raised against purified MIF, 3 lymphocyte activation products were initially identified with molecular weights of 60,000, 45,000 and 30,000, and similar pI of about 5.2. This suggested a common subunit of 15,000 molecular weight and a standard pI of 5.2. Thymosin β4 has a molecular weight of slightly less than 5,000 and a pI of 5.1. The size of these two thymosin polypeptides make it possible to consider that they are the active component of the subunit proposed by Klinkert and Sorg or that they are an even smaller subunit of MIF. Thymosin β3 is slightly larger than 5,000 mol. wt. and has a pI of 5.2.

Isolation of MIF from thymus tissue has been previously reported by Houck, et al. (12). They found that MIF could be demonstrated in the ethanol precipitate of an aqueous extract of thymus tissue from adult animals responding to antigenic challenge. The factor was not present in extracts of thymus tissue from immunologically naive animals. Subsequent work (11) demonstrated that this factor behaved like MIF that had been isolated from stimulated lymphocytes. It had a molecular weight of about 36,000 daltons, it was trypsin sensitive and neuraminidase sensitive, and was thermostable. It is tempting to speculate that Houck's thymus-derived MIF and our thymus-derived thymosin β4 may be closely related, and that they originate from the same molecule. Further investigation into these possibilities are underway.

Although many questions remain to be answered, the fact that we have isolated, sequenced and synthesized a thymic polypeptide that significantly inhibits the migration of macrophages may help to further delineate the structure and function of MIF itself.

ACKNOWLEDGEMENTS

The contribution of various polypeptides by Drs. Patrick Trown and Countney McGregor of Hoffmann-La Roche and by Drs. Harold Ringold and Pamela Burton of Syntex was very helpful in this study. The technical expertise of Cary Seals was invaluable in the MIF assay. This work was supported by Hoffmann-La Roche and by grants CA24974 and CA25017 from the National Cancer Institute.

1. Aiuti, F. and Wigzell, H., editors (1980): Thymus, Thymic Hormones and T Lymphcytes. Academic Press, New York.

2. Bach J. F., Dardenne, M. and Plen, J. M. (1977): Nature 266:55-57.

3. Emeson, E. E. and Thrush, D. R. (1974): J. Immunol 113:1575-1582.

4. Field, E. J. and Shenton, B. K. (1975): Lancet i:49.

5. Goetzl, E. J., Kleickstein, L. B., Watt, K.W.K. and Wintroub, B. U. (1980): Biochem. Biophys. Res. Comm. 97:1097-1102.

6. Goldstein, A. L., Low, T. L. K., McAdoo, M., McClure, J., Thurman, G. B., Rossio, J. L., Lai, C.-Y., Chang, D., Wang, S. S., Harvey, C., Ramel, A. H., Meienhofer, J. and Burns, J. J. (1977): Proc. Natl. Acad. Sci. 74:725-729.

7. Goldstein, A. L., Stater, F. D. and White, A. (1966): <u>Proc. Natl. Acad. Sci.</u> 56:1010-1017.

8. Goldstein, G., Scheid, M. P., Boyse, E. A., Schlesinger, D. H. and Van Wauwe, J. (1979) <u>Science</u> 204:1309-1310.

9. Harrington, J. T. and Slastny, P. (1973): <u>J. Immunol</u> 110:752-759.

10. Hooper, J. A., McDaniel, M. C., Thurman, G. B., Cohen, G. H., Schulof, R. S. and Goldstein, A. L. (1975): <u>Annals N. Y. Acad. Sci.</u> 249:125-144.

11. Houck, J. C. and Chang, C. M. (1975-1976) <u>Inflammation</u> 1:189-200.

12. Houck, J. C., Chang, C. M. and Platt, M. (1973) <u>Proc. Soc. Exp. Biol. Med.</u> (1973) 143:858-861.

13. Klinkert, W. and Sorg C. (1980) <u>Molec. Immunol.</u> 17:555-564.

14. Kersten, M. C. M., Pels, E., De Weger, R. A. and Den Otter, W. (1980): <u>J. Immunol. Methods</u> 33:387-390.

15. Low, T. L. K., Hu, S. K. and Goldstein, A. L. (1981): <u>Proc. Natl. Acad. Sci.</u> 78:1162-1166.

16. Low, T. L. K., Thurman, G. B., McAdoo, M., McClure, J., Rossio, J. L., Naylor, P. H. and Goldstein, A. L. (1979): <u>J. Biol. Chem.</u> 254:981-986.

17. Miller, J. F. A. P. (1961): <u>Lancet</u> ii:748-749.

18. Newman, W., Diamond, B., Flomenberg, P., Scharff, M. D. and Bloom, B. R. (1979): <u>J. Immunol</u> 123:2292-2297.

19. Rowley, D. A., Gowans, J. L., Atkins, R. C., Ford, W. L. and Smith, M. E. (1972): <u>J. Exp. Med.</u> 136:499-513.

20. Schlesinger, D. H. and Goldstein, G. (1975): <u>Cell</u> 5:361-365.

21. Sprent, J., Miller, J. F. A. P. and Mitchell, G. F. (1971): <u>Cell. Immunol.</u> 2:171-181.

22. Stanzl, T. E., Porter, K. A., Andres, G. Groth, C. G., Putnam, C. W., Penn, I., Halgrimson, C. G., Starkie, S. J. and Brettischneider, L. (1970): <u>Clin. Exp. Immunol.</u> 6:803-814.

23. Stuttman, O. (1975): In: <u>Biological Activity of Thymic Hormones</u>, edited by D. W. Van Bekkum, pp. 87-94. Kooyker Scientific Publications, Rotterdam.

24. Thurman, G. B., Marshall, G. D., Low, T. L. K. and Goldstein, A. L. (1979): In: <u>Cell Biology and Immunology of Leukocyte Function</u> edited by M. R. Quastel, pp. 189-199. Academic Press, New York.

25. Thurman, G. B., Rossio, J. L. and Goldstein, A. L. (1977): In: <u>Regulatory Mechanisms in Lymphocyte Activation</u>, edited by D. O. Lucas, pp. 629-631. Academic Press, New York.

26. White, A. (1975): In: Biological Activity of Thymic Hormones, edited by D. W. Van Bekkum, pp. 17-23. Kooyker Scientific Publications, Rotterdam.

27. Wetzel, R., Heyneker, H. L., Goeddel, D. V., Jhurani, P., Shapiro, P., Crea, R., Low, T. L. K., McClure, J. E., Thurman, G. B. and Goldstein, A. L. (1980): Biochem. 19:6096-6104.

Lymphokines and Thymic Hormones: Their
Potential Utilization in Cancer Therapeutics,
edited by A. L. Goldstein and M. A. Chirigos,
Raven Press, New York © 1981.

Lymphokine-Induced Macrophage Proliferation and Activation

J. W. Hadden, A. Englard, J. R. Sadlik, and E. Hadden

*Laboratory of Immunopharmacology, Sloan-Kettering Institute for Cancer Research,
New York, New York 10021*

INTRODUCTION

In the last fifteen years, the role of the macrophage in host resistance particularly to facultative intracellular pathogens and to tumor progression has seen expanded interest and a refocusing. The understanding of the process of macrophage activation and proliferation in vivo has been significantly advanced by the following observations. In in vivo infections with facultative intracellular pathogens, the reticuloendothelial system (RES) undergoes an expansion and activation process which results in enhanced clearance of not only the original pathogen but unrelated pathogens as well (1,35,36,37). The cell responsible for the expression of activation is the macrophage, particularly the mobile population of monocyte-derived macrophages, more than the fixed members of the RES (46,57). The cell responsible for inducing the state of macrophage activation is the thymus-derived lymphocyte (14, 38,39). The process of macrophage activation under these circumstances involves macrophage proliferation, lysosomal enzyme accumulation, increased phagocytosis, secretion, and metabolic activities, and enhanced ability to eradicate pathogens which are otherwise relatively resistant to intracellular killing and degradation by macrophages (2,6,9,12,27). In addition, activated macrophages derived from animals immunized by a variety of means have shown increased activity in killing tumor cells in vitro when compared to macrophages from controls (10,24,25). Increasingly, correlations of macrophage activation and tumor regression have been made (28). We interpret the foregoing to indicate that lymphocyte-mediated macrophage activation occurs and is important in resistance to infection and tumor cell proliferation and that the essential ingredients of macrophage activation involve replication, differentiation, and enhanced microbicidal and tumoricidal activity.

The cellular and molecular basis underlying these processes are in need of elucidation. A large body of evidence indicates that macrophage proliferation and activation induced by T lymphocytes are mediated by soluble substances termed lymphokines (see 5, 8 for review). To date, more than 60 lymphokines have been described (59), and there are many descriptions of *in vitro* biological activies often with little

regard to in vivo relevance and to rigorous purification and characterization relevant to other factors acting on the same target cell.
  A number of factors produced by sensitized thymus-dependent lymphocytes have been shown to act on macrophages. These include:
1)   a macrophage growth factor (MGF$_L$) previously termed macrophage mito-
     genic factor (MMF) which induced mature non-sensitized macrophages
     to replicate (16);
2)   a migration inhibitory factor (MIF) which inhibits macrophage
     migration (3,7);
3)   a macrophage aggregating factor (MAggF) which agglutinates macro-
     phages (34);
4)   a macrophage activating factor(s) which stimulates protein synthe-
     sis and hexose monophosphate shunt activity in macrophages (45) and
     which increases listericidal and tumor cell killing activity of
     macrophages (49);
5)   a macrophage chemotactic factor (MCF) which induced macrophage
     chemotaxis (60);
6)   colony stimulating factors (CSF) which regulate the proliferation
     and differentiation of granulocytes and macrophages from a precur-
     sor colony-forming cell (CFU-c) (41,44,48);
7)   "immune" interferon (γ-IFN) which inhibits viral replication and
     may activate macrophages to kill tumor cells (52,53);
8)   a macrophage fusion factor (MFF) which induces giant cell formation
     (13).
  The present report will focus on the characterization of the macrophage growth factor produced by antigen-stimulated lymphocytes and its
comparison to other lymphokines acting on the macrophage. This factor
is induced by sensitized lymph node lymphocytes from guinea pigs using
standard protocols for producing other lymphokines including MIF. This
lymphokine has been shown to induce mature macrophages to divide (16)
and it was proposed that it is probably responsible for the in vivo
macrophage proliferation shown to occur prior to activation (35,11,29,
46,47).
  It has been independently shown that mature macrohpages can be
induced to proliferate upon stimulation with fibroblast and macrophage
cytokines also termed macrophage growth factors (MGF$_c$) (55). These
MGF's also have been shown to have colony stimulating factor (CSF)
activity, for production of colonies of the macrophage-monocyte lineage.
MGF of fibroblast origin has been purified to homogeneity by Stanley
(56) and the CSF activity has not been dissociated from the MGF activity
indicating that CSF and MGF activities are two actions of the same
molecule.
  Using a modification of the conventional soft agar techniques, by
the addition of indomethacin,we have recently shown that the lymphocyte
produced MGF also contains CSF activity for macrophage but not granulo-
cyte colonies (Sadlik and Hadden, unpublished observation). Similarly,
we found that guinea pig embryo CSF is as active as our MGF as an
inducer of macrophage proliferation in the thymidine incorporation
assay and their dose response profiles are identical. We therefore
have concluded that this lymphokine is a MGF produced as part of the
cellular immune response to antigenic stimulation and we will, therefore, refer to it as MGF$_L$ (not MMF) for the remainder of this report.

MGF$_L$ GENERATION AND ASSAY AND CHARACTERIZATION

Hartley strain guinea pigs (200 to 400 g) are immunized with bovine gamma globulin (BGG) in Freund's complete adjuvant. Regional lymph nodes are harvested 14 to 17 days later and the cells are collected and cultured at a concentration of 1.5 x 10^7/ml in Eagle's minimal essential media with 100 units/ml penicillin and 100 μg/ml streptomycin (referred to hereafter as media) without serum, with or without BGG (1 mg/ml). After incubation at 37°C in a 5% CO_2 and air atmosphere for 24 hr, the cell-free supernatants are collected and antigen is added to the control supernatant. In the subsequent experiments, supernatants preincubated with antigen (P) are compared to those reconstituted with antigen after culture (R). The macrophage migration inhibition assay is performed as described (16).

In the MGF assay Microtest II tissue culture plates (3040, Falcon Division, Beckton, Dickinson & Co., Oxnard, Calif.) are used for assay of tritiated thymidine uptake into monolayers. One-tenth milliliter of a suspension of macrophages (2 x 10^6/ml) in HBSS is added to wells of a microtest plate. Attachment is allowed for only 15 min at 37°C in a CO_2 incubator. Attachment for such a short time circumvents the contamination with fibroblasts that can be seen if longer times are used for attachment. Wells are washed three times with HBSS and 0.2 ml media containing 20% FCS (Microbiological Associates, Bethesda, Md) is added to each well. The culture plates are incubated at 37°C in a humidified atmosphere of 3% CO_2 in air.

Thymidine incorporation at various times is determined by a terminal 24 hr pulse of ^{3}H-thymidine (2.50 μCi/ml, S.A. 20 Ci/mmole, New England Nuclear, Boston, MA). At termination of culture the plate is frozen at -70°C and thawed and refrozen twice before processing with a multiple automatic sample harvester (Otto Hiller Co., Madison, Wis.) and liquid scintillation spectrometry.

The supernatant fluids are assayed for MGF and MIF activity in serial dilution to determine their starting potency. The fluids are then vacuum dialyzed for 24 hrs at 4°C with collodion bags with a 25,000 dalton exclusion limit. The retentates are chromatographed on G-100 superfine Sephadex and eluted with phosphate buffer. MGF activity elutes with molecules of mw between 40,000 and 70,000 daltons as determined by standard markers (Fig. 1). This elution pattern parallels that described for MIF. If supernatant fluids are dialyzed in this manner, the residual MIF activity after Sephadex chromatography is <10% of starting activity and is generally only observed if fractions are concentrated relative to starting fluids. During these steps, MGF$_L$ activity generally increases indicating a relative dissociation between MIF and MGF$_L$ activity. Sephadex chromatography yields an 80 X increase in specific activity per milligram protein. The active non-concentrated fractions eluted from Sephadex G-100 can be utilized at a 1:100 dilution and show significant activity: i.e., >10-fold increase in thymidine incorporation. Most subsequent experiments to be described were performed with Sephadex fractionated MGF-rich preparations with minimal MIF activity.

Work to date has indicated that MGF is stable over a wide pH range (pH2-8). Its activity is recoverable after heating at 56°C for 30 min. It can be frozen and thawed repeatedly. It is also stable at high salt concentrations and precipitates between 40-80% ammonium sulphate

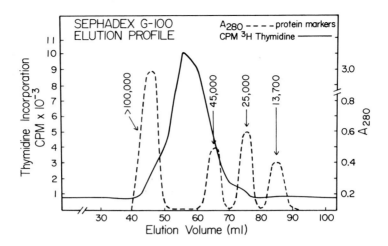

FIG. 1. Sephadex elution profile of MGF$_L$ activity.
Crude supernatant was vacuum dialyzed and applied
to a Sephadex G-100 superfine column as described.
Protein markers BGG (>100,000 m.w.), ovalbumin
(45,000), chymotrypsinogen (25,000), and ribonuclease (13,700) were run in parallel for the purposes of m.w. estimation.

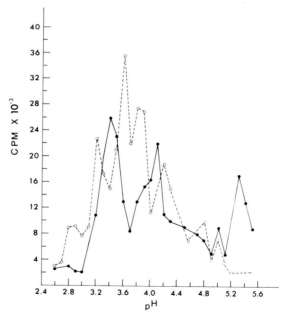

FIG. 2. Isoelectric focusing profile of
guinea pig MGF$_L$ activity (solid line) and
guinea pig fibroblast MGF$_C$ activity
(dotted line).

(pH 7.4), thus removing the bulk of the protein with a 50% loss of MGF activity. This step constitutes a 20x purification. Preparative flat bed isoelectric focusing was used to characterize MGF_L as to its iso-electric point as well as to effect a separation from other biologi-cally active factors.

Figure 2 depicts the isoelectric focusing profile of MGF_L and guinea pig embryo fibroblast MGF showing several peaks of activity between pH 3.0-5.0. Protein content of the active fractions of MGF prepared under these and similar circumstances is less than 5 µg/ml indicating up to a 200-fold purification with respect to original supernatant fluids. These isoelectric profiles are comparable to those obtained utilizing mouse L-cell MGF (56). Mouse L-cell MGF and MGF_L also exhibit similar elution profiles when chromatographed on Sephadex G-100. Guinea pig embryo fibroblast MGF and MGF_L both elute similarly from Sephadex G-100, exhibit less than 10% adsorbtion to AFFI-GEL 202, precipitate out of solution between 40% and 80% saturated ammonium sulfate, and exhibit 10% adsorbtion to columns of Con A Sepharose. Table 1 summarizes the similarities between the lymphocyte produced MGF_L and fibroblast MGF. It is on the basis of such comparisons that we have tentatively concluded that the lymphokine MGF_L and MGF's from several sources are comparable substances chemically and biologically. Complete purification will be essential to confirm this assumption.

TABLE 1.

	MGF_L	Fibroblast MGF_c*
Sephadex M.W.	35,000-70,000	35,000-70,000
pI	3.0-5.0	3.0-4.9
Affi gel 202	<10% adsorption	<10% adsorption
Con A Sepharose	10% adsorption	80% adsorption
Stability		
dialysis	+	+
salt	1M	ND
pH	pH 2	pH 2
temperature	-70°C to 56°C	-70°C to 56°C
Ammonium sulfate		
precipitation	40%-80%	50%-80%
MAF bacteriacidal	+	+
CSF macrophage	+	+
IFN	negative	negative

*From the work of E.R. Stanley, et al. (39) and J.R. Sadlik and J.W. Hadden.

ANALYSIS OF THE ACTION OF THE MITOGENIC FACTOR

Analysis of action of the mitogenic factor on macrophage prolifera-tion in terms of DNA synthesis and cell replication has been carried out (18). The studies presented indicate that MGF_L induces prolifera-tion of both non-immune oil-induced monocyte-derived peritoneal and non-induced alveolar macrophages. Cell counts and nuclear labeling experiments indicate that this proliferation can be effectively assayed under conditions of monolayer culture by tritiated thymidine

incorporation (see Figure 3). High coefficients of correlation
(r's > .90, p's < .01) were obtained between each of these three
separate measures of proliferation. The magnitude and the kinetics of
the proliferative response of macrophages in this system are dependent
upon the concentration and the time of addition of the soluble mediator.
Influences that operate to limit proliferation in this system appear
to be high macrophage density, the production of prostaglandin by
macrophages, and other mediators present in the lymphokine preparation,
such as MIF. A high degree of correlation existed (r = .80, p <.01)
between residual presence of MIF and depressed expression of MGF$_L$. We
found that if MGF$_L$ is added to macrophages after 24 hours of culture,
a time when MIF responsiveness is markedly reduced, or is added to
exudates which have been prepared after 5 rather than 3 days, also a
time of reduced MIF responsiveness (33), MGF$_L$ activity was greater. In
addition, alveolar macrophages which have been shown to lack MIF
receptors (32) are responsive to MGF$_L$, indicating further that the
actions of MIF and MGF appear to be not only unrelated but antagonistic.

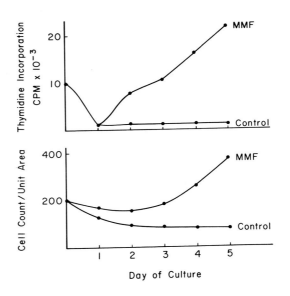

FIG. 3. Upper panel: Kinetics of MGF$_L$
(MMF) induced ^{3}H-thymidine incorporation
in macrophage monolayers incubated for
1 to 5 days in culture. A composite of
10 experiments is depicted.
Lower panel: Cell counts during 5 days
of culture under conditions comparable
to those depicted in the upper panel,
cell number per unit area was determined
in MGF$_L$ (MMF) and control cultures.

PROSTAGLANDIN IN MGF ACTION

We have observed that macrophages produce prostaglandin E_2 (PGE) and thromboxane B_2 during culture (Sadlik, et al., unpublished). Exogenously added PGE inhibits MGF_L-induced proliferation. The addition of indomethacin (10^{-5}M) into the media to inhibit PGE synthesis markedly potentiates MGF_L action but does not increase proliferation of the control monolayers. Indomethacin enhances the MGF_L-induced proliferation at high concentrations of MGF_L and particularly at early times (i.e. before 18 hours of culture) suggesting that effects of indomethacin may be on MIF-related anti-proliferative events (Fig. 4).

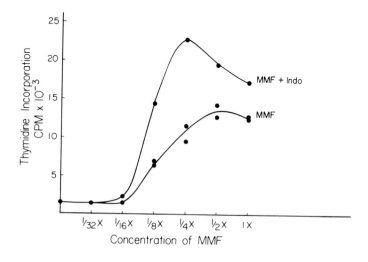

FIG. 4. Dose response profile of MGF_L (MMF) action at 3 days of culture. Effects of inhibition of prostaglandin synthesis by 10^{-5}M indomethacin (Indo) are depicted.

CELLULAR TARGETS OF MGF ACTION

Macrophage population: Both MGF_L and embryo MGF_C induce alveolar macrophage as well as oil-induced peritoneal cells to proliferate in the MGF assay. The response of alveolar macrophages is generally of greater magnitude than that of the oil-induced peritoneal cells and less sensitive to the potentiating effect of indomethacin. This observation indicates that fixed, as well as mobile members of the RES, are targets of MGF_L action and suggests that Kupfer cells, splenic and lymph node reticular cells may show responsiveness. The difference in the response between alveolar and peritoneal cells and the lack of more than 60% labeling of peritoneal cells (even in the presence of indomethacin) suggests that subpopulations of peritoneal macrophages might be responding differently. By separating 3-day exudates on discontinuous albumin gradients as described by Rice and Fishman (51), we

found that the less dense cells (Fractions A-D, comprising 20% of the
total exudate) showed a marked proliferative response to MGF$_L$ with
little potentiation with indomethacin and in contrast, that the more
dense cells (Fraction E, comprising 80% of the total),showed less proliferative response to MGF$_L$ unless indomethacin was present. When a
6-day exudate was employed, which Leu has shown is unresponsive to MIF
(33), 70% of the cells were found in Fraction A-D and showed a marked
response to MGF$_L$. The remaining 30% in Fraction E now showed a pronounced response to MGF$_L$ without indomethacin. These results indicate
that as exudate macrophages mature, they produce less PG's and become
less MIF responsive and less dense and more MGF responsive. Furthermore,
guinea pig blood monocytes are unresponsive to MGF$_L$ as are human blood
monocytes to MGF$_L$ prepared from Con A-stimulated human peripheral blood
lymphocytes (Duncan and Hadden, submitted for publication).

MACROPHAGE ACTIVATION TO KILL LISTERIA MONOCYTOGENES

Employing crude supernatant fluids and Sephadex G-100 (17,20) and
isoelectric focusing fractions containing MGF$_L$ and depleted of MIF, we
examined the effect of MGF on the activation of mineral oil-induced
non-immune guinea pig peritoneal macrophages. In the assay for activation, monolayers of macrophages are exposed to MGF for varying periods
of time in LABTEK chambers, as described for the MGF assay. The monolayers are then subjected to a short exposure to virulent Listeria
monocytogenes organisms at a low ratio of bacteria to macrophage.
Afterwards the monolayers are washed and the number of phagocytized
bacteria is confirmed visually by gram staining. At the onset of incubation, following the pulsed exposure to the bacteria, approximately
30-40% of the macrophages have ingested an average of two organisms;
over the ensuing 6 hrs. of incubation, the ingested bacteria will replicate in the normal macrophage with a doubling time of $\cong$ 2 hrs. When
macrophages have been pre-treated with MGF$_L$-preparation for 4-6 days,
they inhibit this replication of Listeria and proceed to digest them as
judged by disintegration of the bacteria visualized by gram staining
and confirmed by plating and culture of surviving intracellular Listeria.
Based upon a number of criteria including molecular weight estimation,
isoelectric point, stability, etc. we have so far been unable to distinguish MGF$_L$ from this activating factor. We therefore tenatively
ascribe MAF microbicidal activity to MGF$_L$.

Indomethacin does not potentiate MGF$_L$-induced listericidal activity
indicating that constitutive PG production does not play a role in
determining, nor modulating the process. Endotoxin (LPS .05-.5 µg/ml)
is also very effective at activating macrophages in this system whether
added at time 0 or day 5.

MACROPHAGE ACTIVATION TO KILL TUMOR CELLS

Churchill et al. (4) have shown that crude MIF-rich supernatant
fluids and corresponding Sephadex fractions would induce guinea pig
adherent peritoneal macrophages to kill guinea pig hepatoma cells after
72 h of co-incubation. These workers concluded that MAF for tumoricidal
activity was the same as MIF (based on the Sephadex elution profile),
although they noted little correlation between the two activities. In
our studies with the guinea pig (23), we have observed little or no kill
with undialyzed crude lymphokine supernatant fluids or MGF$_L$-rich, MIF-
depleted Sephadex fractions using three different assays (4,40,53),

using as targets line 1 Hepatoma, 3T6, L1210, and MBL-2 cells, and using macrophage at target ratios of 10-50:1. Based on the observations of Hibbs et al. (26), we performed the experiments in the presence and absence of nanogram quantities of endotoxin and still did not see significant or consistent killing during 1-6 days of culture. Our own results and those of Churchill et al. (4) show tumor cell killing by guinea pig macrophages to be inferior to that described in the mouse, perhaps indicating possible deficiencies in the guinea pig assay.

Schultz et al. (53) have reported that in the mouse system interferon induces adherent macrophages to kill tumor cells over 72 h of culture. Unlike the guinea pig system, in which a maximum of 10-20% growth inhibition is observed over 72 h, the mouse system shows tumor cell growth inhibition by interferon stimulated macrophages by 24 h and at 72 h up to 100% kill. We have been able to consistently reproduce these results using the mouse system (Warfel and Hadden, unpublished). These results are in marked contrast to the guinea pig system. A number of interferon inducers will reproduce this effect, as will lymphokine-rich supernatant fluids (which may contain interferon or induce it) (52). Both Meltzer and coworkers (31,43) and Fischer and coworkers (42,30) have characterized a lymphokine that induced killing of tumor cells by adherent mouse peritoneal macrophages. The characteristics of the lymphokine involved do not rule out the possibility that it is indistinguishable from interferon (W.E. Stewart II, personal communication).

From the results of available studies, it appears that lymphocyte-produced interferon is the most likely candidate for a macrophage-activating factor responsible for tumor cell kill. The distinct possibility remains that as an activator it does not preclude other lymphokines other than IFN as MAF's for tumoricidal activity.

OTHER PARAMETERS OF MACROPHAGE ACTIVATION INDUCED BY MGF

Morphological Changes Induced by MGF: Scanning electron microscope studies in MGF-treated and control macrophages after 4 days of culture revealed marked differences in surface morphologies between activated and control macrophages. MGF-treated macrophages were much larger overall than control cells. Activated macrophages exhibited marked spreading on the plastic cover slips, while control cells remained spherical in shape, although attached. MGF-treated macrophages presented a very complex and non-uniform surface morphology including micro blebs, membranous veil-like structures, pseudopodia, and extensive surface convolutions not apparent in the control (Fig. 5).

RELATIONSHIP OF MGF$_L$ TO OTHER LYMPHOKINES ACTING ON THE MACROPHAGE

We have discussed the relationship of MGF$_L$ to other lymphokines or cytokines having action to promote proliferation of macrophages or their precursors. With respect to MIF, in addition to dissociation of biological activity, recent advances in purification of guinea pig MIF (see Sorg this volume) would indicate MIF has multiple molecular weight forms of 15,000, 30,000, 45,000 and 60,000, all of which have their pI at 5.2 and thus differ from MGF$_L$ by these criteria. MCF having a molecular weight of 12,000 (58) and MAggF with a molecular weight >150,000 (15) thus also differ from MGF$_L$. MFF, only occasionally observed in our supernatant fluids and not in Sephadex fractions is also distinct from MGF$_L$ (21,62). We have not observed IFN in either our crude supernatant fluids or Sephadex fractions. While MGF_L can be considered distinct from other lymphokines it is important to remember that lymphokines probably act collectively and in an interacting manner to modify macrophage proliferation and differentiation in vivo.

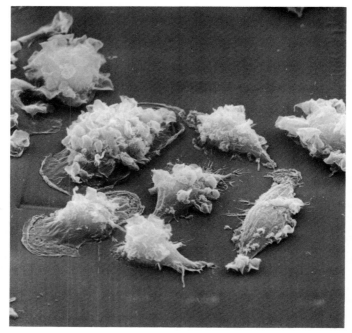

FIG. 5. Scanning electron micrograph of MGF_L activated macrophages.

ACTION OF IMMUNOPOTENTIATING AND ACTIVATING AGENTS ON MACROPHAGES

We have examined a variety of agents in macrophage proliferation, both alone and in the presence of MGF (20,22,54). Agents, like PHA, Con A, and phorbol myristate acetate, have been shown by us to induce directly, macrophage proliferation in the MGF system. Agents like iso-prinosine, levamisole, NPT 15392, azimexone, muramyl dipeptide, and SM1213, were not directly mitogenic. Isoprinosine, NPT 15392, azi-mexone, and to a slight extent levamisole, potentiated the effect of MGF on macrophage proliferation. In no case did indomethacin obviate the effect indicating that none of the agents potentiated the action of MGF by acting as an inhibitor of PG production. MDP, but not a similar compound, SM1213, inhibited MGF-induced proliferation. This effect was partially reversed by indomethacin indicating PG mediation.

Many of these same agents have been examined on macrophage activation to kill Listeria monocytogenes. In addition to MGF_L, endotoxin, MDP, and SM1213, all activated the macrophage to kill Listeria when added to the macrophages 5 days before or at the time of the listericidal assay. Levamisole and isoprinosine had a small effect added at the time of the assay, but none if added 5 days earlier. When added 5 days earlier, in the presence of a suboptimal and an otherwise inactive preparation of MGF$_L$, levamisole and isoprinosine induced full activation characteristic of optimal MGF$_L$. These studies serve to contrast the two classes of agents: One group characterized by MDP and SM1213 directly activates the macrophage without promoting proliferation, while the other characterized by levamisole and isoprinosine has no direct activating or mitogenic effect, yet potentiates the action of MGF on both responses.

ANALYSIS OF MECHANISM OF ACTION

As with mitogens in the lymphocyte, we have observed that MGF$_L$ induces early 3-fold increases of cyclic GMP levels in guinea pig oil-induced macrophages (19). The levels peak at 5-10 minutes and decline to near control levels by 15 minutes. No changes in cyclic AMP levels were observed during the time period. Deletion of calcium in the media reduced the increases indicating their calcium dependence. Under these circumstances, Pick (50) has observed lymphokine (?MGF$_L$) induced calcium influx in peritoneal macrophages. These results directly compare with mitogen action in the lymphocyte (see 17 for review) and suggest a similar mechanism.

We have analyzed a number of agents on macrophage cyclic nucleotide levels. Both muramyl dipeptide and SM1213, which induce macrophage activation but not proliferation, increase cyclic GMP levels. The calcium dependence of this action has not been examined; however, parallel experiments in the lymphocyte would predict that, like cholinergic influences, these changes will not involve calcium influx. In so far as we have probed the macrophage, it appears that mitogenic, chemotactic, and bactericidal activating agents have in common early increases in cyclic GMP. The role of calcium and other membrane-related events remain to be determined in order to sort out the differences between their intracellular signals.

CONCLUSION

In the present report we describe an antigen-induced lymphokine (MGF$_L$) acting to induce colony formation from macrophage precursors, macrophage replication and macrophage activation to kill <u>Listeria monocytogenes</u>. Its partial characterization would indicate that it is related to a family of cytokines having macrophage growth factor and colony stimulating factor activities and that it is distinct from other lymphokines acting on the macrophage including migration inhibition, fusion, aggregating and chemotactic factors and interferon. As a "biological response modifier" promoting macrophage replication and differentiation, MGF$_L$ is a logical candidate to be used immunotherapeutically to enhance the expression of delayed hypersensitivity reactions to cancer and/or pathogens. In the therapy of cancer, it might be employed alone to increase macrophage numbers or in conjunction with other lymphokines and/or immunostimulating agents to promote macrophage activation for tumoricidal activity.

REFERENCES

1. Blanden, R.V., Mackaness, G.B., Collins, M.B., and Collins, F.M. (1966): J. Exp. Med., 124:585-600.
2. Blanden, R.V., Mackaness, G.B., and Collins, F.M. (1966): J. Exp. Med., 124:601-619.
3. Bloom, B.R. and Bennett, B. (1966): Science, 153:80-82.
4. Churchill, W.H., Piessens, C.A. Sulis, and David, J.D. (1975): J. Immunol., 115:781-786.
5. Cohen, S., Pick, E. and Oppenheim, J.J., editors (1979): Biology of the Lymphokines, Academic Press, New York.
6. Coppel, S., and Youmans, G.P. (1969): J. Bacteriol., 97:114-120.
7. David, J.R. (1966): Proc. Natl. Acad. Sci., USA, 56:72-77.
8. DeWeck, A., Kristensen, F., and Landy, M., editors (1980): Biochemical Characterization of the Lymphokines, Academic Press, New York.
9. Dubos, R.J., and Schaedler, R.W. (1957): J. Exp. Med., 106:703-717.
10. Evans, R. and Alexander, P. (1972): Nature, 236:168-170.
11. Forbes, I.J. and Mackaness, G.B. (1963): Lancet, 2:1203-1204.
12. Forbes, I.J. (1965): J. Immunol., 94:37-39.
13. Galindo, B. and Myrivik, Q.N. (1970): J. Immunol., 105:277-287.
14. Girard, G. and Grumbach, F. (1958): C.R. Soc. Biol., 152:280-282.
15. Godfrey, H.P., and Geczy, C.L. (1978): J. Immunol., 121:1428-1431.
16. Hadden, J.W., Sadlik, J.R., and Hadden, E.M. (1975): Nature, 257:483-485.
17. Hadden, J.W. and Englard, A (1977): In: Immunopharmacology, edited by J.W. Hadden, R.G. Coffey, and F. Spreafico, pp. 87-98. Plenum Press, New York, N.Y.
18. Hadden, J.W., Sadlik, J.R., Hadden, E.M. (1978): J. Immunol., 121:231-238.
19. Hadden, J.W., and Englard, A. (1978): In: The Pharmacology of Immunoregulation, edited by G.H. Werner and F. Floc'h, pp. 273-282. Academic Press, London, U.K.
20. Hadden, J.W., Englard, A. Sadlik, J.R., and Hadden, E.M. (1979): Int. J. Immunopharmacol., 1:17-27.
21. Hadden, J.W., Sadlik, J.R., Englard, A., Warfel, A.H. and Hadden, E.M. (1980): In: Biochemical Characterization of Lymphokines, edited by A. L. deWeck, F. Kristensen, and M. Landy, pp. 235-242. Academic Press, New York, N.Y.
22. Hadden, J.W., and Coffey, R.G. (1980): In: Recent Results in Cancer Research, Vol. 75, edited by G. Mathe and F. M. Muggia. Springer Verlag, New York, N.Y.
23. Hadden, J.W., Sadlik, J.W., and Warfel, A.H. (1981): In: Biochemistry of the Lymphokines, edited by J.W. Hadden and W.E. Stewart, II, pp. 39-52. Humana Press, Clifton, N.J.
24. Hibbs, J.B. (1973): Science,180:868-870.
25. Hibbs, J.B. (1974): J. Natl. Cancer Inst.,53:1487-1492.
26. Hibbs, J.B., Taintor, R., Chapman, H, and Weinberg, J. (1977): Science, 197:282-284.
27. Howard, J.G., Biozzi, G., Halpern, B.N., Stiffel, C., and Mouton, D. (1959): Br. J. Exp. Pathol., 40:281-286.
28. James, K., McBride, W., and Stuart, A. (1977): The Macrophage in Cancer. Econoprint, Edinburgh.
29. Khoo, K.K. and Mackaness, G.B. (1964): Aust. J. Exp. Biol. Med. Sci., 42:607-716.

30. Kniep, E.M., Kickhofen, B., and Fisher, H. (1980): In: Biochemical Characterization of Lymphokines, edited by A.L. deWeck, F. Kristensen, and M. Landy, pp.149-154. Academic Press, New York, N.Y.

31. Leonard, E.J., Ruco, L.P., and Meltzer, M.S. (1978): Cell Immunol.,41:347-357.

32. Leu, R.W., Eddleston, A.L.W.F., Hadden, J.W., and Good, R.A. (1972): J. Exp. Med., 136:589-603.

33. Leu, R.W., Woodson, P.D., and Whitely, S.B. (1977): J. Reticulo-endothelial Soc., 22:329-339.

34. Lolekha, S., Dray, S., and Gotoff, S.P. (1970): J. Immunol., 104:296-304.

35. Mackaness, G.B. (1962): J. Exp. Med., 116:381-406.

36. Mackaness, G.B. (1964): J. Exp. Med., 120:105-120.

37. Mackaness, G.B. and Blanden, R.C. (1967): Prog. Allergy, 11:89-140.

38. Mackaness, G.B. (1969): J. Exp. Med., 129:973-992.

39. Mackaness, G.B. and Hill, W.L. (1969): J. Exp. Med.,129:993-1012.

40. McDaniel, M.D., Laludico, R., and Papermaster, B. (1976): Clin. Immunol. Immunopath., 5:91-104.

41. McNeill, T.A. (1973): Nature New Biol., 244:175-177.

42. Meerpohl, H.G., Lohmann-Matthew, M.L., and Fischer, H. (1976): Eur. J. Immunol., 6:213-218.

43. Meltzer, M.S., Wahl, L.M., Leonard, E.J., and Nacy, C.A. (1980): In: Biochemical Characterization of Lymphokines, edited by A. L. deWeck, F. Kristensen, and M. Landy, pp. 161-168. Academic Press, New York, N.Y.

44. Metcalf, D., and Moore, M.A.S. (1971): Haematopoietic Cells., North Holland Publishing Co., Amsterdam.

45. Nathan, C.F., Karnovsky, M.L., and David, J.R. (1971): J. Exp. Med., 133:1356-1376.

46. North, R.J. (1969): J. Exp. Med., 130:315-326.

47. North, R.J. (1970): J. Exp. Med., 132:521-545.

48. Parker, J.W. and Metcalf, D. J. (1974): J. Immunol., 112:502-510.

49. Piessens, W.F., Churchill, W.H., and David, J.R. (1975): J. Immunol., 114:293-299.

50. Pick, E., Seger, M., Honig, S., and Griffel, B. (1979): Annals New York Acad. Sci., 332:378-394.

51. Rice, S.G., and Fishman, M. (1974): Cell Immunol., 11:130-145.

52. Schultz, R.M., Papamatheakis, J.D., and Chirigos, M.A. (1977): Science, 197:674-676.

53. Schultz, R.M. and Chirigos, M.A. (1978): Cancer Res., 38:1003-1007.

54. Simon, L.N., Giner-Sorolla, A., and Hadden, J.W. (1980): Fourth International Congress of Immunology Abstracts, 17-7, Paris, France.

55. Stanley, E.R., Cifone, M., Heard, P.M. and Defendi, J. (1976): J. Exp. Med., 143:631-647.

56. Stanley, E.R., and Heard, P.M. (1977): J. Biol. Chem., 252:4305-4312.

57. Truit, G.L. and Mackaness, G.B. (1971): Am. Rev. of Resp. Dis., 104:829-843.

58. Wahl, S.M., Altman, L.C., Oppenheim, J.J., and Mergenhagen, S.E. (1974): Int. Arch. Allerg. Appl. Immunol., 46:768-784.

59. Wacksman, B.H., and Yuziro, N. (1976): J. Cell. Immunol., 21:161-176.

60. Ward, P.A., Remold, H.G., and David, J.R. (1970): Cell Immunol., 1:162-174.

61. Warfel, A.H., and Hadden, J.W. (1978): Am. J. Pathol., 93:753-770.
62. Warfel, A.H., and Hadden, J.W. (1980): Exp. Mol. Path., 33:153-168.

Lymphokines and Thymic Hormones: Their Potential Utilization in Cancer Therapeutics, edited by A. L. Goldstein and M. A. Chirigos, Raven Press, New York © 1981.

Human Macrophage Activation Factors

Mildred C. McDaniel

Quillen-Dishner College of Medicine, East Tennessee State University, Johnson City, Tennessee 37614

INTRODUCTION

Lymphoid cells in response to stimuli release a variety of molecules (lymphokines) which mediate the immune response and inflammatory reaction. These factors are released into culture medium by antigen or mitogen stimulated lymphocytes or by lymphoid or fibroblast cell lines as a constitutive product(s). Macrophages incubated with lymphokines manifest a variety of morphologic and metabolic changes including increased adherence to glass and plastic, increased membrane ruffling, increased size and protein content, increased or decreased phagocytic activity, increased hexose monophosphate shunt activity and increased or decreased levels of various enzymes (5,6,7,2). There is no data as yet associating any of these parameters with the acquisition of tumoricidal ability. Activated macrophages in this research are defined by a functional assay in which macrophages kill syngeneic tumor cells. The lymphokine mediating this function is called macrophage activation factor or MAF.

METHODS

Cytotoxic Assay

The assay used has been described in detail elsewhere (3). Briefly, peritoneal exudate cells from C57B1/6 mice are induced with thioglycollate. The cells are harvested and plated in microtiter II trays (falcon) at 50,000 cells per well. The adherent cells are washed, and then incubated with MAF fractions for 48 hours. The MAF is then removed and ^{125}I-iododeoxyuridine (IUDr) labelled F10-B16 melanoma cells are added at 5000 cells per well. After incubation for 5 days the cells are washed with saline twice and lysed with 0.1 N NaOH. The residue $^{125}IUDr$ is determined with a gamma counter. The percent cytotoxicity is determined as follows:

$$\% \text{ cytotoxicity} = \left[1 - \frac{\text{cpm target cells with activated macrophages}}{\text{cpm target cells with normal macrophages}} \right] \times 100$$

RESULTS AND DISCUSSION

The source of MAF was the Namalwa cell line, a human Burkitt's lymphoma, which produces MAF as a constitutive product. It has always been a standard practice in lymphokine research to use as little serum as possible during the time period in which the lymphokines are produced to simplify purification. In this instance it was impossible to use serumless media because Namalwa would not survive without fetal calf serum (FCS) for a 24 hour period. MAF supernatants were prepared using 2% FCS - RPMI 1640 (the minimum FCS concentration for viable cells) and 10% FCS - RPMI 1640. The harvested supernatants were desalted on a Sephadex G25 column, and stored as a lyophilized powder at -70°C.

Previous work has shown that MAF copurifies with serum proteins, such as albumin and α-2 macroglobulin (4). A denaturing solvent to reduce adherence was used to chromatograph MAF supernatant. The supernatants were chromatographed on Sepharose 6B-Cl column in 6M guanidine-HCl pH 8.0. The samples were not reduced and alkylated. The guanidine column was standardized with proteins of various molecular weights. A comparison of the size of MAF activity obtained from Namalwa cells cultured in 10% FCS and in 2% FCS indicated a different molecular weight distribution produced in each instance. In 2% FCS the molecular weights of the active fraction were 70,000 ± 7,000, 25,000 ± 2,500, 12,500 ± 1,250 and less than 10,000. Namalwa cells incubated in 10% FCS produced activity at 12,000 daltons and below. As a control FCS at a concentration of 10% in RPMI 1640 was incubated for 24 hours and then chromatographed and tested for MAF activity. No activity was found in any guanidine fraction. To compare MAF from Namalwa cells with MAF from putatively "normal human lymphocytes", supernatant from human tonsil lymphocytes was assayed for MAF activity. The tonsil cells were put into culture without mitogen in serumless media for 48 hours. After chromatography the MAF activity was found at 12,000 daltons and the column void volume. This result is similar to the MAF activity found in Namalwa supernatant. All active fractions were tested for interferon and found not to contain interferon (8). In addition all active fractions were tested for endotoxin by the Limulus assay and found to contain less than 0.05 ng/ml which is considered insignificant (11).

With higher concentrations of serum protein, lower molecular weight molecules containing MAF activity are formed and/or stabilized. The initial product could be a small molecular weight molecule that associates or a large molecular weight product which is cleaved by enzymatic degradation. To test the size of the initial product the following experiment was designed: material from 10% FCS supernatant was purified on the guanidine column and the region of activity below 12,000 daltons was pooled, dialyzed and lyophilized. A portion of the material was then resuspended in 6M guanidine and incubated at 37°C for 24 hours. Another portion of the column fraction was dissolved in 10% FCS-media and incubated for 24 hours at 37°C. Both samples were then re-chromatographed on Sepharose 6B-Cl in guanidine-HCl and all column fractions were assayed for activity. In figure 1 the results of this assay is given. A is the region from which the original sample was taken from the column, and B shows the area of MAF activity from the sample incubated in 6M guanidine supernatant. MAF activity originally chromatographed as a low molecular weight component was eluted at the void volume suggesting the presence of activity of a much higher molecular

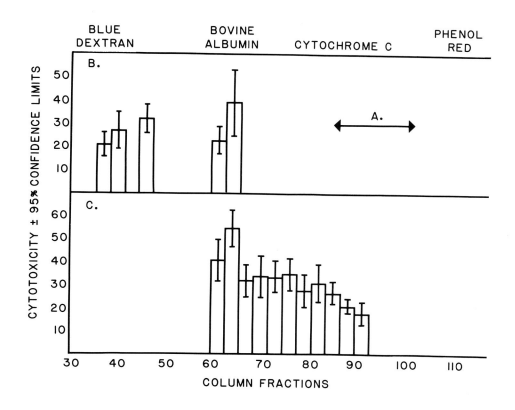

Figure 1. Re-chromatography of active low molecular weight
MAF fractions after incubation at 37°C for 24 hours. See
text for complete explanation. (reproduced from reference 3
by permission of Plenum Publishing Company.)

weight which can be estimated to be greater than 100,000 and at ca.
70,000 daltons at the albumin marker. However, incubation of the original material (A) in 10% FCS media for 24 hours causes it to elute at a
position corresponding to proteins of molecular weight 70,000 to 12,000
daltons (C).

An alternative explanation which might account for these different
molecular sizes of MAF might be found in the chromatography procedure
itself. Denaturation in 6M guanidine-HCl increases the Stokes radii of
molecules, allowing them to be separated by size on a molecular sieving
column. If MAF molecules do not completely denature in 6M guanidine at
room temperature due to the presence of serum protein or its own structure, but do denature at 37°C, this could account for the differences
between samples treated at room temperature and 37°C. However, in 2%
FCS Namalwa cells appear to produce only one component of MAF during
six hours of incubation with cells, as assayed from 6M guanidine column
fractions, not a range of molecular sizes as seen in 24 hour samples.
If this one component denatured stepwise, the same molecular species

should be seen from guanidine chromatography of supernatant harvested in six hour as well as after 24 hour incubation in 2% FCS.

The presence of multiple molecular weights for MAF is not a unique property of this lymphokine. It has been reported by Sorg that guinea pig lymphocytes produce MIF of multiple molecular weights (9). DiSabato found that murine thymocyte-stimulating factor (TSF) has multiple molecular forms (1). The smallest active TSF was 4,000 and 4,700 daltons and these appear to aggregate to give higher molecular forms. In another report in which lymphocyte activating factor, (LAF), was reconstituted with 2% human serum and rechromatographed, it appeared with active higher molecular weight components; thus, it was suggested that a complex of lower molecular weight LAF with serum components had been formed (10).

It appears that MAF may consist of multiple units which form from a low molecular weight unit by some as yet unknown mechanism of association. The actual size of the smallest active component of MAF, and the type of bonding between the smallest active component and the higher molecular weight species of MAF are now under examination in this laboratory.

REFERENCES

1. Altin, M. and DiSabato, G. (1980): Cell. Immun. 54:462-470.
2. Cohen, Z.A. (1978): In:Differentiation of Normal and Neoplastic Hematopoietic Cells, edited by B. Clarkson, P.A. Marks, and J.E. Tell, Vol. 5, pp. 383-392. Cold Spring Harbor Conferences on Cell Proliferation, Cold Spring Harbor Laboratory.
3. McDaniel, M.C. (1980): Inflammation, 4:125-135.
4. McDaniel, M.C., Laudico, R., and Papermaster, B.W. (1976): Clin. Immun. Immunopath. 5:91-104.
5. Morahan, P.S., Edelson, P.J., and Gasa, K. (1980): J. Immun. 125: 1312-1317.
6. Nathan, C.F., Karnovsky, M.L., and David, J.R. (1971): J. Exp.Med. 133:1356-1376.
7. Poulter, L.W. and Turk, J.L. (1975): Cell. Immunol. 20:12-24.
8. Schultz, R.M., Chirigas, M.A., and Heine, W.L. (1978): Cell Immunol. 35:84-91.
9. Sorg, C. and Klinkert, W. (1978): Fed. Proc. 37:2748-2753.
10. Togawa, A., Oppenheim, J.J., Mizel, S.B. (1979): J. Clin. Microbiol. 1:116-117.
11. Weinberg, J.B., Chapman, H.A., and Hibbs, J.B. (1978): J. Immunol. 121:72-80.

Lymphokines and Thymic Hormones: Their
Potential Utilization in Cancer Therapeutics,
edited by A. L. Goldstein and M. A. Chirigos,
Raven Press, New York © 1981.

Pharmacological Modulation of the Interaction Between Lymphokines and Macrophages — Effect of Antioxidants and Thromboxane Synthetase Inhibitors

Edgar Pick, Yona Keisari, Aniela Jakubowski, Yael Bromberg, and Maya Freund

Section of Immunology, Department of Human Microbiology, Sackler School of Medicine, Tel-Aviv University, Tel-Aviv 69978, Israel

INTRODUCTION

The molecular mechanisms by which lymphokines affect the target cells are largely unknown. Because of this, lymphokine action is still mostly expressed in terms of "biological activity" which, frequently, can be the expression of multiple biochemical processes. In the course of the last decade, we have centered our investigative effort on the elucidation of the cellular action mechanism of the lymphokine, macrophage migration inhibitory factor (MIF) and this work was reviewed recently (15). The main proposals for explaining the molecular basis of the inhibition of cellular motility resulting from the action of lymphocyte-derived MIF on macrophages (MPs) are summarized in Table 1.

TABLE 1. Principal models for the mediation of the effect
of MIF on macrophages

A. Mechanistical models (agglutination by multivalent lymphokine, decreased surface charge, loss of glycocalix).

B. Second messenger models (cyclic AMP, cyclic GMP, calcium).

C. Cytoskeleton-mediated models (polymerization of tubulin, actin).

D. Fibronectin-fibrin neomechanistical proposal.

E. Oxidative autotoxicity hypothesis.

F. Arachidonic acid metabolite hypothesis (cyclooxygenase or lipoxygenase product.

The evidence in support of the various models and the inability of most of these to provide an adequate explanation for MIF action was

recently discussed (19). Progress on this area was hampered by the
lack of highly purified MIF preparations and of monospecific antibodies
directed against MIF as well as by the semiquantitative nature of the
migration inhibition assay itself. Additional confusion was generated
by the fact that MIF-containing culture supernatants also exhibit an
even more complex array of effects on MPs, normally referred to as MP
activation. In the absence of strictly characterized lymphokines, it is
yet impossible to determine whether MIF is also the bearer of MP activating activity or whether such activity is the property of a distinct
lymphokine.

MP migration inhibition in the whole animal is essentially a local
phenomenon, possibly meant to assure the prolonged localization of
chemotactically attracted MPs at sites of bacterial, fungal, viral or
parasitic attack. In this sense, the ideal but yet unproven lymphokine
action sequence is chemotaxis, local immobilization and, finally, activation. In addition to the unsettled question of whether MP migration
inhibition and MP activation are caused by the same lymphokine, the
question of whether a chemotactic lymphokine could exhibit a motility
blocking effect at high concentrations has also been raised. We have
recently suggested that, independently of the number and nature of
participating lymphokines, the biochemical events occurring in the MP
going through the "chemotaxis → immobilization → activation" sequence
are tightly linked. The common denominator is the involvement of oxidative burst (OB) products intimately linked to the pathways of arachidonic
acid oxidation (19,7). We now present new experimental evidence in
support of our working model and shall attempt to integrate this new
information within the framework provided by earlier experimental results.
The essence of our model is that MIF induces or facilitates a membrane-
initiated OB in the target MP. A product or products of the OB inflict
a reversible toxic effect on cytoplasmic and/or membrane structures
involved in cell motility resulting in inhibition of migration. This is
followed by the intervention of effective antioxidant feedback mechanisms which allow the resumption of normal cell movement and serve as
background for the subsequent activation stage. MP activation is characterized by an enhanced propensity to respond to certain types of membrane
stimulation by an OB, supported by an enhanced cellular buffering capacity
permitting the massive production of damaging oxygen products while
avoiding autotoxic damage. The experimental evidence for the second
part of this proposal, namely the relation between OB and MP activation,
is well documented by the work of Z. A. Cohn and collaborators (12,10,11).
The evidence for a causal connection between the OB and the inhibition
of cellular motility was, so far, mostly indirect (reviewed in Ref. 19).

EXPERIMENTAL RESULTS

The methodological aspects of these experiments are described in
detail by Jakubowski et al. (6). In brief, guinea pig peritoneal MPs
were elicited by paraffin oil injection and these cells served as targets
for the action of antigen-induced guinea pig lymphocyte MIF, produced as
previously described (17). MP migration inhibition assays were performed
by the conventional capillary tube method using both continuous exposure
of MPs to MIF and pulse exposure to MIF techniques (9). Antioxidant
compounds and drugs interfering with arachidonic acid release or oxidation
were first tested for a direct effect on MP viability and spontaneous
migration over a wide concentration range. Drugs at concentrations

having no detrimental effect on MP viability and motility were then tested for a modulating effect on MP migration inhibition caused by MIF or by the MIF-mimicking agent, phorbol myristate acetate (PMA). We have shown in the past that exposure of MPs to low, nontoxic concentrations of PMA results in massive but reversible inhibition of migration (20) and have linked this effect of PMA to its capacity to elicit an intense OB, as measured by the production of superoxide (O_2^-) and hydrogen peroxide (H_2O_2) (7,16). MPs were preincubated with the various drugs for time intervals varying from 1 to 4 hours and subsequently packed in capillaries. These were placed in migration chambers containing one of the following 4 materials: culture medium; supernatant of immune guinea pig lymphocytes cultured in the absence of antigen (control supernatant); supernatant of immune guinea pig lymphocytes cultured in the presence of the antigen, tuberculin PPD (MIF-containing supernatant), or culture medium containing 20 nM PMA. Control supernatant was supplemented with antigen after culture and both control and MIF-containing supernatants were extensively dialyzed against fresh medium. To the chambers containing capillaries with cells preincubated with a certain drug, the same drug was readded, assuring continuous exposure of MPs to the pharmacological agent both before and in the course of incubation with MIF or PMA. Areas of MP migration were measured after overnight incubation at 37°C and the drug-induced change in migration areas was subjected to statistical treatment. Whenever an effect was seen on MIF or PMA-elicited inhibition of migration, this was compared (and assessed statistically) to the influence of the same drug on migration in culture medium and control supernatant. The major categories of drugs investigated were: enzymes catabolizing O_2^- or H_2O_2, scavengers of O_2^-, H_2O_2, hydroxyl radicals (OH·) or singlet oxygen ($^1O_2$), other antioxidants with less defined sites of action, and inhibitors of phospholipase A_2, cyclooxygenase, lipoxygenase and thromboxane (TXA_2) synthetase. A summary of the effects of individual drugs on MIF and PMA-induced migration inhibition is presented in Tables 2 and 3. A detailed description of these results will be published separately (6).

These results indicate clearly that the inhibitory action of lymphocyte-derived MIF and of the model compound, PMA, on MP migration is reversed by some antioxidant agents and by drugs blocking the enzyme TXA_2 synthetase. The MIF-induced inhibition of motility could be prevented by 3 antioxidants (methionine, histidine and propyl gallate) while only one (methionine) prevented PMA action. Also, all 4 TXA_2 synthesis inhibitors tested prevented MIF action while only 3 out of 4 blocked the effect of PMA. It is not yet possible to say whether these differences are indicative of a basic distinction in the mechanisms by which MIF and PMA act or merely reflect our failure to optimize the conditions required for inhibiting PMA action. It should be made clear at this point that PMA can only serve as a model compound mimicking MIF action while being clearly different from MIF in many respects. The most obvious difference is the ability of PMA to induce rapid and massive O_2^- and H_2O_2 production and release by MPs while MIF lacks such capacity.

DISCUSSION

We have recently reviewed the published evidence compatible with our hypothesis that autotoxic damage of a reversible nature is the mechanism responsible for the effect of MIF on MP motility (19). The principal circumstantial evidence in support of such a proposal is the finding

TABLE 2.   Modulation by antioxidants of the effects of
            MIF and PMA on macrophage migration

Agent	Function	Concen-tration	Effect on: MIF	Effect on: PMA
Ferricytochrome C	O_2^- scavenger	50–200µM	–	–
Superoxide dismutase	O_2^- scavenger	625U/ml	–	–
Catalase[a]	Degrades H_2O_2	1250–2500U/ml	–	–
Catalase[b]	Degrades H_2O_2	3000–7000U/ml	–	–
2,3-dihydroxybenzoic-acid	O_2^-, H_2O_2 scavenger	0.25–1mM	–	–
Mannitol	OH· scavenger	25mM	–	–
Na benzoate	OH· scavenger	2.5–5mM	–	–
L-tryptophan	OH·, $^1O_2$ scavenger	2.5–5mM	–	–
L-methionine	OH·, $^1O_2$ scavenger	10–80mM	R	R
L-histidine	OH·, $^1O_2$ scavenger	20–80mM	R	–
1,4-diazabicyclo-octane (DABCO)	$^1O_2$ scavenger	2.5–5mM	–	–
2,5-dimethylfuran	$^1O_2$ scavenger	1–2mM	–	–
Propyl gallate	Antioxidant	0.12–0.25mM	R	–

– = no effect; R = reverses action of MIF or PMA;
E = enhances action of MIF or PMA

[a] Catalase, purified powder from bovine liver

[b] Catalase, 2 x crystallized from bovine liver

TABLE 3.   Modulation by inhibitors of arachidonic acid
             oxidation of the effects of MIF and PMA on
                        macrophage migration

Agent	Function	Concen-tration	Effect on: MIF	Effect on: PMA
Mepacrine	Phospholipase A2 inhibitor	12.5–25 μM	–	–
ETYA[a]	Cyclooxygenase & lipoxygenase inhibitor	50–100 μM	–	–
Indomethacin	Cyclooxygenase inhibitor	25–100 μM	–	–
Imidazole	TXA_2[d] synthetase inhibitor	1.25–2.5 mM	R	R
Benzylimidazole	TXA_2 synthetase inhibitor	0.25–1 mM	R	–
U-44069[b]	TXA_2 synthetase inhibitor	12.5–100 μM	R	R
U-51605[c]	TXA_2 synthetase inhibitor	50–100 μM	R	R

– = no effect; R = reverses action of MIF or PMA;
E = enhances action of MIF or PMA

[a]5,8,11,14-eicosatetraynoic acid; [b](15S) hydroxy-9α,11α-(epoxymethano) prosta-5Z,13E-dienoic acid (Upjohn Company)

[c](5Z, 9α, 11α, 13E)-9,11-azoprosta-5,13-dienoic acid (Upjohn Company)

[d]TXA_2 = thromboxane A_2

that several chemically unrelated compounds having in common the ability to induce an OB also block MP motility in the concentration range optimal for OB stimulation. PMA, the calcium ionophore A23187, several formylated peptides, such as N-formyl-met-leu-phe (FMLP), and the lectins, concanavalin A (Con A) and wheat germ agglutinin (WGA), exert such an effect on guinea pig MPs. The PMA analog, 4-0-methyl-PMA, which lacks the ability to elicit an OB, is also inactive in the migration inhibition assay. The concentrations of FMLP causing MP immobilization are well correlated with those inducing an OB but are higher than the optimal chemotactic concentration. These results are closely paralleled by recent findings with polymorphonuclear leukocytes (PMNs); concentrations of FMLP higher than the chemotactic optimum were found to inhibit PMN motility, increase cell adhesiveness and stimulate the hexose mono-phosphate shunt (HMPS) in a closely correlated manner (4). It was also found that the formylated peptide-induced inhibition of spontaneous PMN migration is not only correlated with the OB (as shown by the parallel stimulation of the HMPS) but is causally related to it. Thus, PMNs of patients with chronic granulomatous disease (lacking the ability to develop an OB) do not demonstrate a depression in cellular motility upon exposure to N-formyl-met-phe while exhibiting normal chemotactic respon-siveness (13). These observations are in perfect agreement with earlier reports of reduced PMN motility in the presence of H_2O_2 and of the motility enhancing properties of antioxidants, such as catalase, α-tocopherol and 2,3-dihydroxybenzoic acid (1,2). Autotoxicity can reach degrees incompatible with cell survival, as shown by the ability of PMA to cause the death of PMNs in culture by a mechanism which could be antagonized by catalase, methionine, histidine or serum (23). MPs are notoriously resistant to damage by oxygen radicals, probably by virtue of an effective enzymatic scavenging system, the backbone of which is catalase (11). This contrasts with the susceptibility of other target cells, such as erythrocytes, as demonstrated by the massive, OB dependent cytotoxic effect of PMA-stimulated MPs towards syngeneic erythrocytes (8). The resistance of MPs to gross damage nevertheless permits the expression of more subtle aspects of toxicity, such as the impairment of cellular motility. However, inspite of prolonged exposure of MPs to MIF, the inhibition of migration is reversed (the "escape" phenomenon, see Ref. 3), most likely as the result of MIF-induced increases in catalase, glutathione peroxidase and superoxide dismutase (11).

The nature of the toxic oxygen product(s) responsible for the effect on cellular motility as well as the identity of the intracellular target are yet unknown. Methionine and histidine are scavengers of $^1O_2$ and OH· but other agents with related activities (tryptophan, DABCO) did not prevent MIF (and PMA) action. Also, the ability of propyl gallate to reverse MIF action does not shed light on the nature of the oxygen product involved and further work is required for defining the nature of the injurious agent. The most challenging difficulty which will have to be surmounted is the development of methods for the detection of OB products within the cell since, obviously, the measurement of products released by the cells into the culture medium is inappropriate and is unlikely to be relevant to the in vivo reality. A less direct approach is to look for indicators of an oxidative process taking place in MIF-treated cells. Indeed, a rapid increase in the oxidation of SH groups and of NADPH was detected in MIF-treated MPS (21) and we have preliminary evidence for a temporary lessened ability of MPs incubated with MIF for 1 hour to reduce glutathione (M. Freund, Y. Keisari and E. Pick, unpublished.)

An unexpected finding was the capacity of drugs blocking TXA_2 synthesis to prevent MIF and PMA-mediated inhibition of MP migration. The most obvious interpretation of this finding is that TXA_2 synthesis is involved in MIF action as either a causal or a modulating factor. The significance of such a finding is further augmented by the inability of cyclooxygenase inhibitors (indomethacin, ETYA) to affect MIF action. This suggests that the determining factor at this stage of MIF action is not the absolute concentration of TXA_2 but rather the relative levels of the two major cyclooxygenase products in the guinea pig MP, TXA_2 and prostaglandin E_2 (PGE_2). The indiscriminate blocking of the synthesis of both products does not prevent MIF action but the selective inhibition of TXA_2 synthesis, which is accompanied by a simultaneous increase in PGE_2 synthesis (5), blocks MIF action. A preliminary and probably simplistic interpretation of these results is that TXA_2 and PGE_2 have opposite effects or MP motility; TXA_2 inhibits MP migration while PGE_2 prevents this inhibition, probably by a cyclic AMP-dependent process. It has been recently reported that TXA_2 mediates augmented PMN adhesiveness while E-type prostaglandins had an antiadhesive effect (22). Our data seem to indicate a striking similarity between MIF (or PMA)-elicited MP migration inhibition and thrombin-induced platelet aggregation, a process in which TXA_2 is the proaggregatory and prostaglandin, the antiaggregatory mediator.

TXA_2 is the major product of the cyclooxygenase-initiated pathway of arachidonic acid oxidation in guinea pig MPs in short term culture. We have recently found that all agents capable of eliciting an OB in guinea pig MPs (16) are also active inducers of TXA_2 synthesis, PMA being one of the most potent stimulants (Y. Bromberg, unpublished). The effect of MIF on TXA_2 synthesis by guinea pig MPs in being currently investigated in our laboratory.

A key requirement for any new hypothesis is that, in addition to providing an explanation for the new data on which it rests, it should also be compatible with earlier experimental results. The "oxygen auto-toxicity and thromboxane" hypothesis can accommodate the biochemical correlates of MIF action described in the past. Thus, the calcium requirement (17) for MIF activity is in agreement with the key role of this cation in the elicitation of an OB and the activation of the arachidonic acid releasing enzyme, phospholipase A_2. The MIF-induced fall in cyclic AMP levels (14) could well be the result of a TXA_2 or prostaglandin endoperoxide-mediated inhibition of adenylate cyclase. The MIF-related enhanced tubulin polymerization (18) could be the result of the fall in cyclic AMP resulting in a modified cyclic AMP/cyclic GMP ratio. Finally, the MIF antagonizing action of agents elevating cyclic AMP levels (17) is compatible with the blocking effect of cyclic AMP on the induction of an OB and on phospholipase A_2 activity required for arachidonic acid release.

In summary we propose a model for MIF action (Table 4) which involves the participation of unidentified oxygen radicals and TXA_2 in the cessation of cell movement. The relative importance of these two factors cannot be estimated and present; it is possible that the effect of the oxygen radicals is principally on the locomotory apparatus itself while TXA_2 affects mostly membrane properties, such as cell adhesion. The mechanism behind the correlated ability of MIF to stimulate both an OB and TXA_2 synthesis appears to be common to a number of more trivial OB stimulants, such as PMA, zymosan or FMLP and is, most likely, linked to some form of calcium mobilization. In the light of our inability to detect OB products in the culture medium of MPs exposed to MIF, it seems likely that toxic radical generation occurs at an intracellular site and is not associated with extracellular release of either O_2^- or H_2O_2. Escape from migration inhibition is the result of the MPs developing effective antioxidant mechanisms in preparation for the "activation" stage. This is, in essence, characterized by a capacity to mount an intense oxidative burst upon adequate membrane stimulation on a back-ground of augmented cellular antioxidant buffering capacity. The activated MP is geared for extracellular release of the OB products providing effective antimicrobial activity against most pathogens although, occasionally, the cell's own scavenging mechanism might interfere with the destruction of pathogens (11). This working model provides ample opportunities for additional experimental confirmation.

TABLE 4.   Sequential biochemical events in the activation
of macrophages by MIF

A. Early immobilization following chemotaxis (0-2 hours)

1. Direct effect of oxidative burst products (O_2^-, H_2O_2, OH· or (O_x)) on locomotory apparatus or cell membrane.

2. Stimulation of thromboxane A_2 synthesis → increased cell adherence and aggregation.

3. Fall in cyclic AMP (PG endoperoxide, thromboxane or H_2O_2 - mediated?)

B. Transition stage (consolidation of immobilization, shift to activation (2-24 hours))

1. Increase in tubulin polymerization, microtubule generation

2. Enhanced actin polymerization

C. Activation stage (24-72 hours) (Possibly mediated by a distinct lymphokine)

1. Enhanced propensity for oxidative burst upon membrane stimulation but autotoxicity is prevented by:

a) hexose monophosphate shunt stimulation linked to enhanced glutathione peroxidase activity
b) elevated catalase level

2. PGE_2 production replaces thromboxane synthesis

3. Enhanced secretory function (neutral proteases, acid hydrolases, complement components, etc.)

ACKNOWLEDGEMENTS

This research was supported by a grant from the National Council for Research and Development, Israel, and the Deutsches Krebsforschungszentrum, Heidelberg, Germany, and by grant No. 1505 from the U.S.-Israel Binational Science Foundation. We thank Mrs. Carol Oesch for secretarial assistance.

REFERENCES

1. Baehner, R. L., Boxer, L. A., Allen, J. M., and Davis, J. (1977): Blood, 50:327-335.
2. Boxer, L. A., Allen, J. M., and Baehner, R. L. (1978): J. Lab. Clin. Med., 92:730-736.
3. Brostoff, J. (1974): J. Immunol. Methods, 4:27-30.
4. Fehr, J., and Dahinden, C. (1979): J. Clin. Invest., 64:8-16.
5. Gorman, R. R., Bundy, G. L., Peterson, D. C., Sun, F. F., Miller, O. V., and Fitzpatrick, F. A. (1977): Proc. Nat. Acad. Sci. U.S.A., 74:4007-4011.
6. Jakubowski, A., Keisari, Y., and Pick, E., in preparation.

7. Keisari, Y., and Pick, E. (1980): In: <u>Biochemical Characterization of Lymphokines</u>, edited by A. L. deWeck, F. Kristensen, and M. Landy, pp. 113-121, Academic Press, New York.
8. Keisari, Y., and Pick, E. (1981): <u>Cell. Immunol.</u>, (in press).
9. Manheimer, S., and Pick, E. (1973): <u>Immunology</u>, 24:1027-1034.
10. Murray, H. W., and Cohn, Z. A. (1980): <u>J. Exp. Med.</u>, 152:1596-1609.
11. Murray, H. W., Nathan, C. F., and Cohn, Z. A. (1980): <u>J. Exp. Med.</u>, 152:1610-1624.
12. Nathan, C. F., Nogueira, N., Juangbhanich, C., Ellis, J., and Cohn, Z. A. (1979): <u>J. Exp. Med.</u>, 149:1056-1068.
13. Nelson, R. D., McCormack, R. T., Fiegel, V. D., Herron, M., Simmons, R., and Quie, P. G. (1979): <u>Infect. Immun.</u>, 23:282-286.
14. Pick, E. (1977): <u>Cell. Immunol.</u>, 32:329-339.
15. Pick, E. (1979): In: <u>Biology of the Lymphokines</u>, edited by S. Cohen, E. Pick, and J. J. Oppenheim, pp. 59-119. Academic Press, New York.
16. Pick, E., and Keisari, Y. (1981): <u>Cell. Immunol.</u>, (in press).
17. Pick, E., and Manheimer, S. (1974): <u>Cell. Immunol.</u>, 11:30-46.
18. Pick, E., Honig, S., and Griffel, B. (1979): <u>Int. Arch. Allergy</u>, 58:149-159.
19. Pick, E., Keisari, Y., and Bromberg, Y. (1980): In <u>Advances in Allergology and Applied Immunology</u>, edited by A. Oehling, pp. 399-407. Pergamon Press, London.
20. Pick, E., Seger, M., Honig, S. and Griffel, B. (1979): <u>Ann. N.Y. Acad. Sci.</u>, 332:378-394.
21. Poulter, L., and Turk, J. L. (1975): <u>Cell. Immunol.</u>, 20:12-24.
22. Spagnullo, P. J., Ellner, J. J., Hassid, A., and Dunn, M. J. (1980): <u>J. Clin. Invest.</u>, 66:406-414.
23. Tsan, M. F., and Denison, R. C. (1980): <u>Inflammation</u>, 4:371-380.

Lymphokines and Thymic Hormones: Their
Potential Utilization in Cancer Therapeutics,
edited by A. L. Goldstein and M. A. Chirigos,
Raven Press, New York © 1981.

Chemical Characterization of Antigen-Specific Suppressor Lymphokines

D. R. Webb, K. Krupen, *B. Araneo, *J. Kapp, I. Nowowiejski,
C. Healy, K. Wieder, and S. Stein

*Roche Institute of Molecular Biology, Nutley, New Jersey 07110; *Department of Pathology,
The Jewish Hospital of St. Louis, St. Louis, Missouri 63110*

Extensive studies performed over the last few years have established that regulation of the immune response involves soluble mediators which may be either antigen-specific or non-specific (6,8). These soluble factors have not been chemically well characterized since they are found in very low concentrations with very high specific activities. The development of new and more sensitive technology for chemical analysis, as well as the explosive development of new cell culture techniques (e.g. hybridomas) have improved the opportunities for characterizing the mediators which help to regulate immunocompetent cell function. Generally, mediators may be classed into cytotoxins, helper factors, growth regulatory factors and suppressor factors.

While much is not known about the structural details of a majority of immunoregulatory substances, some of the general aspects of their chemistry are established. For example, antigen-specific mediators are probably all glycoproteins (1) while non-specific mediators may be protein, carbohydrate, lipid, fatty acids or nucleic acids (28).

Recently, several groups have focused on the purification and bio-chemical and biological analysis of suppressor factors which are specific for the antigen which induced their synthesis. A description of some of these factors is presented in Table 1. As indicated in the Table, these factors may be specific for the class of antibody which is regulated, the type of response regulated (e.g. antibody versus delayed type hypersensitivity) and for given types of determinants (e.g. carrier versus hapten-specific). Not listed here are factors recently described which are idiotype-specific, i.e., they suppress the appearance of a given idiotype to a specific antigen. The apparent molecular weights of the various factors is quite uniform and most, if not all, bear determinants which react with antisera specific for regions of the H-2 locus. Recently, several laboratories have reported the preparation of T-cell hybrids which constituitively produce some of these suppressor factors (13,18,24,25,26). This represents an important development which will facilitate the purification and analysis of these molecules. Thus far, the hybrid derived factors faithfully represent the chemical and biological properties of those molecules which are found in vivo (see Table II).

187

Table I: Antigen-Specific T Cell Factors that Suppress the Immune Response

TsF	Ref.	Method of Isolation*	M. Wt.	Immune Response	Allogeneic Deter.	Ag. Specificity	Genetic Restrictions	Target
IgE response in rats	(21)	E	35-60,000	Ab (anti-hapten IgE)	-	DNP-Ascaris suum (carrier)	Syngeneic	?
	(22) (23)	E	35-55,000	Ab (2° immuniz.) (2° response)	I-J	KLH	Syngeneic I-J	Ts_2
Carrier specific properties	(17)	S	80,000	Ab (1° response)	I-J	KLH	Syngeneic or Allogeneic	T_H
	(5)	S	45-50,000	Ab (adoptive 2° response)	I-J	HGG (human γ-globulin)	Syngeneic I-J	T_H
Synthetic poly-peptides specificity	(16)	E	45-50,000	Ab (1° immuniz.) (1° PFC)	I-J	GAT (L-glutamic acid 60: L-alanine 30: L-tyrosine 10:)	Non-responder (Syngeneic or allogeneic)	Ts_2
	(27)	E	40-50,000	Ab (1° response)	I-J	GT (L-glutamic acid 50: L-tyrosine 50)	Non-responder (Syngeneic or allogeneic)	Ts_2
Delayed Type Hyper-sensitivity	(29)	S	50,000	DH	I-J	TNP	Syngeneic	M Ø
	(19)	S	-	DH	I-C	DNP	Syngeneic K or D	Immune T cell
	(10)	S	33-68,000	DH	I-J	ABA (P-azobenzenearsonate)	Syngeneic I-J	Ts_2
Tumor Immunity	(9)	E	67,000	Tumor Rejection	I-J	Sarcoma 1509	Syngeneic	T_K

* E = Cell Extract
  S = Supernatant

Table II: T Suppressor Factor Produced by Hybridoma Cell Lines

Antigen	Ref.	Fusion	TsF Activity (Supernatant)	TsF Properties
HGG	(24)	HGG Ts [CBA origin - (H-2^k)] x EL-4 [C57BL/6 - (H-2^b)] lymphoma	First reported T cell hybrids w/ Ts function. Extracts gave specific suppressive activity to HGG in vivo. After 3 months lost CBA parent (chromosome loss).	---
KLH	(18)	KLH-Ts [CBA origin (H-2^k)] x BW5147 (AKR-H-2^k)	Suppression of specific in vitro Ab response to TNP-KLH.	Absorbs to KLH, anti-Ia^k, anti-I-J^k. Does not absorb to anti-mouse Ig. M.W. 50-60,000 daltons.
KLH	(25)	KLH-Ts [C57BL/6 (H-2^b)] x BW5147	Suppression of specific in vitro Ab response against DNP-KLH. Suppress responses of H-2^b and H-2$^{k/b}$ spleen cells but not H-2^k.	Absorbs to KLH, anti-H-2^b anti-I-J. Does not absorb to anti-Ig. M.W. 42-68,000 daltons.
sRBC	(26)	sRBC-Ts [C57BL/10 (H-2^b)] x BW5147	Suppress in vitro primary Ab response to sRBC.	Absorbs to sRBC, anti-H-2^b. Does not absorb to anti-Ig. Does not absorb to anti-I-J. M.W. 200,000 daltons.
GAT	(13)	GAT-Ts [DBA/1 (H-2^q)] x BW5147	Suppress in vitro GAT-specific PFC and GAT-specific proliferation response to GAT-MBSA in non-responder DBA/1 cells.	Absorbs to GAT, absorbs to anti-I (presumed I-J subregion). Does not absorb to anti-Ig. M.W. 24,000 daltons.

The work to be discussed in this paper concerns the purification of a suppressor molecule produced by a T cell hybridoma, whose characteristics have been described in detail (13). Briefly, splenic T cells (nylon wool passed) obtained from DBA/1 mice ($H-2^q$) immunized with the synthetic polypeptide glutamic acid^{60}-alanine^{30}-tyrosine^{10} (GAT) were fused with the AKR lymphoma BW5147 (HGPRT^{-}, Oubain resistant). The fusion products were screened for suppressor production and the positive clones were screened again and recloned to provide lines for further study. Two subclones which originated from the same initial clone (Cl4#4 and Cl4#6) have been used for the analysis of their suppressor product.

The synthetic terpolymer, GAT, has been used by Kapp et al. (2,3,11, 12,13,16,27) to define the role that H-2 linked Ir genes play in regulating humoral immune responses. *In vivo* studies have shown that mice bearing $H-2^{a,b,d,f,j,k,r,u,v}$ haplotypes are responders to GAT whereas mice bearing the $H-2^{p,q,s}$ haplotypes are non-responders, i.e., no antibody or antibody forming cells can be detected. However if GAT is complexed with methylated bovine serum albumin (MBSA), an immunogenic carrier, then both responder and non-responder mice develop antibody responses specific for GAT. The genes which control responsiveness to GAT have been mapped to the I-A - I-B subregions of the H-2 locus.

In vitro studies using the Mishell-Dutton spleen cell culture system have shown that the immune response to GAT is T-cell dependent and requires macrophages. The failure of non-responder mice to make antibody was traced to effects on B cells as a result of the activation of GAT-specific suppressor T cells (12). The GAT-specific suppressor T cell is an Ly 1$^-$, 2$^+$ cell. In studies carried out by Benacerraf and Germain and their associates (4), it appears that suppression involves two suppressor cell populations, Ts_1 and Ts_2, which produce two suppressor factors, Ts_1SF and Ts_2SF. The serological properties of Ts_1SF are identical to the properties of the suppressor factor <u>extracted</u> from suppressor cells from non-responder strains. The evidence currently available suggests that Ts_1SF from non-responder mice functions exclusively to induce Ts_2 cells and cannot directly suppress T-helper activity (4). The biological and serological properties of Ts_1SF extracted from non-responder mice immunized with GAT are identical to those of the partially purified hybridoma product. The factor from both sources binds GAT and GA but not GT, both lack immunoglobulin (Ig) constant region determinants and have I region or I-J subregion determinants, and both appear to have carbohydrate moieties.

Our approach to the study of these substances is to purify the factors to chemical homogeneity and to obtain information on their structure (i.e. amino acid composition and sequence, location of V_H and I region determinants, etc.). We then intend to purify factors obtained from mice bearing different haplotypes and from mice bearing identical haplotypes but immunized with related synthetic polymers such as GT. The various factors will be structurally compared so that we may begin to understand structure-function relationships as well as the genetic relationships among these factors. To date, we have completed the chemical purification of the hybridoma-derived Ts_1SF, which suppresses the response to GAT and whose chemical and biological properties are listed in Table 3. The factor is a protein with a molecular weight estimated to be 24,000 daltons (SDS-polyacrylamide gel analysis). It binds to GAT and to GA, but not GT. Ts_1SF binds to an antisera specific for the q haplotype in the H-2 I region but not to an unrelated H-2 I antisera. The factor is biologically active in that it suppresses the <u>in vitro</u> antibody response to sRBC-coupled GAT but not sRBC alone and it blocks the proliferative response of lymphnode cells from non-responder mice immunized with GAT-MBSA (Krupen et al., in preparation; Kapp et al., in preparation). A second suppressor factor partially purified from a hybridoma in which the fusion partner was of the H-2^S haplotype shows the biological and chemical properties of the H-2^S TsF to be identical to the H-2^q TsF except that they react with different antisera specific for the H-2 haplotype.

Table III: Chemical and Biological Characteristics of GAT-Ts$_1$SF

from a T Cell Hybridoma - Cl4#4

---

1. M.W. = 24,000 daltons as estimated by SDS polyacrylamide gel electrophoresis.

2. Single polypeptide chain under both reducing and non-reducing conditions on SDS-polyacrylamide gels.

3. Binds to GAT and to GA but not to GT.

4. Biological activity is absorbed by sepharose bound anti-H-2I^q antisera; not absorbed by anti-I-J^S antisera.

5. Specifically suppresses the primary immune response to GAT-MBSA in non-responder mice.

In addition to purifying the GAT-specific Ts$_1$SF (q haplotype) from the Cl4#4 hybridoma we have been carrying out experiments which will lead to a genetic analysis of the Ts$_1$SF using recombinant DNA technology. Initial experiments involved the isolation of polyA containing mRNA from the BW5147 parental cell line and the Cl4#4 hybridoma. These mRNA preparations were fractionated on sucrose density gradients and mRNA from each fraction was translated in a cell-free system using rabbit reticulocyte lysates (20). The translated products were then assayed for biological activity. Results show mRNA from Cl4#4 with a size of approximately 16S contains a message which translated biologically active Ts$_1$SF. This message was missing in the 16S mRNA population from BW5147 cells. Using GAT-sepharose and anti-H-2I^q antisera bound to sepharose, we have found 3 major protein bands on SDS polyacrylamide gels which bind both GAT and anti-H-2I^q. These bands have approximate molecular weights of 70,000, 44,000 and 24,000. Other, more faint, bands are present but in greatly reduced quantity. It remains to be determined whether one or all of these bands contain the Ts$_1$SF activity. Future work in this area will be directed towards obtaining molecular probes which may be used to study directly, the genes which code for Ts$_1$SF.

A direct examination of the gene(s) coding for Ts$_1$SF should be of great interest. Previous studies from Taniguchi et al. (25) and from Cantor and coworkers (7) have suggested a rather different structure for TsF. The different proposed structures are indicated in Fig. 1. Studies by Taniguchi et al. have suggested that the H-2 determinant was present on a peptide different from that of the antigen-binding site (25). This makes the translation and processing steps much simpler since one could hypothesize that an immunoglobulin variable region gene could code for the antigen binding peptide. Many suppressor factors, including GAT-specific Ts$_1$SF, react with anti-idiotypic or anti-V$_H$ region specific antisera. Thus, one need hypothesize only one more gene under the control of the I region (specifying the second peptide) to complete the minimum number of genes required for Ts_1SF. However, the results obtained in our studies showed that both the antigen-binding site and I region determinant were present on a single 24,000 dalton protein. It is not known whether V_H genes or "V_H-like" genes are expressed in the H-2 region. Thus, we must consider a model which includes the processing of a minimum of two gene products - one bearing the antigen-binding site and the other bearing the I region determinant and possibly controlling the biological function - to yield a secreted product consisting of a single polypeptide chain. So far, analysis of C14#4 Ts_1SF under both reducing and non-reducing conditions gives the same result - a single peptide. This would indicate a non-sulfhydryl covalent link between the V_H gene product and the I region gene product. Future studies should help us to understand how the genes for antigen binding and the I-region interact to give these interesting biological entities.

Fig. 1. Possible models of TsF structure

(See references 25; 7; Krupen et al., in preparation)

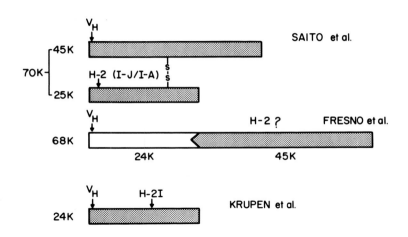

REFERENCES

1. Altman, A., and Katz, D.H. (1980): J. Immunol. Meth. 38:9-41.

2. Araneo, B.A., and Kapp, J.A. (1980) J. Immunol. 124:1492-1498.

3. Araneo, B.A., and Kapp, J.A. (1980) J. Immunol. 125:118-123.

4. Benacerraf, B., and Germain, R. (1979) Fed. Proc. 35:2053-2057.

5. Chaovat, G. (1978) Cell. Immunol. 36:1-14.

6. De Weck, A.L., Kistensen, F., and Landy, M., editors (1980) Biochemical Characterization of Lymphokines: Academic Press, New York.

7. Fresno, M., Nabel, G., McVay-Boudreau, L., and Cantor, H. (1980) Fourth Internat. Congr. Immunol. Abstr. 5.4.02.

8. Friedman, H., editor (1979) Subcellular Factors in Immunity. Ann. N.Y. Acad. Sci. 332.

9. Greene, M.I., Fujinato, S., Sehon, A.H. (1977) J. Immumol. 119:757-764.

10. Green, M.I., Bach, B.A., and Benacerraf, B. (1979) J. Exp. Med. 149:1069-1083.

11. Kapp, J.A. (1978) J. Exp. Med. 147:997-1006.

12. Kapp, J.A., and Araneo, B.A. (1980) In: Macrophage Regulation of Immunity, edited by E. Warner and A.S. Rosenthal, pp. 141-151. Academic Press, New York.

13. Kapp, J.A., Araneo, B.A., and Clevinger, B.L. (1980) J. Exp. Med. 152:235-240.

14. Kapp, J.A., Pierce, C.W., and Benacerraf, B. (1973) J. Exp. Med. 138:1107-1120.

15. Kapp, J.A., Pierce, C.W., Benacerraf, B. (1977) J. Exp. Med. 145:828-838.

16. Kapp, J.A., Pierce, C.W., DeLa Croix, F., and Benacerraf, B. (1976) J. Immunol. 116:305-309.

17. Kontaiainen, S. and Feldman, M. (1977) Eur. J. Immunol. 7:310-315.

18. Kontaiainen, S., Simpson, E., Bohrer, F., Beverly, P.C.L., Herzenberg, L.A., Fitzpatrick, W.C., Vogt, P., Torano,A., McKenzie, F.F.C., and Feldman, M. (1978) Nature 274:477-479.

19. Moorhead, J. (1977) J. Immunol. 119:315-321.

20. Pelham, H.R.B., and Jackson, R.J. (1976) Eur. J. Biochem. 67:247-256.

21. Tada, T., Okumura, K., and Taniguchi, M. (1973) J. Immunol. 111:952-958.

22. Tada, T., Taniguchi, M., and David, C.S. (1976) Cold Spring Harbor Symp. Quant. Biol. 41:119-127.

23. Taniguchi, M., Hayakawa, K., and Tada, T. (1976) J. Immunol. 116:542-548.

24. Taniguchi, M., and Miller, J.F.A.P. (1978) J. Exp. Med. 146:373-379.

25. Taniguchi, M., Saito, T., and Tada, T.(1979) Nature 278:555-557.

26. Taussig, M.J., and Holliman, A. (1979) Nature 277:308-310.

27. Theze, J., Waltenbough, C., Dorf, M.E., and Benacerraf, B. (1977) J. Exp. Med. 146:287-292.

28. Waksman, B.H., and Namba, T. (1976) Cell. Immunol. 21:161-168.

29. Zembala, M., and Asherson, G.L. (1974) Eur. J. Immunol. 4:799-804.

*Lymphokines and Thymic Hormones: Their
Potential Utilization in Cancer Therapeutics,*
edited by A. L. Goldstein and M. A. Chirigos,
Raven Press, New York © 1981.

Structure and Mechanism of Action of the Lymphokine, Soluble Immune Response Suppressor

Carl W. Pierce and Thomas M. Aune

*Department of Pathology and Laboratory Medicine, The Jewish Hospital of St. Louis and Departments of
Pathology and Microbiology and Immunology, Washington University School of Medicine,
St. Louis, Missouri 63110*

INTRODUCTION

Suppression of immune responses in many situations is mediated by T lymphocytes. These T lymphocytes may be antigen-specific or nonspecific and usually mediate suppression through the release of a soluble factor which also may be antigen-specific or nonspecific (13-15). Over the past few years, we have investigated the mechanism of action concanavalin A (con A)-activated suppressor T cells. Activation of murine T cells with mitogenic concentrations of con A leads to the development of a population of suppressor T cells which inhibit a variety of immune responses, including IgM and IgG plaque forming cell responses to a variety of T cell-dependent and T cell-independent antigens, the generation of cytotoxic T cells and spleen cell proliferative responses to alloantigens and mitogens (11,13,15,16). These suppressor T cells are Ly 1^-, 2^+ and after induction suppressive activity is radio-resistant (7,13,15). Kinetic analysis shows that antibody and cytotoxic T cell responses develop normally for the first 3 days of culture in the presence of suppressor T cells, but prematurely terminate and are suppressed on day 4 and 5 (11,13,17).

MECHANISM OF ACTION

Suppressor T cells, activated by con A, act via a soluble mediator, soluble immune responses suppressor (SIRS) (12-15,17). SIRS effectively suppresses antibody responses, T and B cell DNA synthetic responses to mitogens and T cell responses to alloantigens (2,12-15,17). Production of SIRS does not require DNA synthesis, but does require protein synthesis (15). SIRS is a protein with an apparent mol. wt. of 50,000-55,000 daltons; it is stable at 56°C, but is inactivated at 70°C and pH <3. SIRS activity is also lost following treatment with chymotrypsin or trypsin, but not after treatment with RNase or DNase. Supernatant fluids with SIRS activity also contain MIF activity and these two activities have not been dissociated. It is conceivable that they represent different biological expressions of the same molecule (13-15,21).

195

   We have recently generated and cloned a T cell hybridoma (393.D2.6)
which produces SIRS constitutively (2,4,12). A dilution analysis
comparing suppressive activity from culture fluids of con A-activated
spleen cells and the SIRS-producing T cell hybridoma is shown in
Figure 1.

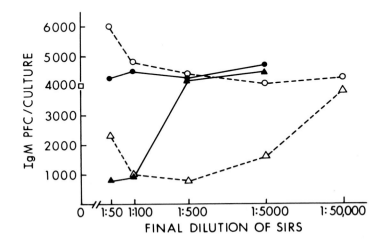

FIG. 1. Comparison of suppression of day 5 PFC responses to
SRBC by conventional and hybridoma-derived SIRS added at
culture initiation. ▲——▲ conventional SIRS; △——△
hybridoma-derived SIRS (393.D2.6); ●——● conventional
control fluid; o——o hybridoma-derived control fluid
(394.C4.5).

Suppression of PFC responses by conventional SIRS was maximal at
dilutions of 1:50 or 1:100, but was not observed at dilutions of 1:500 or
greater. By contrast, hybridoma-derived SIRS still yielded greater than
50% suppression at dilutons of 1:5000. Figure 1 also shows that
supernatant fluids from another fusion product had no suppressive
activity throughout the range of dilutions tested. SIRS suppresses PFC
responses with a characteristic kinetic pattern; PFC responses initiate
normally for the first three days of culture, and prematurely terminate
such that up to 90% suppression is observed on day 5. Both conventional
SIRS (1:50 dilution) and hybridoma-derived SIRS (1:500 dilution) mediate
the same kinetic pattern of suppression (Figure 2).

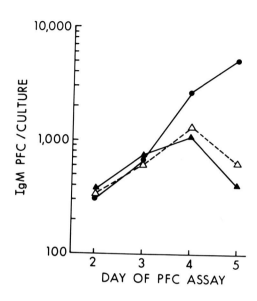

FIG. 2 Comparison of kinetics of suppression of PFC responses
to SRBC by conventional and hybridoma-derived SIRS added at
culture initiation. ▲——▲ conventional SIRS (1:50 final
dilution); △——△ hybridoma-derived SIRS (1:500 final
dilution); ●——● conventional control fluid (1:50 final
dilution).

The target of SIRS activity is the macrophage (Mø) (1,14,19). Kinetic
analysis of antibody responses in cultures with SIRS-treated Mø shows a
pattern of suppression identical to that shown in Figure 2 (1,12,19,20).
SIRS does not inactivate Mø function; suppression by SIRS-treated Mø is
an active, but reversible, process mediated by a soluble factor,
macrophage derived suppressor factor (Mø-SF) (1,3,12,20). Mø-SF is
released by Mø 24-72 hr after a 2 hr exposure to SIRS and can act by
inhibiting B cell proliferation and/or differentiation into
antibody-producing cells and can also act by directly interfering with
antibody secretion by mature B cells (3,12).

These observations are compatible with this sequence of events in
SIRS-mediated suppression of antibody responses. Macrophages in culture
rapidly become refractory to the effects of SIRS, explaining why SIRS
must be added at culture initiation to mediate suppression. SIRS-treated
Mø require 48-72 hr to release Mø-SF. Therefore, responses can develop
in a normal manner during the first three days of culture until Mø-SF is
present in sufficient quantity to inhibit both B cell proliferation and
antibody secretion (12).

PROPERTIES OF Mø-SF

Mø-SF can be obtained from Mø treated with conventional or hybridoma-derived SIRS (2). Mø-SF can also be obtained following treatment of the Mø-like cell line RAW 264.7 (but not several other Mø cell lines) with SIRS (1,12). Mø-SF is a protein with an apparent mol. wt. of 50,000–55,000 daltons; biological activity is lost following treatment with chymotrypsin, at pH 3 or temperatures greater than 70°C. Activity is also lost after reaction with sulfhydryl reagents (2-mercaptoethanol, dithiothreitol or cysteine, 10^{-9}M), sodium borohydride (10^{-9}M), certain amines (taurine, ethanolamine and alanine (10^{-4}–10^{-2}M) and iodide (10^{-7}M), but not thiocyanate, bromide or chloride (10^{-3}M) (1,12).

Inactivation of Mø-SF by sulfhydryl reagents could suggest that Mø-SF has a critical disulfide group essential for biological activity. However, the low concentration of sulfhydryl necessary to inactivate Mø-SF and the fact that amines and iodide also inactivate Mø-SF argue against this interpretation. Each of the above reagents can also serve as electron acceptors suggesting that an active moiety on Mø-SF may be an oxidizing equivalent, which when reduced by an appropriate substrate leads to loss of biological activity. These properties further suggest that the suppressive properties of Mø-SF may be due to its ability to oxidize cellular componenets essential for either cell division or antibody secretion (1–3,12).

MECHANISM OF Mø-SF PRODUCTION

Release of Mø-SF by SIRS-treated Mø is not sensitive to inhibitors of protein synthesis (puromycin or cycloheximide) or inhibitors of prostaglandin synthesis (indomethacin) (6,22) indicating that Mø-SF is not a newly synthesized product or a prostaglandin. By contrast, catalase or cyanide completely inhibit generation of Mø-SF indicating that peroxide is necessary for Mø-SF formation (catalase sensitivity) and that a hemoprotein may be necessary at some stage in the process (cyanide sensitivity) (18). Since SIRS and Mø-SF have many similar properties a possible interpretation of these results is that peroxide produced by Mø converts SIRS to Mø-SF (2,4,12). To test this possibility hybridoma- or conventionally-derived SIRS was treated with various concentrations of H_2O_2 and Mø-SF activity determined. Reaction of SIRS with 10^{-12} – 10^{-13}M H_2O_2 at 4°C for 15–20 min yields Mø-SF. Conversion of SIRS to Mø-SF by H_2O_2 is inhibited by catalase or cyanide, but once formed, Mø-SF is not inactivated by either reagent (2,4,12). This suggests the following reaction sequences:

$$\text{SIRS} + \text{Mø} \longrightarrow \text{Mø-SF or SIRS} + H_2O_2 \longrightarrow \text{Mø-SF}$$

Thus, Mø appear to serve only as a source of peroxide (8–10) and Mø-SF appears to be modified SIRS (2,4,12).

The ability of SIRS to combine with H_2O_2 in a cyanide-sensitive fashion suggests that SIRS may have certain peroxidase-like properties. To further explore this possibility and to compare Mø-SF produced by SIRS-treated Mø and the SIRS + H_2O_2 reaction, different peroxidase substrates were tested for their ability to inactivate Mø-SF. The following peroxidase substrates inactivated Mø-SF by approximately 50%

at the concentrations indicated: phenylenediamine (10^{-8}M); iodide and hydroquinone (10^{-7}M); pyrogallol (10^{-6}M); o-dianisidine, p-amino-benzoic acid and tyrosine (10^{-5}M); and ascorbic acid (10^{-4}M) (4,12). All reagents tested inactivated both sources of Mø-SF at concentrations, indicated, but none of these reagents inactivate SIRS at these concentrations. Finally, those reagents which inactivate Mø-SF or prevent its formation should block SIRS-mediated suppression of antibody responses. To test this possibility, SIRS was added to cultures on day 0 and the putative reversing agents were added on day 3 of culture when conversion of SIRS to Mø-SF was maximal. Iodide, 2-mercaptoethanol, catalase and to a lesser extent tyrosine, ascorbic acid and p-aminobenzoic acid effectively reversed or prevented SIRS-mediated suppression (4,12).

MECHANISMS OF Mø-SF ACTION

Mø-SF nonspecifically suppresses all types of immune responses tested in a dose dependent fashion. These include antibody responses to T cell-dependent and T cell-independent antigens, mixed lymphocyte and cytotoxic lymphocyte responses to alloantigens, DNA synthetic responses to T and B cell mitogens and, in addition, proliferation of several tumor cell lines (MOPC-315, EL-4, P815, and L929) (3,12). Since Mø-SF is active in each of these systems, it is important to note that one strain of mouse, DBA/1, appears to be resistant to Mø-SF. Spleen cells from DBA/1 mice produce both SIRS and Mø-SF, but antibody responses and proliferative responses to T cell or B cell mitogens are not suppressed by Mø-SF. Furthermore, responses by B10.Q (B10 background, H-2^q) spleen cells are suppressed by SIRS, whereas D1.LP (DBA/1 background, H-2^b) spleen cell responses are not suppressed indicating that susceptibility is not controlled by major histocompatibility complex genes. This system should be useful in determining how Mø-SF acts.

In contrast to SIRS, where suppression of antibody responses is apparent only on days 4 and 5, Mø-SF suppresses responses throughout the culture period when added at culture initiation. Under appropriate conditions, suppression can be reversed up to 72 hr of culture by 10^{-4}M 2-mercaptoethanol or dithiothreitol, but not by taurine or cysteine. Additionally, Mø-SF suppresses antibody responses when added late in the culture period. Expression of antibody responses can be inhibited by greater than 80% by Mø-SF added as late as 2 hr before assay. Similar rapid effects of Mø-SF have been observed in inhibition of T cell responses and tumor cell division (3,12).

Studies on inhibition of tumor cell proliferation have provided considerable insight into the mechanism of action of Mø-SF and have strengthened our working hypothesis that Mø-SF is a reversible, general inhibitor of cell proliferation. Proliferation of the plasmacytoma cell line, MOPC-315, is reproducibly completely inhibited by small amounts of Mø-SF and has been used in the following studies. Complete inhibition of proliferation by more rapidly dividing cell lines (EL-4 and P815) requires larger amounts of Mø-SF, approximately 5 times that required for MOPC-315, although repeated addition of the smaller amounts of Mø-SF will also result in complete inhibition of proliferation (3). Mø-SF inhibits division of MOPC-315, as reflected by cell number, very rapidly (within 4 hr), whereas, significant decreases in thymidine incorporation into DNA are not apparent for 8-16 hr after addition of Mø-SF (Figure 3) (3,12).

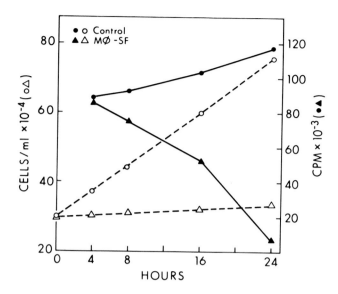

FIG. 3. Dissociation of inhibition of cell proliferation from
inhibition of DNA synthesis in nonsynchronous MOPC-315
plasmacytoma cells exposed to Mɸ-SF at time 0. DNA synthesis
was assessed by incorporation of ^{3}H-thymidine into DNA (CPM
X 10^{-3}) during a 2 hr pulse, cell proliferation was assessed
by viable cell counts (cells/ml X 10^{-4}).

    This dichotomy suggests that Mɸ-SF inhibits cell division directly,
and that decreases in DNA synthesis are secondary to this event. To
determine at what point in the cell cycle Mɸ-SF acts, MOPC-315 cells were
synchronized with a double thymidine block (3,5,12); under these
conditions the cells divide 6-7 hr after release from the thymidine block
and go through two cycles of synchronous division. Mɸ-SF was added at
various times after release as indicated in Figure 4.
    Mɸ-SF added at any point before the onset of cell division completely
inhibits any increase in cell number. When Mɸ-SF is added during the
cell division period, no further increase in cell number is observed.
However, addition of 10^{-3} M 2-ME to the completely inhibited MOPC-315
population leads to an immediate and almost complete reversal of the
block in cell division induced by Mɸ-SF (3,12). These data suggest that
Mɸ-SF does not interfere with the processes leading up to cell division,
but has a direct effect on mitosis which can be reversed by 2-ME.
Further studies with nonsynchronous MOPC-315 cells exposed to Mɸ-SF
demonstrate that these cells collect at a stage just prior to cell
division and can be released into mitosis with 2-ME within 1 hr (3,12).

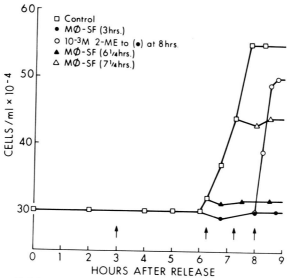

FIG. 4.   Inhibition of proliferation of synchronized MOPC-315 plasmacytoma cells by MØ-SF and reversal of the inhibition by 2-mercaptoethanol (2-ME). MOPC-315 cells were synchronized by a double thymidine block; MØ-SF was added at the indicated times after release and cells were enumerated at the indicated times thereafter.

CONCLUSION

The mechanism of action of soluble immune response suppressor (SIRS), as currently perceived is presented schematically in Figure 5.

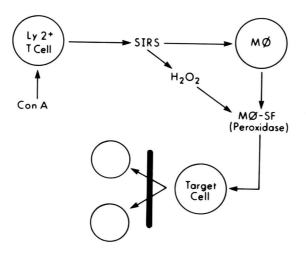

FIG. 5.   Pathways for inhibition of cell proliferation or immune responses by soluble immune response suppressor (SIRS), a product of concanavalin A-activated suppressor T cells.

Concanavalin A (Con A) activates Ly 2^+ T cells which function as nonspecific suppressor T cells. One mechanism of action of these cells is the production of SIRS, a glycoprotein with a mol wt of approximately 55,000 daltons which nonspecifically suppresses T cell and B cell responses. SIRS acts via macrophages which release macrophage–derived suppressor factor (M∅–SF) which appears to be a potent and rapid but reversible inhibitor of cell division. This pathway accounts for all phenomenology related to the action of SIRS. Moreover, the function of macrophages in this pathway appears to involve only the release of peroxide. The reaction of peroxide with SIRS, which has properties of a hemoprotein with peroxidase-like activity, generates M∅–SF, the oxidized counterpart of SIRS which is capable of inhibiting mitosis presumably by oxidizing cellular components essential for this process.

The applicability of this pathway to immunosuppression and to inhibition of cell division in general remains to be elucidated, as does the usefulness of SIRS/M∅–SF-like molecules in cancer therapy. It is worth considering that nonspecific inhibitors of immune responses, such as interferon and BCG, may act via a SIRS/M∅–SF mechanism either directly or indirectly. These inhibitory factors may themselves have SIRS–like properties, or may induce formation of SIRS. Considerable evidence is available demonstrating production of peroxides by macrophages (8–10), an essential step in this pathway. The small quantity of peroxide required to efficiently convert SIRS to M∅–SF suggests that this pathway could be a common denominator in the mechanism of action of nonspecific immunosuppressive factors and inhibitors of proliferation. The further investigation of the SIRS/M∅–SF pathway could provide fundamental information on regulation of cell division. This investigation and any potential application to cancer therapy will be facilitated once the structure and amino acid composition and sequence of SIRS are known. The availability of hybridomas constitutively producing large quantities of SIRS should make this a reality in the near future.

SUMMARY

The mechanism of action of soluble immune response suppressor (SIRS), a product of concanavalin A–activated murine Ly 2^+ T cells, which nonspecifically suppresses immune responses in vitro is discussed. Macrophages, after exposure to SIRS, release macrophage–derived suppressor factor (M∅–SF), a potent inhibitor of proliferation of T cells, B cells and several tumor cell lines. The effects of M∅–SF on cell division are rapid, but reversible, and several observations suggest that M∅–SF may be an oxidizing agent. Generation of M∅–SF by macrophages is insensitive to inhibitors of protein and prostaglandin synthesis, but is blocked by catalase suggesting that peroxide is necessary. SIRS and M∅–SF are proteins (mol wt ~ 55,000 daltons) with similar properties; M∅–SF appears to be modified SIRS and peroxide produced by macrophage converts SIRS to M∅–SF. Reaction of SIRS with H_2O_2 generates M∅–SF; this reaction is blocked by cyanide and catalase and a variety of peroxidase substrates effectively inactivate M∅–SF. Collectively, these data strongly suggest that SIRS is a peroxidase which is converted by macrophages or H_2O_2 to M∅–SF, an oxidizing agent whose biological activity appears to be mediated by oxidation of cellular components essential for cell division. The availability of T cell hybridomas producing SIRS will greatly facilitate its purification, characterization and determination of mechanism of action.

ACKNOWLEDGMENTS

This investigation was supported by USPHS Research Grants AI-13915 and AI-15353. Dr. Aune is supported by USPHS Training Grant AI-07163.

Figures 1 and 2 are reproduced from "Monoclonal Soluble Immune Response Suppressor (SIRS) Derived from T Cell Hybridomas" by T.M. Aune and C.W. Pierce in <u>Monoclonal Antibodies and T Cell Hybridomas</u>, G.J. Hammerling, U. Hammerling and J.F. Kearney, editors, Elsevier Publishing Corp., NY with permission of the publishers. Figures 3, 4, 5 are reproduced from "Mechanism of Action of Soluble Immune Response Suppressor (SIRS)" by C.W. Pierce and T.M. Aune in <u>Advances in Immunopharmacology</u>, J. Haddon, P. Mullen, L. Chedid and F. Spreafico, editors, Pergamon Press Ltd., Oxford, with permission of the publishers.

REFERENCES

1. Aune, T.M., and Pierce, C.W. (1981): <u>J. Immunol.</u> (In press).
2. Aune, T.M., and Pierce, C.W. (1981): In: <u>Monoclonal Antibodies and T Cell Hybridomas</u>, edited by G.J. Hammerling, U. Hammerling and J.F. Kearney, Elsevier Publishing Corp., New York (In press).
3. Aune, T.M., and Pierce, C.W. (1981): <u>J. Immunol.</u> (In press).
4. Aune, T.M., and Pierce, C.W. (1981): <u>Proc. Nat. Acad. Sci. (USA)</u> (In press).
5. Byars, N., and Kidson, C. (1970): <u>Nature</u> 226:648-650.
6. Humes., J.L., Borney, R.J., Pelus, L., Dahlgre, M.E., Sadowski, S.J., Kuehl, F.A., and Davies, P. (1977): <u>Nature</u> 269:149-151.
7. Jandinski, J., Cantor, H., Tadakuma, T., Peavy, D.L., and Pierce, C.W. (1976): <u>J. Exp. Med.</u> 143:1382-1390.
8. Metzger, Z., Hoffeld, J.T., Oppenheim, J.J. (1980): <u>J. Immunol.</u> 124:983-988.
9. Nathan, C.F., and Root, R.K. (1977): <u>J. Exp. Med.</u> 146:1648-1662.
10. Nathan, C.F., Silverstein, S.C., Brukner, L.H., Cohn, Z.A. (1976): <u>J. Exp. Med.</u> 149:84-99.
11. Peavy, D.L., and Pierce, C.W. (1974): <u>J. Exp. Med.</u> 140:356-369.
12. Pierce, C.W., and Aune, T.M. (1981): In: <u>Advances in Immunopharmacology</u>, edited by J. Hadden, P. Mullen, L. Chedid and F. Spreafico, Pergamon Press Ltd., Oxford (In press).
13. Pierce, C.W., and Kapp, J.A. (1976): <u>Contemp. Top. Immunobiol.</u> 5:91-144.
14. Pierce, C.W., and Kapp, J.A. (1981): In: <u>Molecular Mediators of Cellular Immunity</u>, edited by J.W. Hadden and W.E. Stewart, The Humana Press, Inc., Clifton, NJ (In press).
15. Pierce, C.W., T. Tadakuma (1977): <u>Prog. Immunol.</u> III:405-412.
16. Rich, R.R., and Pierce, C.W. (1973): <u>J. Exp. Med.</u> 137:649-659.
17. Rich, R.R., and Pierce, C.W. (1974): <u>J. Immunol.</u> 12:1360-1368.
18. Schonbaum, G.R., and Chance, B. (1976): In: <u>The Enzymes</u>, vol. XII, 3rd ed., edited by P.D. Boyer, pp. 363-408, Academic Press, NY.
19. Tadakuma, T., and Pierce, C.W. (1976): <u>J. Immunol.</u> 117:967-972.
20. Tadakuma, T., and Pierce, C.W. (1978): <u>J. Immunol.</u> 120:418-426.
21. Tadakuma, T., Kuhner A.L., Rich, R.R., David, J.R., and Pierce, C.W. (1976): <u>J. Immunol.</u> 117:323-330.
22. Webb, D.R., Jamisson, A.J., and Nowowiejski, I. (1976): <u>Cell Immunol.</u> 24:45-47.

Lymphokines and Thymic Hormones: Their Potential Utilization in Cancer Therapeutics, edited by A. L. Goldstein and M. A. Chirigos, Raven Press, New York © 1981.

Characterization of an Inhibitor of Monocyte Function in Effusions of Cancer Patients

George J. Cianciolo and Ralph Snyderman

Laboratory of Immune Effector Function, Howard Hughes Medical Institute, Division of Rheumatic and Genetic Diseases, Departments of Medicine and Microbiology and Immunology, Duke University Medical Center, Durham, North Carolina 27710

INTRODUCTION

Approaches to the development of cancer immunotherapy have generally focused on either the stimulation of immune responses to specific tumor antigens or on the non-specific activation of the host's immune system. Biological response modifiers (BRM) capable of stimulation of cells of the reticuloendothelial system have been extensively investigated during the last several years. Efforts to enhance the function of macrophages or monocytes have paralleled the growing awareness that these cells may play an important role in the restriction of growth or destruction of neoplasms (1). Indeed, previous investigations have shown that macrophages can destroy tumor cells both in vivo and in vitro (7, 17, 21). Immunotherapy directed at systemic, non-specific activation of the mononuclear phagocyte system has not, however, resulted in reproducible, clear-cut benefits to the tumor-bearing host. However, any effort to stimulate the tumoricidal capacity of the macrophages in tumor-bearing hosts should recognize that the tumor itself may locally and/or systemically abrogate the effects of the immunotherapeutic approaches. Several years ago this and other laboratories made the observation that the chemotactic responsiveness of monocytes was depressed in patients with cancer (3, 5, 14, 20, 24). An intriguing finding which emerged from these studies was that surgical removal of the tumor usually resulted in normalization of the patient's monocyte chemotactic response (23, 28) (Table 1). This observation suggested that the tumor itself was responsible for the defect in monocyte function in tumor-bearing individuals, perhaps by the release of a soluble mediator.

Initial efforts to isolate and characterize human tumor-associated inhibitors of monocyte function were hindered by the lack of a suitable assay. In vitro monocyte chemotaxis assays can give spurious results when materials tested for their effects on leukocyte function are not highly purified and contain both chemotactic and inhibitory activities. A murine system was therefore developed in order to assess the in vivo effects of intact tumor cells and tumor cell products on macrophage function. We showed that tumor cells, low molecular weight extracts thereof, or the plasma and urine of tumor-bearing mice were all capable of

TABLE 1. Effect of tumor removal on monocyte chemotactic responsiveness

| Patient | Neoplasm | Chemotactic Response[a] (±SE) | |
		Pre-Op	Post-Op
G.W.	Renal Adenocarcinoma	21.3±4.2	83.3±5.6
A.G.	Renal Adenocarcinoma	20.9±2.6	86.9±7.6
T.W.	Renal Adenocarcinoma	58.2±2.9	74.3±1.7
C.F.	Renal Adenocarcinoma	57.6±5.0	91.9±5.2
M.B.	Carcinoma Breast	49.2±0.9	78.3±1.3
C.M.	Carcinoma Breast	25.9±1.9	54.9±3.6
V.P.	Carcinoma Breast	37.6±5.4	52.6±5.0
M.P.	Carcinoma Breast	32.6±1.7	81.2±0.7
M.S.	Carcinoma Breast	48.2±2.6	69.2±1.9
M.W.	Carcinoma Breast	32.9±3.5	40.6±9.4
M.W.	Carcinoma Breast	46.6±3.6	114.2±3.9
A.W.	Carcinoma Breast	51.9±0.7	69.3±3.6
	Mean ± 1 SEM	40.6±3.7	74.2±5.5
		($p < 0.005$)	
Mean of Six Non-Cancer Patient Controls		69.9±10.3	70.9±4.9
		($p > 0.2$)	

[a]Mononuclear cell suspensions were obtained from the heparinized venous blood of patients by dextran sedimentation and Ficoll-Hypaque density gradient centrifugation of the leukocyte-rich plasma. The cells were washed and resuspended to 1.5×10^6 monocytes/ml in GBSS, pH 7.0. Two-tenths ml of this cell suspension was placed in the upper compartment of a modified Boyden chemotaxis chamber. The upper compartment was separated from the lower compartment, which contained 20% (v/v) of lymphocyte-derived chemotactic factor (LDCF), by a polycarbonate filter with 5.0 µm diameter pores. The chambers were incubated for 90 min at 37°C, the filters removed, fixed, and stained. The number of cells which had migrated through the filter was determined for each of twenty oil immersion (1000X) fields and averaged.

depressing macrophage accumulation at inflammatory sites (10, 22, 26). Other laboratories have also reported similar defects in macrophage function in tumor-bearing animals (6, 13, 18, 19, 27). In addition, we demonstrated that low molecular weight extracts of certain oncogenic murine leukemia viruses could also inhibit macrophage migration (9). In these studies we reported that one of the structural components of the virus envelope, $P_{15}(E)$, depressed macrophage accumulation in mice.

Our recent development of an assay which measures one of the early responses of monocytes to chemotaxins (11), i.e., their change in shape from a round to an elongated, triangular, "polarized" configuration (Fig. 1), has allowed us to study the effects of various fluids from humans with cancer on monocyte function. Using this assay we have found that human cancerous effusions contain novel and potent inhibitors of monocyte responses to chemotaxins and that these inhibitors are recognized by monoclonal antibody reactive to the type C retroviral protein,

$P_{15}(E)$.

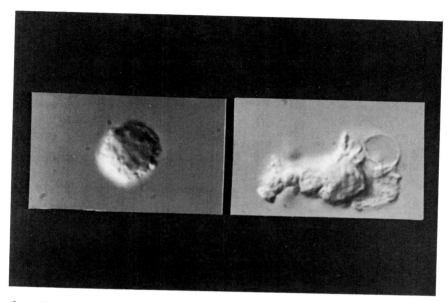

FIG. 1. Change in morphology of human peripheral blood monocytes exposed to FMLP. Cells were suspended at a concentration of 1 x 10^6 peroxidase positive cells/ml in GBSS and then incubated for 20 min at 37°C with either GBSS (left) or 10 nM FMLP (right), fixed, and then examined. Nomarski interference contrast optics X800.

METHODS AND RESULTS

The monocyte polarization assay was used as previously described (11). Briefly, mononuclear cells were isolated from heparinized venous blood (10 units/ml; Upjohn Co., Kalamazoo, Mich.) of healthy volunteers by sedimentation at room temperature for 30 min with dextran followed by Ficoll-Hypaque density gradient centrifugation of the leukocyte-rich supernatant (4). The cells were then washed twice in Gey's balanced salt solution (GBSS, pH 7.0; Flow Laboratories, McLean, Va.) containing sodium bicarbonate and 2% bovine serum albumin and resuspended to 1.6 x 10^6 peroxidase positive (16) cells per ml. The cell suspension was then incubated in polypropylene tubes for 10 min at 37°C with either buffer alone or buffer containing the material being tested. A chemotactic stimulant, either the synthetic peptide N-formyl-methionyl-leucyl-phenylalanine (FMLP; Sigma Chemical Co., Saint Louis, Mo.), zymosan-activated human serum (AHS) (25), or lymphocyte-derived chemotactic factor (LDCF) (2), was then added at a concentration sufficient to induce maximal polarization. The cells were incubated an additional 7.5 min, fixed by the addition of ice-cold 10% formaldehyde (0.01 M PO_4, pH 7.2), and 200-400 cells examined using phase contrast microscopy (400X). The percentage of monocytes polarized was calculated as

$$\% \text{ monocytes polarized} = \frac{\% \text{ total cells polarized}}{\% \text{ peroxidase positive cells in cell suspension}} \times 100$$

Percent inhibition of monocyte polarization was calculated as

$$\% \text{ Inhibition} = 1 - \frac{(\% \text{ Polarized to Chemotaxin})_{Tx} - (\% \text{ Polarized to GBSS})}{(\% \text{ Polarized to Chemotaxin}) - (\% \text{ Polarized to GBSS})} \times 100$$

where Tx represents cells treated with effusion or some fraction thereof.

Polymorphonuclear leukocyte (PMN) polarization was performed in a similar fashion but at pH 7.2.

Effusions were obtained from patients with a variety of types of neoplasms or non-cancerous diseases. These diagnoses and other chemical information regarding these patients are more fully described elsewhere (15) but included patients with: adenocarcinoma of the pancreas, ovary, lung, breast, or colon; hepatoma; melanoma; lymphoma; squamous cell carcinoma of the lung; melanosarcoma; liposarcoma; renal cell carcinoma; undifferentiated carcinoma of the lung; and acute myelocytic leukemia. Non-cancerous diseases included: cirrhosis; endometriosis; uremia; congestive heart failure; pulmonary embolus; lupus serositis; bacterial empyema; bacterial peritonitis; and fibrocystic breast disease. Effusions were standardized using absorbance at 280 nm and the pH adjusted to 7.0 for compatibility with the assay conditions.

Incubation of cancerous effusions with human monocytes resulted in the inhibition of their subsequent polarization to the synthetic chemotactic peptide FMLP (Fig. 2). At the highest concentration tested the average inhibition by the cancerous effusions (n=16) was 55.9 ± 12.7% while the non-cancerous fluids (n=17) inhibited only 6.2 ± 4.2%. The inhibitory activity in the cancerous effusions appeared to affect the monocyte rather than the chemotactic factor. Preincubation of the cells with effusion (10 min) followed by exposure to the chemotactic factor resulted in inhibition of polarization. If the chemotactic factor was preincubated with the effusion (10 min) followed by the addition of cells, monocyte polarization was normal (15). In addition, preincubation of monocytes with cancerous effusion, followed by extensive washing of the cells, still resulted in inhibition of polarization (15).

The inhibitory activity for monocyte polarization in cancerous effusions did not affect PMNs (12, 15). Incubation of PMNs with cancerous effusions for varying lengths of time did not affect their subsequent polarization to several different doses of chemotactic factors. This specificity for the monocyte is identical to that observed for the defect in chemotactic responsiveness in cancer patients in that their monocyte but not PMN responses are abnormal (30). In addition to inhibiting monocyte polarization to the synthetic chemotactic peptide FMLP, cancerous effusions also inhibited polarization to the naturally-derived chemotactic factors present in zymosan-activated human serum or in Con-A stimulated lymphocyte culture supernatants (12, 15).

Fractionation of cancerous effusions using high-pressure liquid chromatography and a gel-filtration system suggested that there are three peaks of inhibitory activity with approximate molecular weights of ≥ 200,000 daltons, ca. 40-60,000 daltons, and ca. 10-25,000 daltons (15). Fractionation of effusion from patients with non-cancerous diseases revealed only a single peak of inhibitory activity with an approximate

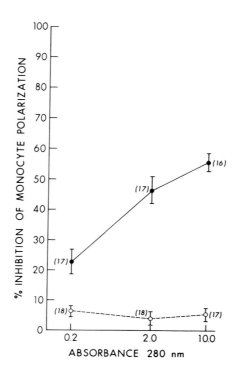

FIG. 2.   Effect of cancerous (●) or non-cancerous (○) effusions on monocyte polarization.   Effusions were incubated at the indicated concentrations with normal human peripheral blood monocytes for 10 min at 37°C.
FMLP (10 nM) was added, the cell suspensions incubated an additional 7.5
min, fixed, and 200 cells examined using phase contrast microscopy (400X).
Percent inhibition of polarization was calculated as

$$\% \text{ Inhib.} = 1 - \frac{(\% \text{ Polarized to FMLP})_{\text{Tx}} - (\% \text{ Polarized to GBSS})}{(\% \text{ Polarized to FMLP}) - (\% \text{ Polarized to GBSS})} \times 100$$

where Tx = cells treated with effusion.

molecular weight of $\geq$ 200,000 daltons (15).   Characterization of the low
molecular weight inhibitory activity of cancerous effusion obtained by
their ultrafiltration through Amicon CF_{25} centriflo cones (normal M.W.
cutoff of 25,000 daltons) indicated that the activity was stable at 56°C
for 30 min and trypsin-sensitive (12).
    Since studies in mice had suggested that the retroviral structural
component $P_{15}(E)$ was capable of inhibiting macrophage accumulation in
vivo we tested the effect of monoclonal antibody reactive to $P_{15}(E)$ on
the inhibitory activity for monocyte polarization contained in human cancerous effusions.   Monoclonal antibody (7.5 μg)of was incubated for 15
min at 22°C with 500 μl of effusion or ultrafiltrate of effusion.   The
antibody was then removed by incubation for 12 min at 22°C with formalin-

fixed Staphlococcus aureus followed by centrifugation. The absorbed effusion was then tested as previously described. The inhibitory activity
contained in the ultrafiltrates of eight different cancerous effusions
was removed by absorption with monoclonal anti-P_{15}(E) while 7 different
monoclonal antibodies had no effect (12). Table 2 is a representative
example of the effects of absorption with monoclonal anti-P_{15}(E). As a
control, a low molecular weight extract of Rauscher leukemia virus (RLV),
a virus known to contain P_{15}(E), was used. Monoclonal antibody to P_{15}
(E) but not monoclonal anti-GP70 or murine IgG_{2a} was capable of removing
almost all of the inhibitory activity.

TABLE 2.   Effect of absorption by monoclonal anti-P_{15}(E) on inhibitory
activity of ultrafiltrates of cancerous effusions[a]

Effusion[b]	% Inhibition ($\pm$SE) of Monocyte Polarization after Preincubation with[c]			
	Buffer	aP_{15}(E)	aGP70	IgG_{2a}
A	58.4±4.3	4.3±1.2	50.0±0	56.7±12.0
B	67.6±1.1	9.4±0	63.0±12.3	63.0±0
C	46.5±8.6	7.9±1.5	52.4±9.0	57.9±9.0
RLV	60.6±2.1	0.8±1.3	55.5±7.2	55.5±3.1

[a]Five-tenths ml of ultrafiltrate was incubated for 15 min at 22°C
with 10 μl of GBSS or GBSS containing 7.5 μg of the indicated antibody.
Twenty-five μl of formalin-fixed Staph. a. was added, the mixture incubated an additional 12 min at 22°C, and the Staph. a. removed by centrifugation.

[b]Ultrafiltrates were prepared from (A) pleural fluid, squamous carcinoma of the lung, (B) ascites fluid, melanoma and (C) pleural fluid, metastatic carcinoma of unknown origin or from (RLV) sonicated Rauscher leukemia virus (2 mg/ml).

[c]One-tenth ml of absorbed ultrafiltrate was incubated for 10 min at
37°C with 0.3 ml of cell suspension containing 4.8 x 10^5 peroxidase-pos-
itive mononuclear cells. One-tenth ml of GBSS or 50 nM FMLP in GBSS was
then added to each of duplicate tubes, the tubes incubated an additional
7.5 min at 37°C, the cells fixed and the percent of polarized monocytes
determined. The percent inhibition of polarization was calculated as

$$\% \text{ Inhib.} = \frac{1-(\% \text{ Polarized to FMLP})_{Tx}-(\% \text{ Polarized to GBSS})}{(\% \text{ Polarized to FMLP}) -(\% \text{ Polarized to GBSS})} \times 100$$

where Tx = cells treated with ultrafiltrates.

An affinity column was prepared by coupling 5 mg of monoclonal anti-
P_{15}(E) to 1 gm of cyanogen-bromide activated Sepharose 4B. This affinity column was then used to absorb cancerous and non-cancerous effusions.
Fifty ml of four different cancerous effusions and three benign effusions
were individually passed through the affinity column. The column was
washed extensively and bound material eluted by lowering the pH. Significant inhibitory activity for monocyte polarization could be detected at
dilutions of up to 1:8000 in the eluates of the four cancerous effusions

while no activity was detected in the eluates of the benign effusions (12). Since the protein concentration required to attain 50% inhibition of polarization was ca. 5 mg/ml with the unfractionated cancerous effusions and <50 ng/ml with the affinity column eluates this procedure resulted in a >100,000-fold increase in specific activity of the inhibitory factors.

DISCUSSION

The recent development of a rapid, quantitative assay to measure monocyte responsiveness to chemotactic stimuli has allowed us to begin investigating the mechanisms of the monocyte chemotactic defect in cancer patients. Of the seventeen cancerous effusions thus far tested, all contained significant inhibitory activity for monocyte polarization while none of the 17 benign effusions tested had inhibitory activity (15). The inhibitory activity for monocytes in cancerous effusions does not affect the polarization of PMNs. This is identical to the cell specificity previously observed for the chemotactic defects in cancer patients and tumor-bearing mice (26, 30). Preliminary characterization of the inhibitory activity from cancerous effusions indicates that a significant portion of it is of low molecular weight, is relatively heat stable and is, at least in part, proteinaceous (12). Furthermore, monoclonal antibody reactive to the $P_{15}(E)$ component of type C retroviruses is capable of specifically absorbing the inhibitory activity from cancerous effusions. Use of anti-$P_{15}(E)$ affinity columns on a large scale basis should allow purification of the inhibitory factors in quantities sufficient to complete their characterization.

The significance of an antibody reactive to a retroviral protein being capable of absorbing the inhibitory activity from human cancerous effusions is not yet clear. Our earlier murine studies had indeed suggested that $P_{15}(E)$ played a role in the ability of retrovirus extracts to inhibit macrophage function (9). Furthermore, data suggested that both viral and murine tumor-derived inhibitors of macrophage accumulation shared several physiochemical and antigenic characteristics (8). Studies by Thiel et al. (29) have recently shown that $P_{15}(E)$ of many species is broadly cross-reactive. Therefore, the inhibitory factors in human cancerous effusions could be $P_{15}(E)$. However, the possibility exists that malignant transformation induces the production of a protein which is not $P_{15}(E)$ but merely is antigenically similar to it.

It is too early to determine whether isolation and characterization of the monocyte polarization inhibitor will have practical implication for the immunotherapy of various neoplasms but this could be the case. Evidence thus far accumulated suggests, however, that screening for the inhibitor might serve as a useful diagnostic tool. Indeed, in our initial studies three fluids were examined before a diagnosis had been made and in each case the polarization data correctly predicted whether the cancer was present (15).

SUMMARY

The development of a new assay which measures one of the early respones of monocytes to chemotaxins, their change in shape from round to an elongated, polarized configuration, has allowed us to determine if the fluids of cancer patients contained substances which inhibit monocyte chemotactic responsiveness. We have found inhibitory activity in all of

17 cancer fluids tested thus far but in none of 17 non-cancerous fluids. Much of the inhibitory activity was of low (<25,000 daltons) molecular weight, relatively heat stable and trypsin-sensitive. Monoclonal antibody reactive to the $P_{15}(E)$ component of type C retroviruses was capable of absorbing the inhibitory activity from cancerous effusions. Use of an immunoabsorbent column prepared with monoclonal anti-$P_{15}(E)$ has resulted in the isolation of inhibitory material with a greater than 100,000-fold increase in specific activity. The diagnostic and therapeutic implications of these findings await further investigation.

REFERENCES

1. Adams, D.O. and Snyderman, R. (1979): J. Natl. Cancer Inst., 62: 1341-1345.
2. Altman, L.C., Snyderman, R., Hausman, M.S., and Mergenhagen, S.E. (1973): J. Immunol., 110:801-810.
3. Boetcher, D.A. and Leonard, E.J. (1974): J. Natl. Cancer Inst., 52: 1091-1099.
4. Boyum, A. (1968): Scand. J. Clin. Lab. Invest., 21 (Suppl. 97):77-89.
5. Brosman, S. (1976): In: Neoplasm Immunity: Mechanisms, edited by R.G. Crispen, pp. 149-156. ITR, Chicago, Illinois.
6. Brozna, J.P. and Ward, P.A. (1979): J. Clin. Invest., 64:302-311.
7. Cerottini, J.C. and Brunner, K.T. (1974): Adv. Immunol., 18:67-132.
8. Cianciolo, G.J., Bolognesi, D.P., and Snyderman, R. (1980): Fed. Proc., 39(3):478A.
9. Cianciolo, G.J., Matthews, T.J., Bolognesi, D.P., and Snyderman, R. (1980): J. Immunol., 124:2900-2905.
10. Cianciolo, G.J., Herberman, R.B., and Snyderman, R. (1980): J. Natl. Cancer Inst., 65:829-834.
11. Cianciolo, G.J. and Snyderman, R. (1981): J. Clin. Invest., 67:60-68.
12. Cianciolo, G.J. and Snyderman, R. (submitted for publication).
13. Fauve, R.M., Hevin, B., Jacob, H., Gaillard, J.A., and Jacob, F. (1974): Proc. Natl. Acad. Sci. USA, 71:4052-4056.
14. Hausman, M.S., Brosman, S., Snyderman, R., Mickey, M.R., and Fahey, J. (1975): J. Natl. Cancer Inst., 55:1047-1054.
15. Hunter, J., Cianciolo, G., Silva, J., Haskill, J.S., and Snyderman, R. (submitted for publication).
16. Kaplow, L.S. (1965): Blood, 26:215-219.
17. Levy, M.H. and Wheelock, E.F. (1974): Adv. Cancer Res., 20:131-163.
18. Normann, S.J., Schardt, M., and Sorkin, E. (1979): J. Natl. Cancer Inst., 63:825-833.
19. North, R.J., Kirstein, D.P., and Tuttle, R.L. (1976): J. Exp. Med., 143:559-573.
20. Rubin, R.H., Cosimi, A.B., and Goetzl, E.J. (1976): Cell. Immunol. Immunopathol., 6:376-388.
21. Shin, H.S., Hayden, M., Langley, S., Kaliss, N., and Smith, M.R. (1975): J. Immunol., 114:1255-1263.
22. Snyderman, R. and Cianciolo, G.J. (1979): J. Reticuloendothel. Soc. 26:453-458.
23. Snyderman, R., Meadows, L., Holder, W., and Wells, S. Jr. (1978): J. Natl. Cancer Inst., 60:737-740.
24. Snyderman, R. and Pike, M.C. (1977): Am. J. Pathol., 88:727-739.
25. Snyderman, R. and Pike, M.C. (1978): In: Leukocyte Chemotaxis,

edited by J.I. Gallin and P.G. Quie, pp. 73-78, Raven Press, New York.

26. Snyderman, R., Pike, M.C., Blaylock, B.L. and Weinstein, P. (1976): J. Immunol., 116:585-589.

27. Snyderman, R., Siegler, H., and Meadows, L. (1977): J. Natl. Cancer Inst., 58:37-41

28. Stevenson, M. and Meltzer, M.S. (1976): J. Natl. Cancer Inst., 57: 847-852.

29. Thiel, H.J., Broughton, E.M., Matthews, T.J., Schäfer, W., and Bolognesi, D.P. (1981): Virology (in press).

30. Wilson, J. and Snyderman, R. (1978): Clin. Res., 26:378A.

Lymphokines and Thymic Hormones: Their Potential Utilization in Cancer Therapeutics, edited by A. L. Goldstein and M. A. Chirigos, Raven Press, New York © 1981.

Macromolecular Synthesis in Lymphokine-Producing and Responding Cells

Luigi Varesio, Howard T. Holden, and Donatella Taramelli

Laboratory of Immunodiagnosis, National Cancer Institute, National Institutes of Health, Bethesda, Maryland 20205

Upon activation, lymphocytes undergo a complex series of changes, which lead to the acquisition of many immunologically relevant activities such as proliferation, cytotoxicity, antibody synthesis and lymphokine production (for review see 16). The production of lymphokines (LK) is one of the earliest events associated with the activation of lymphocytes, either by mitogens or antigens, with LK becoming detectable in culture supernatants 4-6 hr after stimulation (24).

Lymphokines seem to play an important role in resistance to parasitic and bacterial infections, as well as in antitumor responses (15). Moreover, detailed studies in vitro showed that LK have a variety of stimulatory effects on lymphoid and other cells such as macrophages, lymphocytes, fibroblasts, granulocytes and osteoclasts (4). Macrophages (MØ) treated in vitro with LK undergo a series of metabolic and functional changes. They show increased production of proteolytic enzymes, such as elastase, proteases and collagenases (3,8,11). They have an increased release of hydrogen peroxide and superoxide (12,13). In addition, LK-treated MØ are more phagocytic, killing bacteria and protozoa more efficiently, and are both cytolytic and cytostatic against tumor cells (2,17). Since MØ recovered from tumor bearing hosts, or from animals affected by inflamatory processes show characteristics similar to those of LK-activated MØ, it has been suggested that LK could act in vivo as physiological mediators (6,9,15).

The production of LK, as well as other immune responses, can be negatively regulated by suppressor cells. It has been shown that impaired production of LK occurs in tumor-bearing mice and this has been attributed to the presence of suppressor MØ (22). Indeed, MØ taken from animals bearing tumors or injected with immunoadjuvants such as Corynebacterium parvum (C. parvum) are able to suppress the production of LK (22,23).

Recently, we have demonstrated that lymphokines themselves are involved in the generation of suppressor cells. We have shown that upon in vitro stimulation of elicited MØ by LK, they developed the ability to suppress the production of lymphokines by activated lymphocytes (19) as well as to kill tumor cells. This suggests a LK-dependent, feed-back mechanism of control between MØ and lymphocytes.

A model of this regulatory system is outline in Fig. 1. Lymphocytes upon stimulation are triggered to produce a variety of soluble mediators

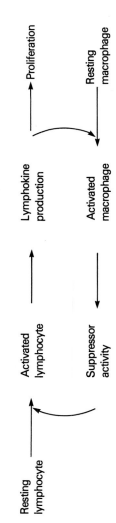

CELLULAR REGULATION OF LYMPHOKINE PRODUCTION

Resting lymphocyte → Activated lymphocyte → Lymphokine production → Proliferation

Activated lymphocyte → Suppressor activity → Activated macrophage → Resting macrophage

Figure I

which can affect different subpopulations of immunocompetent cells. Some lymphokines, operationally defined as macrophage activating factor, interact with resting MØ and induce these cells to perform a variety of effector and immunoregulatory functions. LK-treated MØ acquire the capacity to inhibit lymphokine production by activated lymphocytes. This process would limit the amount of LK produced in response to a stimulus. The consequent shortage of lymphokines would in turn limit the complete range of LK-dependent lymphocyte and MØ functions. Such a self-limiting system could represent an important homeostatic control mechanism during inflammatory processes and ensure a rapid recovery to normal conditions.

In such a model, little is known about the mechanisms of the reactions or the exact biochemical and metabolic events occurring within different cell populations. Since most changes in cell phenotype are dictated by the intracellular macromolecular synthesis and by the extracellular environment, we reasoned that an analysis of RNA and protein synthesis of lymphocytes and of macrophages, during their activation processes and during their interactions, could give interesting information about the mechanisms of activation and regulation.

Three different phases of the regulatory circuit outlined above were studied. First, we analyzed the RNA and protein synthesis required by lymphocytes during the production of LK in vitro. Second, since LK production is susceptible to the suppressor activity of MØ, we studied whether activated MØ could interfere with the intracellular events associated with lymphocyte activation. Third, since LK can dramatically affect the phenotype of MØ, we investigated the changes in RNA and protein synthesis of MØ undergoing stimulation and we compared these events with the acquisition of tumoricidal capacity by MØ.

The changes in RNA and protein synthesis associated with the in vitro activation of MØ and lymphocytes were evaluated by measuring the incorporation of ^{3}H-leucine and ^{3}H-uridine into TCA-precipitable material after a 2 hr pulse, as previously described (23). MØ activation was monitored by their ability to kill ^{51}Cr labeled RL♂1 lymphoma target cells in an 18 hr microcytotoxicity assay (18). As a parameter of lymphocyte activation, we studied their production of LK after stimulation with Concanavalin A (Con A). Two LK were tested: migration inhibition factor (MIF) and macrophage activation factor (MAF), using respectively the microdroplet and microcytotoxicity assays as detailed elsewhere (18,22).

It has previously been reported that RNA and protein synthesis are required for lymphocyte proliferation and for the production of LK (5,10). However, there was no detailed information as to when these functions were required during the development of the response. In order to examine these issues, lymphocytes were treated at different times during activation with a reversible inhibitor of protein synthesis, puromycin, or an irreversible inhibitor of RNA synthesis, actinomycin D.

As shown in Fig. II, treatment of lymphocytes with puromycin during the first two hrs of Con A stimulation completely prevented MIF and MAF production. In contrast, exposure of the lymphocytes to puromycin for the same length of time, between 4 and 6 hrs after the beginning of the culture, had no effect. If puromycin was not removed from the culture, LK production was inhibitied regardless of whether the drug was added at the initiation of culture or 6 hr later (data not shown) (27).

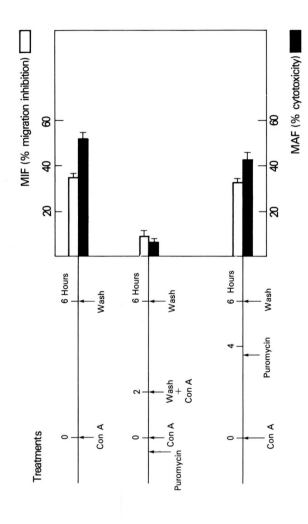

Figure II. Normal spleen cells were treated with Con A (2.5 ug/ml) and puromycin (20 ug/ml) as indicated. The lymphokine activity was measured on supernatants harvested at 18 hr.

Treatment of lymphocytes at the beginning of culture with actinomycin D, an irreversible inhibitor of RNA synthesis, also blocked MIF and MAF production (Fig. III). In contrast, treatment at 5 hr was ineffective. These data suggest that a critical protein which is required for subsequent production of lymphokines is synthetized during the first few hours of stimulation. After this special early requirement, however, continued protein synthesis is needed for lymphokine production. In contrast, the RNA required for MIF and MAF production seems to be completely synthesized within 4 to 6 hr of stimulation.

We have previously shown that early proteins synthesized during the first hr of Con A stimulation, are absolutely required for the full lymphoproliferative response (22). It is of interest to note that LK production shares the requirement of early protein synthesis with the lymphoproliferative response, even though MIF and MAF production is a proliferation-independent phenomenon (1,22). This suggests the existance of a common protein synthesis-dependent step that is required for the development of both functions. Any agent or signal which could interfere with such a "key step" in the activation process would alter either in a positive or negative manner the subsequent development of the response.

TABLE 1.   Inhibition of lymphocyte protein synthesis by C. parvum-activated macrophages[a]

Responder Cells	Material used to elicit Macrophages	Percentage of Macrophages Added			
		0	5	10	20
NSC + Con A	LMO	41 (100)[b]	43 (106)	40 (98)	38 (94)
NSC + Con A	C. parvum	32 (100)	23 (84)	22 (68)	12 (37)
NSC	LMO	22 (100)	24 (108)	28 (126)	26 (120)
NSC	C. parvum	18 (100)	18 (100)	12 (66)	6 (33)

[a]Normal spleen cells (NSC) were mixed with macrophages from animals inoculated three days earlier with light mineral oil or 9 days earlier with Corynebacterium parvum and incubated with Con A or medium. The cultures were pulsed with ^{3}H-leucine for 6 hours and TCA-precipitable material was harvested.

[b]CPM x 10^{-3} [Difference between ^{3}H-leucine incorporation of mixed cultures of MØ and NSC, and macrophages alone] (% Response [compared to control without macrophages])

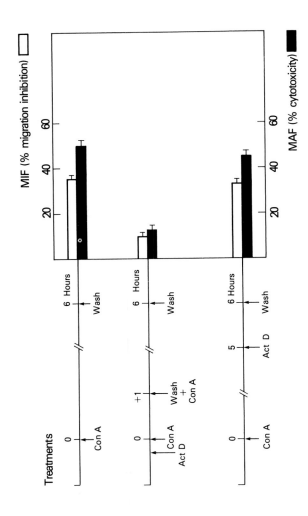

Figure III. Normal spleen cells were treated with Con A (2.5 ug/ml) and Actinomycin D (1 ug/ml) as indicated. The lymphokine activity was measured on supernatants harvested at 18 hours after exposure to Con A.

MØ are one type of cell that appear to be able to regulate the immune response. They can inhibit proliferation-independent immune functions, such as LK production, as well as the proliferation of lymphocytes. Moreover, suppressor MØ exert their inhibitory activity only if added to cultures of lymphocytes at the beginning of the stimulation (22). This suggests that suppressor MØ affect an early step absolutely required for lymphocyte activation. In addition, MØ-dependent suppression always has been associated with functions which are dependent on protein synthesis. Thus, we decided to investigate the effects of suppressor MØ on lymphocyte protein synethesis. Peritoneal MØ induced by injection of either light mineral oil (LMO) or C. parvum were cultivated for 6 hr with resting or Con A-stimulated normal spleen cells (NSC) from C57BL/6 mice (Table I). The incorporation of ^{3}H-lecine into TCA-precipitable materials of mixed cultures of MØ and lymphocytes was then evaluated. We found that the protein synthesis of resting or Con A-stimulated NSC was depressed within 6 hr of culture by the addition of C. parvum MØ, but was unaffected by LMO-MØ. Similar data were obtained when activated MØ, recovered from tumor bearing mice were used (25). Several experimental results suggested that the protein synthesis of T cells, was depressed in cultures of activated MØ and normal spleen cells (data not

TABLE II.   Effect of lymphokine on the macromolecular synthesis and tumor cytotoxicity of proteose peptone-induced macrophages from mice[a]

Macrophage Treatment	RNA Synthesis		Protein Synthesis		Tumoricidal Activity
	CPM x 10^{-3} (+SE)	Percent Response	CPM x 10^{-3} (+SE)	Percent Response	Percent Cytotoxicity[b] (+SE)
Lymphokine Supernatant[c]	4.5 (0.2)	49	8.7 (0.6)	111	38.6 (2.1)
Control Supernatant[d]	9.1 (0.8)	100	7.8 (0.2)	100	3.2 (1.2)

[a] Macrophages were treated for 16 hours with a 1:5 dilution of lymphokine and then pulsed for 2 hours with either ^{3}H-uridine (RNA synthesis) or ^{3}H-leucine (protein synthesis).

[b] Tumor cytotoxicity was measured against RL♂1 in an 18 hr ^{51}CR release assay.

[c] Lymphokine supernatant was obtained from C57BL/6 spleen cells, immune to H-2^k and restimulated in vitro with the same alloantigen.

[d] Control supernatant was obtained from unstimulate C57BL/6 spleen cells, immune to H-2^k incubated in culture.

shown). Therefore since C. parvum MØ, but not LMO MØ are able to suppress the production of LK and lymphocyte proliferation, and since both these functions are absolutely dependent on early protein synthesis, we hypothesize the MØ suppress lymphocyte functions by their early inhibition of protein synthesis. Moreover, finding only C. parvum MØ and not LMO MØ were able to suppress protein synthesis of lymphocytes, suggests that development of suppressor activity occurs along with the acquisition of tumoricidal activity or with the alterations in their metabolic and secretory capacities.

Because of the complex modifications seen in MØ response to either in vivo or in vitro stimuli, we next asked whether changes in macromolecular synthesis of MØ themselves were associated with their activation. We analyzed the changes in RNA and protein synthesis of MØ undergoing in vitro stimulation with LK.

As shown in Table II, RNA synthesis (as measured by ^{3}H-uridine incorporation) of proteose-peptone induced MØ treated for 18 hr with LK was strongly depressed in comparison with pMØ treated with medium alone. In contrast there was only a slight decrease in protein synthesis. The LK-treated MØ were also highly cytotoxic against R1ð1 tumor target cells. The range of suppression of RNA synthesis of LK-treated MØ varied among different experiments between 40 and 70% induced by concentrations of LK optimal for tumoricidal activation. As shown in Table III the decrease of RNA synthesis of LK-treated MØ was not evident at 2 hr after treatment with LK, but it was very strong after 16 hr.

TABLE III. Macromolecular synthesis and tumor cytotoxicity of proteose peptone-induced MØ from C57BL/6 mice treated with LK for different lengths of time[a]

MØ Treatment	Time of harvest (hr)	RNA synthesis CPM x 10^{-3} (+SE)	Percent Response	Protein synthesis CPM x 10^{-3} (+SE)	Percent Response	Tumoricidal Activity[b] % Cytotoxicity (+SE)
LK[c]	4	14.7 (.3)	113	8.5 (.8)	111	4.5 (0.9)
CS		13.0 (.2)	100	7.6 (.4)	100	1.4 (1.9)
LK	18	5.9 (1.1)	44	7.8 (1.6)	81	28.9 (2.1)
CS		13.2 (.5)	100	9.6 (.7)	100	2.6 (1.3)

[a] MØ were tested for 2 or 16 hr with a 1:5 dilution of LK or control supernatant and then pulsed for 2 hr with either ^{3}H-uridine or ^{3}H-leucine.

[b] Tumor cytotoxicity was measured against ^{51}CR labeled R1ð1 tumor target cells in an 18 hr microcytotoxicity assay.

[c] LK supernatant was obtained from C57BL/6 spleen cells stimulated 24 hr with Con A. CS was from C57BL/6 spleen cells without stimulation.

Parallel results were obtained when the same MØ population was tested for tumor cytotoxicity. As previously shown incubation of MØ with LK for only 2 hrs was not sufficient to trigger MØ to become cytotoxic, whereas high levels of cytolytic activity were observed after 18 hr incubation (Table III) (17,20). Similar kinetic studies with Poly I:C, a strong inducer of MØ cytotoxic activity (24), indicated RNA synthesis of MØ started to decrease by 8 hrs after treatment and by 24 hr was 30-40% of the untreated controls. The protein synthesis was also decreased but only at 24-26 hr after stimulation (data not shown). Pulse chase experiments ruled out the possibility that this was due to an increased turnover of RNA. Thus, it seems that the acquisition of a cytotoxic phenotype by MØ is associated with an early decrease in RNA synthesis.

In support of the hypothesis that a decrease in RNA synthesis was associated with MØ activation, we found that MØ activated in vivo by inoculation on C. parvum also showed a depression of RNA synthesis as compared to resident MØ. The level of depression was similar to that observed with MØ treated in vitro with LK. The same population of C. parvum MØ was also highly cytotoxic and able to suppress the production of LK, whereas resident MØ were neither tumoricidal nor suppresive (data not shown). Therefore, it appears that the dramatic decrease in RNA synthesis of both in vivo and in vitro activated MØ correlates with the ability of MØ to exert various effector and regulatory functions.

CONCLUSIONS

We analyzed the macromolecular events associated with the activation of lymphocytes and macrophages, and with the suppression of lymphocyte function by macrophages. We have found that upon treatment of lymphocytes with either mitogens or antigens, an early protein synthesis-dependent step is absolutely required for activation. This key step seems to be one of the targets for regulatory signals from suppressor macrophages since they can inhibit the protein synthesis of lymphocytes during this early critical time after stimulation. We postulate that activated MØ suppress lymphocyte function through an inhibition of lymphocyte protein synthesis. This is supported by the observation that various immune functions which require protein synthesis are sensitive to MØ-dependent suppression (26) whereas protein synthesis-independent functions such as T cell-dependent cytotoxicity (21) are not.

The inhibitory effect of MØ on a common biochemical event associated with the activation of lymphocytes could account for the lack of specificity of the suppressor MØ and the ability of MØ to suppress both proliferation-independent and proliferation-dependent immune functions (13). However, we cannot rule out the possibility that there are other earlier steps required for lymphocyte activation and that these also might be affected by suppressor MØ. Thus, inhibition of protein synthesis may be the result of even earlier modification of the metabolism of lymphocytes by suppressor MØ. Suppressor MØ are a multifunctional type of immunoregulatory cell which acquire the ability to suppress immune responses after undergoing in vitro and in vivo activation. Besides their immunosuppressive functions, MØ also display new effector functions such as tumor cell killing or complex biochemical modifications which result in increased enzyme production. From the analysis of the changes in the macromolecular synthesis of MØ activated in vitro to a cytotoxic stage, we found that treatment of MØ with LK induced a rapid decrease in RNA synthesis of MØ followed by a later decrease in protein synthesis. The degree of alteration of ^{3}H-uridine incorporation was related to the dose of LK used and the level of tumor cytotoxicity exerted by the same MØ. This phenomenon seems to be quite general since MØ treated in vitro with different stimulatory agents or in vivo with C. parvum show similar degrees of depression of RNA synthesis.

These results suggest that activation of MØ is closely related with a reduction in macromolucular synthesis. Therefore, the decrease in RNA synthesis could be a pre-requisite for subsequent MØ activation. Thus, it seems important to consider the possible effects on the immune system by using in vivo antimetabolic drugs such as antitumor agents. Many of these drugs interfere directly with the macromolecular synthesis of the cells with practically no selectivity between tumor or normal target cells. Therefore, the final effect of an anticancer therapy might depend on the balance between the antitumor effect of a given compound and its ability to interfere with the macromolecular synthesis of immuno-competent cells, modulating their functions in a positive or negative way.

Abbreviations Used

LK = lymphokine, MØ = macrophages, C. parvum = Corynebacterium parvum, Con A = Concanavalin A, MAF = macrophage activation factor, MIF = migration inhibition factor, LMO = light mineral oil, NSC = normal spleen cells, CS = control supernatant

REFERENCES

1. Bloom, B.R., Gaffney, J., and Jimenez, L. (1972): J. Immunol., 109:1395-1402.

2. Buchmiller, Y., and Marvel, J. (1979): J. Exp. Med., 150:359-370.

3. Cohn, Z. (1978): J. Immunol., 121:813-816.

4. David, J.R., and Remold, H.G. (1979): In: Biology of Lymphokines, edited by S. Cohen, E. Pick, and J.J. Oppenheim, pp. 121-140, Academic Press, New York.

5. Henney, C.S., Gaffney, J., and Bloom, B.R. (1974): J. Exp. Med., 140:837-852.

6. Herberman, R.B., Holden, H.T., Varesio, L., Taniyama, T., Puccetti, P., Kirchner, H., Janson, J., White, S., Keisari, Y., and Haskill, J.S. (1980): In: Contemporary Topics in Immunobiology, Vol. 10, edited by I.P. Witz and M.G. Hanna, pp. 61-78. Plenum Press, New York.

7. Herberman, R.B., Bonnard, G.D., Brunda, M.J., Domzig, W., Fagnani, R., Goldfarb, R.H., Holden, H.T., Ortaldo, J.R., Reynolds, C., Riccardi, C., Santoni, A., Taramelli, D., and Varesio, L. (1981): In: The Biological Significance of Immune Regulation, edited by M.E. Gershwin and L.N. Ruben, in press. Marcel Dekker, New York.

8. Karnovsky, M.L., and Lazdins, J.K. (1978): <u>J. Immunol.</u>, 121:809-813.

9. Kirpke, M., Budmer, M.B., and Fidler I. (1977): <u>Cell. Immunol.</u>, 30:341-352.

10. Milner, J. (1978): <u>Nature</u>, 272:628-629.

11. Nathan, C.F., Karnosky, M.L., and David J.R. (1971): <u>J. Exp. Med.</u>, 133:1356-1376.

12. Nathan, C., Silverstein, S., Brukner, L, Cohn, D. (1979): <u>J. Exp. Med.</u>, 149:84-99.

13. Nathan, C., Silverstein, S., Brukner, L., Cohn, D. (1979): <u>J. Exp. Med.</u>, 149:100-113.

14. Oehler, J.R., Herberman, R.B., and Holden, H.T. (1978): <u>Pharmac. Ther.</u>, 2(A):551-593.

15. Pick, E., Cohn, S., and Oppenheim, J.J. (1979): <u>In: Biology of Lymphokine</u>, edited by E. Pick, S. Cohen and J.J. Oppenheim, Academic Press, New York.

16. <u>Cell Biology and Immunology of Leukocyte Function</u>, edited by M.R. Quastel, Academic Press, New York (1979).

17. Ruco, L.P., and Meltzer, M.S. (1978): <u>J. Immunol.</u>, 120:1054-1062.

18. Taramelli, D., Holden, H.T., and Varesio, L. (1980): <u>J. Immunol. Methods</u>, 37:225-232.

19. Taramelli, D., Holden, H.T., and Varesio, L. (1981): <u>J. Immunol.</u>, in press.

20. Taramelli, D., and Varesio, L. (1981): <u>J. Immunol.</u>, in press.

21. Thorn, R.M. and Henney, C.S. (1976): <u>J. Immunol.</u>, 116:146-149.

22. Varesio, L., Herberman, R.B., Gerson, J.M. and Holden, H.T. (1979): <u>Int. J. Cancer</u>, 24:97-102.

23. Varesio, L. and Eva, A. (1980): <u>J. Immunol. Meth.</u>, 33:231-238.

24. Varesio, L., and Holden, H.T. (1980): <u>Cell. Immunol.</u>, 56:16-28.

25. Varesio, L., and Holden, H.T. (1980): <u>J. Immunol.</u>, 125:1694-1701.

26. Varesio, L., and Holden, H.T. (1980): <u>J. Immunol.</u>, 124:2288-2294.

27. Varesio, L., Holden, H.T., and Taramelli, D. (1980): <u>J. Immunol.</u>, 125:2810-2817.

Lymphokines and Thymic Hormones: Their
Potential Utilization in Cancer Therapeutics,
edited by A. L. Goldstein and M. A. Chirigos,
Raven Press, New York © 1981.

In Vivo Development and Regulation of Cytolytic T Cells Specific for Altered Self Antigens

Henry L. Wong and Jack R. Battisto

Department of Biology, Case Western Reserve University and Department of Immunology, Cleveland Clinic Foundation, Cleveland, Ohio 44106

INTRODUCTION

Control of Induction of Cytolytic T Cells to Altered Self By Non-specific Suppressor Cells

For some time it has been known that cytolytic-T cells directed toward hapten-modified syngeneic H-2 antigens can be generated in vitro. This has not, however, been possible in vivo without deleting cells. Subcutaneous injection of hapten-modified syngeneic cells (25, 23) or epicutaneous application of hapten (26) does not cause development of primary hapten-specific cytotoxic T cells (CTLs). The absence of CTLs under these conditions has been ascribed to the presence of non-specific T suppressor cells. Elimination of such suppressor cells by pre-administering cyclophosphamide, however, allows cytolytic T cells to be generated to hapten-altered self (23, 26).

Apparently the sensitization of pre-cytolytic cells to the hapten-modified syngeneic H-2 antigens is not controlled by the cyclophospha-mide-sensitive T regulatory cell. When draining lymph nodes are removed from normal mice three days following subcutaneous injection of hapten-modified cells and cultured in vitro for 48 to 72 hours without further antigenic stimulation, hapten-specific CTLs are generated (25). Presumably, the suppressor T cell which controls development of hapten-specific CTLs in vivo becomes inactive early during the in vitro culture period thereby allowing marked cellular proliferation.

Circumvention of Suppressor Cell Control

Recently, we have described a new method for inducing cytolytic T cells in vivo to hapten-altered syngeneic cells (6-9; 27). To generate such killer cells a stimulus for the host's helper T cells is provided in the form of a disparate minor histocompatibility locus (Mls) antigen on an auxiliary cell (CBA/J) that is otherwise compatible with the host (C3H/HeN) at the major histocompatibility locus (both strains have H-2^k antigens, see Figure 1). The auxiliary cells (20x10^6) are injected into the hind paws of host mice along with the hapten-modified syngeneic cells (20x10^6). The latter act as the stimulator for the pre-cytolytic cell. In this manner, the pre-CTLs receive the requisite inputs to differentiate into mature killer T cells that are recoverable after five days from draining popliteal lymph nodes. Such cytolytic T cells have been found to be hapten-specific and genetically restricted (7). Furthermore, by limiting the auxiliary and stimulator cells to splenic B cells, the host's lymphoid cells and not the injected cells were shown to be the source of both helper T and cytolytic T cells (7).

FIGURE 1. VISUALIZATION OF METHOD FOR GENERATING
CYTOLYTIC T CELLS TO ALTERED SELF <u>IN VIVO</u>

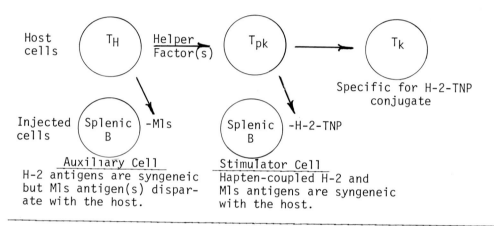

Regulation of CTL Generation At The Helper Cell Level

In prior communications (7), we hypothesized that this system for generating CTLs might be regulated at the level of the helper T cell which experiences the Mls stimulus on the auxiliary cells. We went on to show that this is, indeed, possible by inducing tolerance for the Mls antigen (see Table I). This was accomplished by a method established by others (15, 16). For this purpose, host animals were injected intravenously 7 or 14 days prior to sensitization for CTLs with splenic cells from the F₁ offspring of matings between the host-strain animals (C3H/HeN) and auxiliary cell-strain animals (CBA/J). Spleen cells from tolerized mice displayed mixed lymphocyte culture (MLC) responses toward the Mls antigen(s) that were slightly less than half of the controls. Host animals that were hyporesponsive to the auxiliary cell antigen(s) were found to be unable to generate a significant hapten-specific killer T cell response. In this way the <u>in vivo</u> hapten-specific killer T cell response was shown to be controllable at the point where helper T cells of the host recognize antigens of the auxiliary cell (cf. 7).

TABLE 1. <u>Effect of various tolerizing regimens on the generation of</u>
          <u>CTLs to hapten-altered self in vivo</u>

Tolerization directed to	Method for tolerance induction	Method for detecting tolerance	Presence of CTLs in the draining popliteal lymph nodes following sensitization
Mls antigen	Intravenous injection of Mls-bearing F₁ splenic cells into host on days (-7) or (-14).	Reduced MLC between host and auxiliary splenic cells.	0
Hapten	Intravenous injection of nascent hapten on day (-7).	Reduced DTH to hapten.	0
Hapten	Intravenous injection of hapten-conjugated syngeneic spleen cells on day (-7).	Reduced DTH to hapten.	+

Use of Hapten-Specific Tolerance To Probe CTL Regulation

Earlier we had also proposed (8, 9) that the appearance of CTLs might be controlled at the level of the pre-killer T cell's interaction with hapten-conjugated self antigens. To examine this aspect, two methods for inducing tolerance toward the hapten were used (see Table 1). Mice were injected intravenously with either 5 mg of soluble hapten (trinitrobenzene sulfonic acid, TNBS) or with hapten-(trinitrophenyl, TNP)-coupled spleen cells (50x10⁶). After seven days, all mice, including untreated control animals, were subjected to sensitization to induce either hapten-specific delayed-type hypersensitivity (DTH) or hapten-specific CTL responses.

Pretreating animals with either soluble hapten or hapten conjugated spleen cells abrogated their ability to develop TNP-specific DTH responses as has been abundantly shown in the past (1, 5, 10-12, 14, 19, 24). However, a difference between the two tolerance inducing methods was seen relative to generating CTLs. Pretreating mice with TNBS rendered them unable to develop CTLs, but injecting mice with TNP-spleen had no effect. The latter formed CTLs as well as did non-tolerized control animals.

Inability of Hapten-specific Suppressor Cells or Their Product(s) To Control CTLs

Since pretreatment of host animals with TNBS rendered them unable to generate CTLs in vivo, we wished to determine whether this unresponsiveness was adoptively transferable to naive hosts. Others have successfully transferred tolerance that is directed toward DTH responses (4, 28, 20, 22). The regulation of DTH in this manner has been ascribed to the induction of hapten-specific suppressor T cells. In our experiments, mice pretreated intravenously with TNBS were found to be unresponsive for both DTH and for CTL generation. Spleen cells from these tolerant donors, upon adoptive transfer, diminished the DTH response in naive hosts, but could not suppress the generation of CTLs. Thus, the suppressor cells that arise in the spleen after administering a tolerizing dose of hapten regulate hapten-specific DTH responses but are ineffective in controlling the CTL response (8, 9).

FIGURE 2. SOLUBLE SUPPRESSOR FACTOR DOES NOT SUPPRESS EFFECTOR FUNCTION OF HAPTEN-SPECIFIC CYTOTOXIC T LYMPHOCYTES

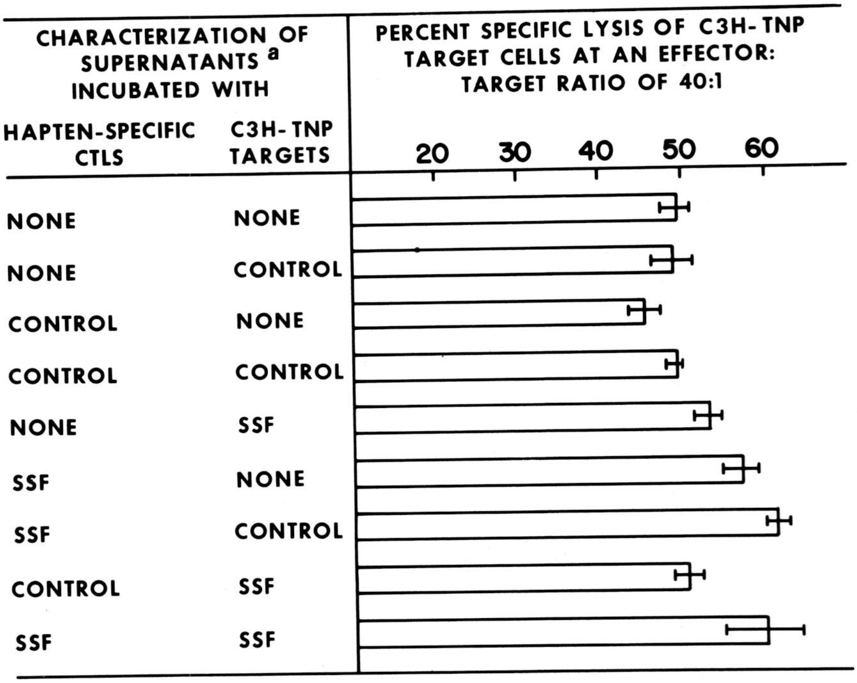

CHARACTERIZATION OF SUPERNATANTS [a] INCUBATED WITH		PERCENT SPECIFIC LYSIS OF C3H-TNP TARGET CELLS AT AN EFFECTOR: TARGET RATIO OF 40:1
HAPTEN-SPECIFIC CTLS	C3H-TNP TARGETS	20 30 40 50 60
NONE	NONE	⊢50
NONE	CONTROL	⊢50
CONTROL	NONE	⊢45
CONTROL	CONTROL	⊢48
NONE	SSF	⊢53
SSF	NONE	⊢55
SSF	CONTROL	⊢58
CONTROL	SSF	⊢48
SSF	SSF	⊢58

[a]SSF AND CONTROL SUPERNATANTS WERE TESTED FOR SUPPRESSOR ACTIVITY BY DTH ASSAY. THEREAFTER, THEY WERE INCUBATED WITH THE APPROPRIATE CELLS AT 10×10^6 CELLS/ml AT 37° C FOR 1 Hr.

Despite this lack of control shown by spleen cells from TNP-toler-
ant mice over the generation of TNP-specific CTLs, we thought to examine the effectiveness of the soluble suppressor factor (SSF) that is
produced by hapten tolerant T cells (9, 6). SSF has been shown to depress both DTH and antibody responses (29, 2, 3, 21, 13, 17, 18). The
effect of TNP-specific SSF (made according to Zembala and Asherson,
2, 3) upon CML was determined by: 1) incorporating it into the effector phase with CTLs that had been generated in vitro and 2) administering it in vivo to determine whether it altered the afferent or
inductive phase of generating hapten-specific CTLs. In the effector
phase, pre-incubating SSF with either effector CTLs and/or TNP-modi-
fied target cells did not reduce specific lysis below control levels
(Figure 2). In fact, pre-incubating CTLs with SSF appeared to enhance
the degree of lysis slightly (Figure 2, bars 6, 7 and 9).

Although incubating hapten-specific SSF with hapten-coupled target
cells did not cause a reduction of cell mediated cytolysis by effector
cells, we thought to reduce the number of haptenic groups on the target cells while keeping the SSF concentration unchanged. In this way,
SSF might become more readily detectable. The hapten concentrations
used to conjugate the target cells were reduced by two ten-fold steps
to the point where they were almost incapable of acting as suitable
targets (Figure 3). Incubating such target cells with SSF, control
supernatants, or simply medium (at 10^7 cells/ml for one hour at 37°C)
prior to use in the effector assay, resulted in no diminution or enhancement of cytolysis (Figure 3).

FIGURE 3.   SUPPRESSION OF CELL MEDIATED CYTOLYSIS BY SOLUBLE
            SUPPRESSOR FACTOR REMAINS UNDETECTABLE
     DESPITE TITRATION OF EPITOPE DENSITY ON TARGET CELLS

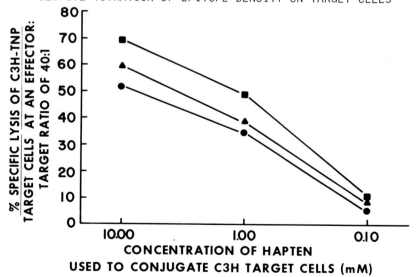

THE TARGET CELLS WERE INCUBATED WITH SSF (■),
CONTROL SUPERNATANTS (▲) OR RPMI 1640 MEDIUM (●)
AT 10×10^6 CELLS/ml FOR 1 Hr. AT 37° C.

For the in vivo test, SSF was given to mice (a total of 6 ml, see Figure 4) just prior to and during sensitization for DTH and CML. While it caused a 50% reduction in the ability of mice to mount DTH responses, it did not suppress (but actually enhanced slightly) the generation of hapten-specific CTLs (Figure 4).

FIGURE 4

SOLUBLE SUPPRESSOR FACTOR INHIBITS DELAYED-TYPE HYPERSENSITIVITY RESPONSES BUT DOES NOT ALTER THE GENERATION OF HAPTEN-SPECIFIC CYTOTYTIC T LYMPHOCYTES

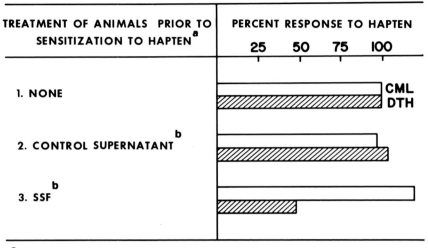

a IN EACH EXPERIMENTAL GROUP; RANDOM MICE WERE EITHER SENSITIZED FOR DTH OR CML.

b A TOTAL OF 6.0 ml OF SUPERNATANT WAS GIVEN EACH MOUSE (2.0 ml ON DAYS 0,1 AND 2) WITH SENSITIZATION ON DAY 0. OF THE 2.0 ml, 0.4 ml WAS GIVEN I.V. AND THE REMAINING 1.6 ml WAS GIVEN I.P.

Site At Which Nascent Hapten Controls CTL Development in Vivo

What, then, is the mechanism that prevents the appearance of CTLs in animals made tolerant with soluble hapten? Knowing that intravenously introduced hapten conjugates spontaneously, we reasoned that pre-cytolytic T cells as well as helper T cells would have hapten on their membrane surfaces. Furthermore, receptors present on these cells would be expected to be blocked by the presence of abundant hapten-protein conjugates. Either or both of the cellular participants might not function properly under these conditions.

To determine first whether pre-killer splenic cells from hapten-injected mice were capable of becoming hapten-specific cytolytic cells, spleens were taken seven days following an intravenously administered tolerizing dose of TNBS (5 mg/mouse). Cells from these animals were placed in culture (10×10^6/ml) for five days with syngeneic, TNP-coupled (50×10^6 cell per ml of 10 mM TNBS) heat-treated ($45°C$ for one hour) thymic cells (10×10^6/ml).

To the cultures was added exogenously produced helper factor-containing supernatant (from one-way 48-hour mixed lymphocyte reaction between 20×10^6 C3H/H$_e$N spleen cells and 20×10^6 X-irradiated Balb/c spleen cells) to a concentration of 50% of the culture volume. The heat-treated TNP-coupled thymic cells are known to serve well as stimulators of pre-cytolytic cells but do not trigger helper cells to synthesize and release helper factors. The addition of excess helper factor supernatant to the cell cultures is essential because the limiting variable in the experimental protocol must be the pre-cytolytic cell and not the helper cell. After five days of in vitro culturing at 37°C in a 5% CO_2 atmosphere the viable cells were harvested and placed in the effector phase with TNP-coupled, mitogen-transformed, ^{51}Cr-labelled T cell targets.

As may be seen in Table 2, the splenic cells derived from hapten-pretreated mice were as capable as splenic cells from non-treated mice to develop hapten-specific cytolytic cells. In fact, the injection of the TNBS may prime the animal toward the hapten since the response was increased by about 40% over controls. Furthermore, a comparison of lines 1 and 2 in Table 2 shows that TNP-C3H heat-treated thymocytes do not stimulate helper cells to produce the requisite second signal but that they do act as adequate stimulators of precytolytic cells in the presence of pre-formed, added helper factor(s).

Table 2. Suppression of the generation of cytolytic T lymphocytes by pre-injecting nascent hapten intravenously is not directed at the pre-effector cell

TNP-C3H Thy$^\Delta$ stimulators[a] co-incubated with spleen cells from C3H mice pre-treated with	Helper factor[b] added to the cultures	% specific lysis of TNP-C3H target cells at an effector to target ratio of:		
		10:1	20:1	40:1
1. Nothing	-	0.0	0.0	0.0
2. Nothing	+	22.7	31.7	40.6
3. 5 mg TNBS (day-7)	-	6.2	12.2	17.1
4. 5 mg TNBS (day-7)	+	48.5	55.7	57.6

[a]Following conjugation with TNP, the thymic cells were heated at 45°C for one hour to prevent them from stimulating helper cells.

[b]Helper supernatant, prepared from a 48-hour MLC between C3H spleen cells and x-irradiated Balb/c spleen cells, was added to the experimental cultures so that it constituted 40-50% of the final volume.

From these data we were able to conclude that the injection of nascent hapten had no depressive effect upon pre-cytolytic cells that could be detected seven days later.

To determine whether tolerance induction using nascent hapten alters the helper cells, we again utilized the spleens of animals seven days following intravenously administering hapten. In this instance, however, the splenic cells were used for the production of helper factor which was to be assayed in a separate in vitro system. Thus, both tolerant and non-tolerant C3H spleen cells were cultured alone (20 x 10^6/ml) as well as with CBA/J splenic B cells (20 x 10^6 ml) that had been mitomycin-treated. We purposely used only the B cells from CBA/J spleens since these possess the Mls antigen required to stimulate helper T cells but cannot themselves be a source of helper factor. After 48 hours the supernatants from these cultures were incorporated in an experimental assay system where the presence of helper factor controls the appearance of cytolytic T cells. This in vitro assay system consisted of C3H spleen cells (10^7 responders) co-incubated with Balb/c heat-treated thymocytes (10^7 stimulators). The heat-treated thymocytes provide the allogeneic antigenic stimulus required by pre-cytolytic T cells but do not stimulate helper T cells. Thus, the system is dependent upon helper factor present in the supernatants that are added to the cultures (40 to 50% of the culture fluid). At the end of a 5 day incubation interval the viable effector

Table 3. Soluble Killer Cell Helper Factor is Produced by Spleen Cells from Mice Made Tolerant with Nascent Hapten

Source of supernatants[a] incubated with C3H responders and BALB/c thymocytes[b]	% Specific lysis of BALB/c targets at effector: target ratios of:	
	8:1	16:1
1. None (negative control)	-2.4	-0.2
2. C3H spleen (negative control)	0.0	-2.7
3. Tolerant C3H spleen (negative control)	-4.2	-3.6
4. C3H spleen x CBA/J splenic B cells[mc] (positive control).	25.0	32.7
5. Tolerant C3H spleen x CBA/J splenic B cells[mc]	33.7	47.1

[a]To prepare these, 20 x 10^6 of each type of cell were mixed in 6 ml of RPMI 1640 supplemented with 10% fecal calf serum, 2-ME, $NaHCO_3$, Hepes and pen-strep and incubated at 37°C, 5% CO_2 for 48 hours. Supernatants were collected by centrifugation, passed through 0.45 millipore filters, and stored at -20°C until used.
[b]Thymocytes were heat treated at 45°C for 1 hour.

cells were harvested and used in the effector assay with mitogen-transformed ^{51}Cr-labelled Balb/c T lymphoblasts as targets (8:1 and 16:1 E:T ratios). As may be seen in Table 3 only minimal background cytolytic values were obtained when no supernatant was added or when supernatants from C3H normal or tolerant splenic cells cultured alone were added to the sensitization phase. The positive control supernatant from C3H spleen cells co-cultured with mitomycin-C treated CBA/J splenic B cells caused the appearance of cytolytic T cells. In a similar way, splenic cells from hapten-tolerized C3H mice that had been co-cultured with mitomycin-C treated CBA/J splenic B cells were able to synthesize measurable helper factor. The percent specific lysis achieved by the latter supernatants compared favorably with those achieved by positive control supernatants (lines 4 and 5 of Table 3). Thus, the tolerization procedure that is accomplished by intravenously introduced nascent hapten does not alter the helper T cell's capability to produce helper factor.

The explanation for the way in which nascent hapten prevents appearance of cytolytic T cells _in vivo_ is not dependent upon the interaction of hapten directly with either helper or pre-cytolytic T cells. The hapten must be causing an effect at another step or stage in the development of cytolytic T cells which in turn could alter the function of helper, pre-cytolytic and/or fully matured cytolytic T cells. We are presently engaged in elucidating what that effect might be.

SUMMARY

The new method we have previously described for inducing cytolytic T cells _in vivo_ to hapten-altered syngeneic cells has been used to examine the development and regulation of this form of cell-mediated immunity. The method consists of stimulating the host's helper T cells with an Mls-disparate auxiliary cell at the same time that hapten-altered syngeneic spleen cells trigger precursor cytolytic cells. Injected together into the hind paws of mice, these cells cause hapten-specific CTLs to appear in the draining popliteal lymph nodes. Inducing tolerance toward the Mls antigens prevents the generation of killer T cells in this system. Inducing tolerance with cell membrane coupled hapten reduces DTH but does not affect CML. Inducing tolerance with soluble hapten prevents DTH and the generation of hapten-specific cytolytic T cells. Although hapten-specific suppressor T cells that are active to depress DTH responses arise when nascent hapten is given intravenously, they have no regulatory effect upon the generation of CTLs. Furthermore, the hapten-specific soluble suppressor factor (SSF) that such cells make has no depressive effect either at the efferent or afferent ends of the CML response.

The nascent hapten methodology apparently has no detrimental effect upon helper cells. Spleen cells removed from hapten-tolerant mice were fully able to make killer cell assisting factor when confronted _in vitro_ with Mls antigen.

Furthermore, the nascent hapten methodology has no effect upon pre-killer T cells. Splenic cells from hapten-tolerant mice developed cytolytic T cells *in vitro* toward hapten-specific syngeneic stimulators to the same extent as splenic cells from normal mice. Since both helper and pre-cytolytic T cells appear to be functional *in vitro*, the nascent hapten must be exerting its primary effect elsewhere *in vivo*.

Acknowledgements

The authors thank Ms. Michael Hart for expert preparation of the manuscript. This work was supported by Grant AI-12468 from the National Institute of Allergy and Infectious Diseases, National Institutes of Health and by a Training Award to H. L. Wong from the National Institutes of Health Training Grant 5-T-32-GM 07225.

REFERENCES

1. Asherson G.L. and Ptak W. (1970): Immunol. 18, 99-106.

2. Asherson, G.L. & Zembala, M. (1974a): Proc. R. Soc. Lond. B. 187, 329-348.

3. Asherson, G & Zembala, M. (1974b): Eur. J. Immunol. 4, 804-807.

4. Asherson, G., Zembala, M. & Barnes, R.M. (1971): Clin. Exp. Immunol. 9, 111-121.

5. Battisto, J.R. & Bloom, B.R. (1966a): Fed. Proc. 25, 152-159.

6. Battisto, J.R., Butler, L.D. and Wong, H. L., (1980): In: Immunological Reviews; Unresponsiveness To Haptenated Self Molecules, edited by G. Möller, 50:47-70, Munksgaard, Copenhagen.

7. Butler, L.D. & Battisto, J.R. (1979a): J. Immunol. 122, 1578-1581.

8. Butler, L.D. & Battisto, J.R. (1979): In ann. N.Y. Acad. Sci. Subcellular factors in immunity, edited by H. Friedman, 332:524-530.

9. Butler, L.D., Wong, H.L. & Battisto, J.R. (1980): J. Immunol. 124: 1245-1250.

10. Claman, H. (1976): J. Immunol. 116, 704-709.

11. Claman, H. & Miller, S.D. (1976): J. Immunol. 117, 480-485.

12. Claman, H.N., Miller, S.D. & Sy, M.S. (1977): J. Exp. Med. 146, 49-58.

13. Greene, M.I., Pierres, A., Dorf, M.E. & Benacerraf, B. (1977b): J. Exp. Med. 146, 293-296.

14. Greene, M.I., Sugimoto, M. & Benacerraf, B. (1977a): J. Immunol. 120, 1604-1611.

15. Jacobsson, H., Lilliehook, B. & Blomgren, H. (1976): Cell. Immunol. 22, 53-65.

16. Lilliehook, Blomgren, B., Jacobsson, H. & Anderson, B. (1977): Cell. Immunol. 29, 223-231.

17. Long, C.A. & Scott, D.W. (1977a): Eur. J. Immunol. 7, 1-6.

18. Long, C.A. & Scott, D.W. (1977b): Fed. Proc. 35, 788.

19. Miller, S.D. & Claman, H.N. (1976): J. Immunol. 117, 1519-1526.

20. Moorhead, J. (1976): J. Immunol. 177, 802-806.

21. Moorhead, J. (1977): J. Immunol. 119, 315-321.
22. Moorhead, J. & Scott, D.W. (1977): Cell. Immunol. 28, 443-448.

23. Rollinghoff, M., Starzinski-Powitz, A., Pfizenmaier, K. & Wagner, H. (1977): J. Exp. Med. 145, 455-459.

24. Scott, D.W. & Long, C.A. (1976): J. Exp. Med. 144, 1369-1373.

25. Starzinski-Powitz, A., Pfizenmaier K., Rollinghoff M., & Wagner, H. (1976): Eur. J. Immunol. 6, 799-805.

26. Tagart, V., Thomas, W.R. & Asherson, G.L. (1978): Immunology 34, 1109-1116.

27. Wong, H.L., Butler, L.D. and Battisto J.R. (1981): In Cellular and Molecular Mechanisms of Immunological Tolerance, edited by T. Hraba, 000, Marcel Dekker, N.Y.

28. Zembala, M. & Asherson, G. (1973): Nature 244, 227-228.

29. Zembala, M. & Asherson, G. (1974): Eur. J. Immunol. 4, 799-804.

Lymphokines and Thymic Hormones: Their
Potential Utilization in Cancer Therapeutics,
edited by A. L. Goldstein and M. A. Chirigos,
Raven Press, New York © 1981.

Immune Interferon as an Antitumor Agent

S. Baron, W. R. Fleischmann, Jr., and G. J. Stanton

University of Texas Medical Branch, Galveston, Texas 77550

The interferon system is well established as a natural defense against virus infections (2). Interferon also may exert significant antitumor action in many systems including virus-induced tumors, carcinogen-induced tumors, and spontaneous tumors (16). The degree of antitumor action of interferon varies greatly among the tumors tested. Although complete remission of certain experimental tumors can be caused by interferon, most tumors are retarded in their progression to varying degrees and some tumors are not affected at all.

The mechanisms of antitumor action by interferon, those demonstrated and those possible, are listed in Table 1. Interferon may directly inhibit cell division and thus more profoundly effect the rapidly dividing tumor cells (16). The degree of this inhibition and the time of onset varies greatly among the cell types tested. For example, the multiplication of some tumor cells is inhibited within 24 hours, but the multiplication of mouse embryo cells may not be affected until one week after initiation of treatment and some cell types may not be inhibited at all (4). Cellular DNA synthesis is inhibited in the affected cells, but the primary biochemical mechanism of inhibition has not been determined.

TABLE 1. Antitumor Actions of Interferon.

Demonstrated
Direct Inhibition of Cell Division
Activation of: Sensitized T Lymphocytes
NK Cells
ADCC Null Cells
Macrophages
Possible
Regulation of Immune Sensitization
Hormonal Effects
Direct Cell Killing

Interferon may also activate many cells in the leukocyte series that in turn may affect tumors. Leukocytes activated by interferon include the sensitized T lymphocyte, NK cells, ADCC effector cells, macrophages, and polymorphonuclear leukocytes (3,19).

A portion of the antitumor action of interferon conceivably could result from the several effects of interferon on the immune response as schematized for immune interferon in Figure 1 (18). A single small dose

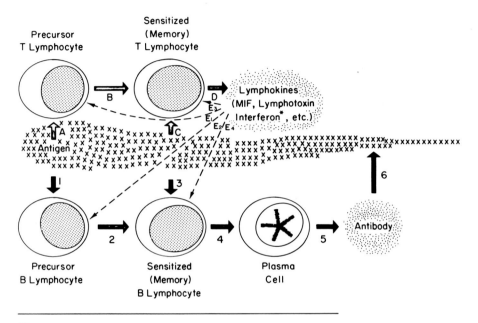

Time ➔

Fig. 1. Cellular events in the induction and immunosuppressive action of interferons. Antigen comes into contact with a precursor T lymphocyte (A), which undergoes differentiation to a sensitized T lymphocyte (B). This cell, driven by antigen (C), may become a memory cell or it may release mediators known as lymphokines (D). Among the mediators produced by the T lymphocyte is antigen-type interferon*. Antigen also reacts with a precursor B lymphocyte (1), which undergoes differentiation to a sensitized B lymphocyte (and memory B cell) (2). The sensitized B cell is further driven by antigen (3) to become a plasma cell (4), which is responsible for most of the antibody (5) that is produced. This antibody reacts with the specific antigen (6). Both antigen- and virus-induced interferons are capable of suppressing precursor T (E_1) and B (E_2) lymphocytes as well as sensitized T (E_3) and B (E_4) lymphocytes. As differentiation progresses, in part as a result of continued antigen presence, it becomes progressively more difficult to inhibit lymphocyte function by interferons. Plasma cell production of antibody is resistant to inhibition by interferon. The macrophage is not included in the figure, but interferons may exert their immunosuppressive effects via a required macrophage function in the immune response. The diagrammatic scheme does not necessarily imply, therefore, a direct effect of the interferons on the lymphocytes.

of interferon may enhance the antibody response. Larger and continued doses of interferon inhibit most B and T cell functions except for the production of antibody by the fully differentiated plasma cell. Another possible antitumor mechanism of interferon is through its hormone-like actions (1,7,8). More recently a possible direct cell-lytic effect of immune interferon preparations on certain tumor cells has been observed and will be discussed below (24).

Three major types of interferon have been identified and are listed along with the major producer cell type and the main stimuli for their induction in Table 2. The fibroepithelial (β) type of interferon was first described by Isaacs as a response by most body cell types to the presence of foreign viral and other nucleic acids (17). The (α) type of interferon may be a response by null and B lymphocytes as well as macrophages to the presence of foreign cell types (including bacteria, virus-altered cells, and transformed cells) as well as to the presence of B cell mitogens (see references in 3). Immune (γ) or type 2 interferon appears to be produced mainly by the sensitized T lymphocyte in response to the presence of a specific foreign antigen or the mimicking T cell mitogen. These three types of interferon are antigenically distinct and are coded for by different genes. Fibroepithelial and leukocyte interferons, studied by purification and genetic cloning techniques, have been found to have a number of subtypes, each specified by different genes (15,23). Immune interferon has not been studied in this manner as yet.

Interferons have many biological and biochemical effects and these are listed in Tables 3 and 4 (see references in 3). Noteworthy is the possible relatedness of interferons to certain hormones and the ability of interferon and certain hormones to cross activate one another, as well as the apparent co-production and binding of certain hormones and leukocyte interferon during production (7). It seems possible that the many biological and biochemical actions of interferon may derive from interferon triggering a set of cellular reactions including many normally triggered by hormones. To date, none of these specifically induced biochemical actions of interferon have been causally correlated with any of the biological actions of interferon.

TABLE 2. Interferon Types.

Interferon Type	Stimulus for Production	Major Producer Cells
Leukocyte (α)	Viruses Bacteria Foreign Cells Mitogens for B Lymphocytes	Null Lymphocytes B Lymphocytes Macrophages
Fibroblast (β)	Viruses Polynucleotides	Fibroblasts Epithelial cells
Immune (γ)	Foreign Antigens Mitogens for T Lymphocytes Galactose Oxidase Calcium Ionophores	T Lymphocytes

TABLE 3. Biological Actions of Interferon[a]

Antiviral
Immunoregulatory
Antitumor
Cell growth
Alteration of cell membranes
Macrophage activation
Enhancement of cytotoxicity of lymphocytes
Influence of subsequent production of interferon
Hormone-like
Maturation of cells

---

[a] for references see 3

TABLE 4. Biochemical Effects of Interferon[a]

Induction of new cellular proteins including:
    dsRNA-activatable protein kinase that phosphorylates
      ribosome-associated proteins and eIF-2
    Protein phosphatase
    2'-phosphodiesterase
Alteration of initiation factor eIF-2
Induction of 2',5'-oligoadenylic acid synthetase
Activation of endonuclease by 2',5'-oligoadenylic acid
Alteration of tRNA concentrations
Changes in glycosyl transferase
Membrane transport and binding alterations

---

[a] for references see 3

DISTINCTIVE PROPERTIES OF IMMUNE INTERFERON

Immune interferon manifests major differences in comparison with
fibroepithelial and leukocyte interferons. Some of these differences
make immune interferon particularly attractive as a possible anticancer
agent. The properties which distinguish immune interferon from the
other interferons are included in Table 5. Immune interferon, both in
the crude and more highly purified state, has been reported to exert a
greater antitumor action relative to its antiviral action than do the
other two types of interferon (20,6). The anticellular action of immune
interferons is from 10 to 50 times greater than that of the other two
interferons.

Marked potentiation of the antiviral and antitumor actions of fibroepithelial or leukocyte interferon can be brought about by the mixture of small amounts of immune interferon with either of the other two types of interferon. The potentiation of antitumor action against the P388 lymphoma in mice is shown in Figure 2 (11,13). Attempts to potentiate the currently available supplies of interferon being used in human cancer would seem to be appropriate.

Another distinctive property of immune interferon is its slow activation of cells (9). Although fibroepithelial and leukocyte interferon may activate cells within minutes, immune interferon activation requires several hours. The slower activation of cells by immune interferon appears to be due to the requirement for induction of an intermediary cell protein before induction of the antiviral proteins, whereas the other two types of intererferon induce the antiviral proteins directly. The differences in mechanisms of cell activation by the different interferons may account for the susceptibility to immune interferon of cells that are resistant to the anticellular action of the other types of interferon (10). Immune interferon has also been reported to have a 20 fold greater immunoregulatory effect than do the other two interferons (21). A recent finding suggests that partially purified γ interferon preparations may exert a direct cell killing effect (as opposed to a cytostatic effect) in some murine tumors, but definitive separation of this activity from lymphotoxin is required (24).

A potent inhibitor of the action of interferon has been found in mitogen-induced preparations of immune interferon (12). This inhibitor is highly potent and is produced somewhat later than immune interferon. It may represent a new lymphokine activity.

TABLE 5. <u>Properties which Distinguish Immune IFN from Leukocyte and Fibroblast IFNs</u>

Property	Interferon		
	α	β	γ
Antigenic	α	β	γ
Microenvironment of Production	Inflammation	Viral	Immune
Immune Effects	++	++	++++
Anticellular Activity	++	++	++++
Kinetics of Production	Rapid	Rapid	Slow
Kinetics of Action	Rapid	Rapid	Slow
Induction of Cell Antiviral Proteins	1 step	1 step	2 steps
Potentiates Interferon Type	γ	γ	α,β

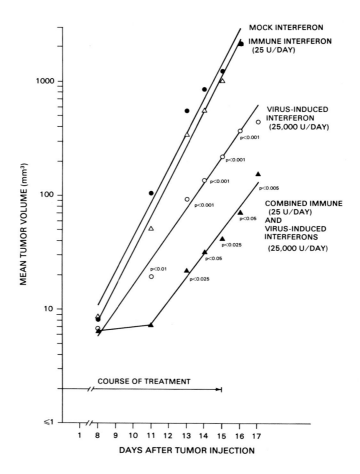

Fig. 2. Effect of combined immune and virus-induced interferons on the rate of P388 tumor development in DBA/2 mice. Each mouse was inoculated sc with 10^5 P388 tumor cells, and they were then divided into 4 groups of 18-20 each. Mice were inoculated 3 hr before tumor injection and daily for 15 days thereafter at the approximate site of tumor injection with mock interferon ( ), immune interferon ( ), virus-induced interferon ( ), or a combination of immune and virus-induced interferons ( ). Volume of the primary tumor was determined for each mouse on the indicated days after tumor cell injection. Data are plotted as $\log_{10}$ increase in mean tumor volume. Probabilities cited for the virus-induced interferon treatment curve compare the virus-induced interferon treatment with the mock interferon treatment. Probabilities cited for the combined-interferon treatment curve compare the combined interferon treatment with the virus-induced interferon treatment.

CELL TO CELL TRANSFER OF INTERFERON ACTION

Interferon-activated cells may transfer their activation to other cells with which they are in direct contact (5-9). Leukocytes which may be activated by interferon they produce or from other sources can in principle migrate throughout the body, attach to target cells, and transfer the interferon activated state to the target cell (22). This is a potentially important antitumor mechanism which merits further study.

CONCLUSIONS

Interferon, one of the body's first defenses against viruses, manifests a number of biological and biochemical actions. Some of these effects of interferon lead to inhibition of certain tumors. Preliminary studies in humans encourage further controlled clinical trials (14). Immune interferon has major differences from fibroepithelial and leukocyte interferons. Some of these differences (greater anticellular effect, potentiation, effects on immunity) make immune interferon particularly attractive for study as an antitumor agent and perhaps for eventual application to humans.

REFERENCES

1. Baron, S. (1966): The biological significance of the interferon system. In: Interferon, N. Finter (ed.), pp. 268-293. North Holland Publishing Co., Amsterdam.

2. Baron, S. (1979): The interferon system. Am. Soc. Microbiol. News, 45:358-366.

3. Baron, S., and Dianzani, F., eds. (1977): The interferon system: a current review to 1978. Tex. Rep. Biol. Med., 35:1-573.

4. Baron, S., Merigan, T.C., McKerlie, M.L. (1966): Effect of crude and purified interferons on the growth of uninfected cells in culture. Proc. Soc. Exp. Biol. Med., 121:50-52.

5. Blalock, J.E., and Baron, S. (1977): Interferon-induced transfer of viral resistance between animal cells. Nature, 269:422-425.

6. Blalock, J.E., Georgiades, J.A., Langford, M.P., Johnson, H.M. (1980): Purified human immune interferon has more potent anticellular activity than fibroblast or leukocyte interferon. Cell Immunol., 49:390-394.

7. Blalock, J.E., and Smith, E.M. (1980): Human leukocyte interferon: Structural and biological relatedness to adrenocorticotropic hormone and endorphins. Proc. Natl. Acad. Sci., 77:5972-5974.

8. Blalock, J.E., and Stanton, G.J. (1980): Common pathways of interferon and hormonal action. Nature, 283:406-408.

9.   Dianzani, F., Zucca, M., Scupham, A., and Georgiades, J. (1980):
     Immune and virus-induced interferons may activate cells by
     different derepressional mechanisms. Nature, 280:400-402.

10. Falcoff, E., Wietzerbin, J., Stefanos, S., Lucero, M., Billardon,
     C., and Catinot, L. (1980): Properties of mouse immune T-
     interferon (type II). Ann. N.Y. Acad. Sci., 350:145-156.

11. Fleischmann, W.R., Jr., Georgiades, J.A., Osborne, L.C., and
     Johnson, H.M. (1979): Potentiation of interferon activity by
     mixed preparations of fibroblast and immune interferon. Infect.
     Immun., 26:248-253.

12. Fleischmann, W.R., Jr., Georgiades, J.A., Osborne, L.C., Dianzani,
     F., and Johnson, H.M. (1979): Induction of an inhibitor of
     interferon action in a mouse lymphokine preparation. Infect.
     Immun. 26:949-955.

13. Fleischmann, W.R., Jr., Kleyn, K.M., and Baron, S. (1980):
     Potentiation of antitumor effect of virus-induced interferon by
     mouse immune interferon preparations. JNCI, 65:963-966.

14. Galasso, G.J., and Dunnick, J.K. (1977): Interferon, an antiviral
     drug for use in man. Tex. Rep. Biol. Med., 35:478-485.

15. Goeddel, D.V., Leung, D.W., Dull, T.J., Gross, M., Lawn, R.M.,
     McCandliss, R., Seeburg, P.H., Ullrich, A., Yelverton, E., and
     Gray, P.W. The structure of eight distinct cloned human leukocyte
     interferon cDNA. Nature 290:20-26.

16. Gresser, I. (1977): Antitumor effects of interferon. In: Cancer:
     a comprehensive treatise. F. Becker (ed.,), vol. 5. Plenum Press,
     New York.

17. Isaacs, A., Baron, S. and Allison, A.E. (1961): as referenced in
     Interferon. Sci. Am., 204:51.

18. Johnson, H.M., and Baron, S. (1976): Interferon: effects on the
     immune response and the mechanism of activation of the cellular
     response. CRC Crit. Rev. Biochem., 4:203-227.

19. Pak, C., Imanishi, J., Kishida, T., and Matsuo, A. (1980):
     Increased nitroblue tetrazolium dye reduction by human neutrophils
     stimulated by interferon in vitro. Microbiol. Immunol., 24:717-
     723.

20. Salvin, S.B., Youngner, J.S., Nishio, J., Neta, R. (1975): Tumor
     suppression by a lymphokine released into the circulation of mice
     with delayed hypersensitivity. J. Natl. Cancer Inst., 55:1233-
     1236.

21. Sonnenfeld, G., Mandel, A.D., and Merigan, T.C. (1977): The
     immunosuppressive effect of type II mouse interferon on antibody
     production. Cell Immunol., 34:193-206.

22. Stanton, G.J., Weigent, D.A., Langford, M.P., and Blalock, J.E. (1980): Human leukocyte transfer of viral resistance to heterologous cells. In: Interferons: Properties and Clinical Uses, edited by A. Kahn,, N.O. Hill and G. Dorn. Wadley Institute of Molecular Medicine, Dallas, Texas.

23. Streuli, M., Nagata, S. and Weissmann, C. (1980): At least three human type α interferons: structure of 2. Science, 209:1343-1347.

24. Tyring, S., Fleischmann, W.R., Jr., and Baron, S. (1980): Personal communication.

Lymphokines and Thymic Hormones: Their
Potential Utilization in Cancer Therapeutics,
edited by A. L. Goldstein and M. A. Chirigos,
Raven Press, New York © 1981.

Effects of Combined Cyclophosphamide and Thymosin Treatment on Tumor Growth and Host Survival in Mice Bearing a Syngeneic Tumor

Marion M. Zatz, *Moshe Glaser, Cary M. Seals, and Allan L. Goldstein

*Department of Biochemistry, George Washington University School of Medicine, Washington, D.C. 20037; *National Cancer Institute, National Institutes of Health, Bethesda, Maryland 20034*

INTRODUCTION

Recent clinical trials utilizing thymosin fraction 5, in combination with other modes of therapy, have suggested a beneficial effect of thymosin on prolonging survival of patients with small cell carcinoma of the lung(3). In view of the use of thymosin in past and ongoing clinical trials of cancer patients, it is imperative that in vivo animal models be available to test: 1) protocols for thymosin administration (time and dose), either alone or in conjunction with chemotherapy; 2) biological activity of different clinical lots of thymosin fraction 5 and the purified component polypeptides of fraction 5; 3) the mechanisms whereby thymosin potentiates host resistance to tumor growth.

In this study we present an animal model using the growth of the MOPC-315 plasmacytoma in its syngeneic Balb/c host, which permits us to address these problems.

METHODS

Animals

Male, Balb/c mice, 6-8 weeks of age, obtained from Charles River, were used.

Tumors

MOPC-315 tumor cells, of Balb/c origin, were passaged as a solid subcutaneous (s.c.) tumor. Tumors were rendered into single cell suspensions (>90% viable), which were then inoculated s.c. into the flank of Balb/c mice at a dose of 10^6 cells/mouse.

Tumor growth was monitored by palpation 2-3 times per week and animal deaths were recorded. Tumors were graded by size on a scale of 1-4 as follows: 1 = <0.5 cm; 2 = <1 cm; 3 = <2 cm; 4 = >2 cm. In presenting mean tumor size data, a score of 5 was used to indicate host death.

Drugs

Cyclophosphamide (Mead-Johnson) was administered intraperitoneally (i.p.) on a mg/kg basis when tumors first became palpable; this time

was generally 9 days after cell injection. All animals were weighed
and doses calculated on the day of cyclophosphamide injection.

Thymosin fraction 5, clinical grade and endotoxin free, was prepared and supplied by Hoffmann–La Roche, New Jersey. It was injected
i.p. in seven doses over a two week period, beginning one week after
cyclophosphamide treatment.

The experimental protocol is shown in Figure 1.

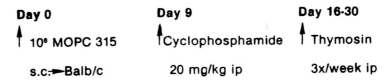

Day 0   **Day 9**   **Day 16-30**

10⁶ MOPC 315   Cyclophosphamide   Thymosin

s.c.➤Balb/c   20 mg/kg ip   3x/week ip

Monitor: Tumor size, death, CMC Response

FIG. 1. Experimental protocol.

RESULTS

Several doses of cyclophosphamide were initially employed, either
alone or in combination with thymosin fraction 5, in an effort to
retard tumor growth and enhance long-term survival in tumor-bearing
animals. As previously reported (6), MOPC-315 is a cyclophosphamide
sensitive tumor. Untreated (no cyclophosphamide) tumor-bearing
animals were all dead four weeks after inoculation of tumor cells
(Fig. 2b). Doses of 20 mg/kg cyclophosphamide per mouse resulted in
slower reappearance of the tumors than did 10 mg/kg (Fig. 2a and b,
Table 1); a dose per mouse of 50 mg/kg cyclophosphamide alone was
curative (Fig. 3, Table 2).

Thymosin fraction 5, given at the lowest doses of both 12.5 and 25
ug per injection per mouse, was effective in combination with cyclophosphamide at 20 mg/kg, in retarding tumor reappearance and in
increasing host survival. At the lower dose of cyclophosphamide
(10 mg/kg), thymosin fraction 5 was ineffective at all doses tested.
(Figs. 2a and b, Table 1)

Thymosin fraction 5, given at the same doses as shown in Fig. 2.,
without prior cyclophosphamide treatment, was also ineffective in
prolonging survival (data not shown).

In another experiment, two separate clinical lots of thymosin
fraction 5 were tested in conjunction with cyclophosphamide (20 mg/kg).
Lot C23/80 was effective at even lower doses than C100496 (used in
previous studies) in preventing tumor growth. Further studies are in
progress to ascertain the minimum effective doses of thymosin fraction

TABLE 1.   EFFECT OF CYCLOPHOSPHAMIDE AND THYMOSIN FR. 5 ON SURVIVAL

Cyclophosphamide (mg/kg)	Treatment*	% Survival**	n
10	Saline	0	0/15
10	12.5 μg	0	0/11
10	25 μg	0	0/11
10	50 μg	0	0/11
10	100 μg	0	0/11
10	200 μg	0	0/11
20	Saline	0	0/15
20	12.5 μg	90.9	10/11
20	25 μg	90.9	10/11
20	50 μg	9.1	1/11
20	100 μg	9.1	1/11
20	200 μg	9.1	1/11

*Thymosin Fr. 5 clinical lot C100496 was used.
**Survival evaluated at 44 days post tumor injection in 10 mg/kg group.
Survival evaluated at 73 days post tumor injection in 20 mg/kg group.

TABLE 2.   EFFECT OF THYMOSIN FR. 5 ON SURVIVAL

Cyclophosphamide (mg/kg)	Treatment	% Survival	n
0	Saline	8.3	1/12
50	Saline	87.3	14/16
20	Saline	26.7	4/15
20	12.5 μg*	64.7	11/17
20	25 μg*	25.0	4/16
20	6 μg**	80.0	12/15
20	12.5 μg**	31.2	5/16
20	25 μg**	12.5	2/16
20	50 μg**	40.0	8/20

*Clinical lot C100496 of thymosin fr. 5 was used.
**Clinical lot C23/80 of thymosin fr. 5 was used.
Survival was evaluated 76 days after tumor cells had been injected.

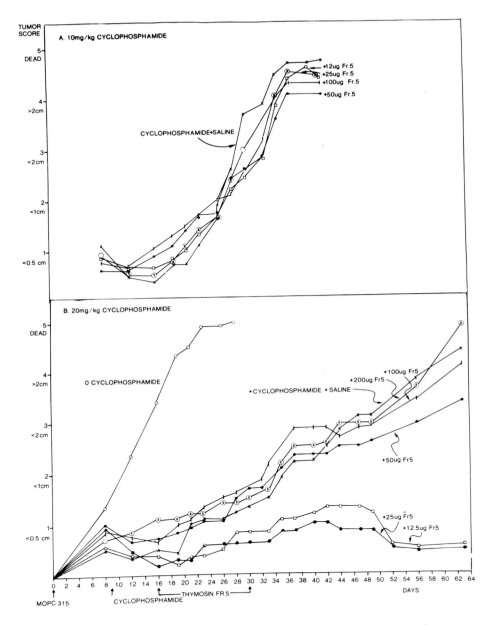

FIG. 2. Combined Effects of Cyclphoshphamide and Thymosin Fraction 5 on MOPC-315 Tumor Growth in Syngeneic Balb/c mice.

Thymosin fraction 5 was given in the same experiment 9 days after A. 10 mg/kg cyclophosphamide, or B. 20 mg/kg cyclophosphamide, injected i.p. The tumor growth curve for the control group (0 cyclophosphamide, -0-) is shown in 2B.

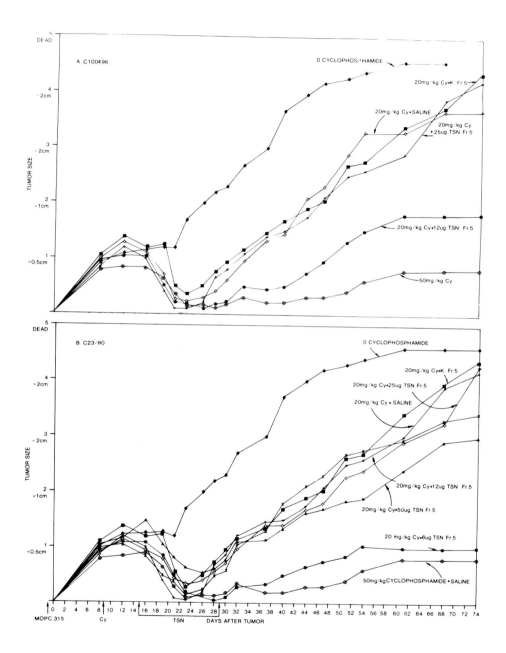

FIG. 3. Comparison of Effects of Two Clinical Lots of Thymosin Fraction 5 on Tumor Growth and Host Survival.

5 which can be used in this model (Figs. 3a and b, Table 2).

All animals without reappearance of tumor by day 75 remained tumor free indefinitely. Some survivors were rechallenged with 10^6 MOPC-315 cells s.c. 6 months following the initial challenge. Tumor cells were also given to age matched normal control mice as well as young control animals. None of the thymosin treated animals surviving the initial tumor inoculation showed any tumor growth upon second challenge (6/6 mice) whereas 100% of the control animals, both young and old, developed tumors and died (7/7).

Thus, appropriate doses of thymosin fraction 5, given one week following 20 mg/kg cyclophosphamide per mouse, resulted in long term survival and immunity to the MOPC-315 tumor.

DISCUSSION

The experimental syngeneic tumor model used in this study was designed to correspond as much as possible to clinical conditions. Thus treatment with a tumoricidal agent, cyclphosphamide, at a dose which is comparable to that used in human patients, was utilized; the thymosin therapy was instituted after the tumor burden had been reduced. Thymosin administered simultaneously with cyclophosphamide, or in a single injection 1 week following cyclophosphamide, was ineffective in preventing reappearance of the tumor (data not shown). As in other studies, both the time and dose of cyclophosphamide(6) and thymosin (2) administration proved to be critical in enhancing survival.

Additional varations of the experimental design need to be tested in order to determine an optimal protocol for use of thymosin fraction 5 in preventing syngeneic tumor growth. The effects of tumor resection, as well as administration of thymosin in fewer doses, need to be investigated.

It was of interest to note that higher doses of thymosin fraction 5 (>25 μg. per injection per mouse) given to cyclophosphamide-treated mice, were ineffective in preventing reappearance of the tumor. While it is unknown at the present time why higher doses of thymosin fraction 5 are less effective, there are several possible explanations: 1) Since fraction 5 is a composite of several biologically active peptides (4), selective peptides at lower doses may be enhancing tumor immunity, while at higher doses, additional peptides may be counteracting these effects by suppressing tumor immunity. It is known that fraction 5 contains peptides with both helper and suppressor function (1,8-10); 2) A single peptide at lower doses may activate a population involved in enhancing tumor immunity, while at higher doses the same peptide may activate cells which suppress immunity and/or activate tumor growth (5,6).

Studies are now underway to test the biological activity of several of the fraction 5 component peptides which have been isolated, purified and characterized (4). These studies are being conducted with the synthetic peptides where available. Hopefully, results of these studies will help to answer some of the questions posed by the dose effects observed with thymosin fraction 5.

It is worth noting that different lots of thymosin fraction 5 were effective at different doses. Lot 23/80CF, which was effective at a lower dose than lot C100496, also proved to have more biological activity in the *in vitro* MIF assay (11, and published observations). Since thymosin α_1 is the only thymosin peptide known to be specifically biologically active in this assay, these results may imply that thymosin α_1 is the component of fraction 5 which is biologically active in this tumor model.

The question of how thymosin fraction 5 or its component peptides, in conjunction with cyclophosphamide, acts to enhance host resistance to tumor growth, remains to be answered. It is likely that the cyclophosphamide treatment both serves to reduce the tumor burden and to reduce a suppressor cell population (5,6). By the time that thymosin is given, it is also likely that at least some of the suppressor cell population has returned (9). In fact, it is possible that high doses of thymosin fraction 5 accelerate the return of this population.

Preliminary experiments have been performed to assess the level of T-cell mediated tumor cell killing generated in co-cultures containing mitomycin C treated MOPC-315 tumor cells and spleen cells from experimental animals. Thus far, the data (not shown) give no evidence for enhanced T-cell cytotoxic activity in the groups showing prolonged survival. These studies need to be extended; it also will be necessary to examine the tumoricidal activity of macrophages and NK (7) cells in thymosin treated animals. Chirigos (2) demonstrated enhanced killing of tumor cells by macrophages from mice transplanted with a lymphoid leukemia, following thymosin treatment.

SUMMARY

Administration of thymosin fraction 5, in multiple microgram doses over a two week period, 9 days following cyclophosphamide treatment, resulted in long term survival of Balb/c mice bearing the syngeneic MOPC-315 tumor. The dose of thymosin fraction 5, as well as the dose of cyclophosphamide, was critical in preventing reappearance of the tumor. Those animals which rejected the tumor following thymosin and cyclophosphamide treatment, were completely resistant to a second challenge with the same dose of tumor cells.

ACKNOWLEDGEMENTS

This work was supported in part by grants from the NIH (CA 24974, CA 25017, and CA 17161), and Hoffmann- La Roche, Inc.

REFERENCES

1. Ahmed A., Wong, D.M., Thurman, G.B., Low, T.L.K., and Goldstein, A.L., (1979): Ann. N.Y. Acad. Sci 332:81.

2. Chirigos, M.A., (1978): Progr. in Cancer Research and Therapy, 7:305.

3. Cohen, M.H., Chretien, P.B., Ihle, D.C., Fossicek, P.E., Makuch, G., Bunn, P.A., Johnston, A.V., Shackney, S.E., Matthews, M.J., Lipson, S.D., Kennedy, D.E., and Minna, J.P., (1979): J.A.M.A., 241:1833.

4. Goldstein, A.L., Low, T.L.K., Thurman, G.B., Zatz, M.M., Hall, N., Chen, J., Hu, S.-K., Naylor, P.B., and McClure, J.E., Recent Progress in Hormone Research. In press.

5. Green, M.I., (1980): Contemp. Top. Immunobiol, 11:81.

6. Hengst, J.C.D., Mokyr, M.B., and Dray, S. (1980): Cancer Res., 27:305.

7. Herberman, R., and Holden, H.T., (1978): Adv. Cancer Res., 40:2135.

8. Horowitz, S., Borcherding, W., Moorthy, A.V., Chesney, R., Schulte-Wisserman, H., and Hong, R., (1977): Science, 197:999.

9. Marshall, G.D., Thurman, G.B., and Goldstein, A.L. (1980): Immunopharmacol, 2:301.

10. Marshall, G.D., Thurman, G.B., Rossio, J.L., and Goldstein, A.L., (1981); J. Immunol, 126:741.

11. Thurman, G.B., Low, T.K., Rossio, J.L., and Goldstein, A.L., (1981): These Proceedings

*Lymphokines and Thymic Hormones: Their
Potential Utilization in Cancer Therapeutics,*
edited by A. L. Goldstein and M. A. Chirigos,
Raven Press, New York © 1981.

Biologic Modification of Immunologic Parameters in Head and Neck Cancer Patients with Thymosin Fraction V

W. M. Wara, M. H. Neely, A. J. Ammann, and D. W. Wara

*Departments of Radiation Oncology and Pediatrics, University of California,
San Francisco, California 94143*

The disease-free interval and ultimate survival of patients with advanced squamous cell carcinoma of the head and neck region are low. Previous studies performed by our group have demonstrated that standard irradiation utilized for these patients' treatment has resulted in marked suppression of cell-mediated immunity (18,19). The severity, duration, and kinetics of this phenomenon, and its impact on disease-free interval and survival, were not possible to predict from these preliminary analyses (16).

These hypotheses, and the recognition of the thymus gland as an endocrine organ which produces humoral factors necessary for normal immunologic competence, have prompted the evaluation of a group of head and neck cancer patients receiving immunosuppressive irradiation. In an attempt to modify this immunosuppression, thymosin fraction V, a preparation containing approximately 20 peptides (4), which can modify the immune response in pediatric immunodeficiency disease and malignancy, was chosen for administration (2,5,7,11,17). The drug was randomly added to the standard local irradiation treatment to determine whether it would modify radiation-induced suppression, disease-free interval and/or survival.

MATERIALS AND METHODS

Patients with the histologic diagnosis of squamous cell carcinoma of the head and neck who were referred for irradiation of their disease to the Department of Radiation Oncology, University of California, San Francisco, were randomly assigned over the last four years to receive standard irradiation with and without thymosin fraction V (supplied by Hoffman-La Roche, Inc., Nutley, New Jersey, USA). To provide quality control for our laboratory values, immunologic evaluation was obtained in over 250 adult controls and 75 patients with cancer. Patients were evaluated with complete blood counts, E and EAC lymphocyte rosette formation, immunization with pneumococcal polysaccharide vaccine (PPS), lymphocyte stimulation with phytohemagglutinin (PHA), and in mixed leucocyte culture (MLC) using previously described methods (15,18,19). Serial prospective samples were obtained preirradiation, postirradiation, and at three-month intervals for one year.

There was no significant difference in stratification for either treatment regimen in regard to sex or age. As seen in Table 1, essentially the same number of patients with each site of primary lesion and stage of disease were assigned to the two regimens. Those that received thymosin had intradermal skin testing of 1 mg of thymosin fraction V, a bovine extract, to test for allergic reaction. The thymosin patients were scheduled to receive 60 mg/m^2 of thymosin x 10 and then twice weekly for 50 weeks.

TABLE 1.   Thymosin F5 - head and neck stratification

	Stage 2	Stage 3	Stage 4	Total
Thymosin F5	6/2[a]	12/0	6/7	24/9
Control	12/0	4/7	11/9	27/16
Total	18/2	16/7	17/16	51/25

[a]Oral cavity - larynx/pharynx.

RESULTS

As demonstrated in Table 2, all patients prior to local field irradiation had normal lymphocyte numbers with essentially no difference between the control and thymosin groups. Postirradiation, marked lymphopenia was noted for both groups (P < .01). There is some recovery at one year, but both groups continue to remain abnormal.

TABLE 2.   Thymosin F5 - head and neck total lymphocyte count

	Preirradiation	Postirradiation	1 Year
Thymosin F5	1714 ± 800 (33)[a]	743 ± 374 (29)	1113 ± 598 (11)
Control	1689 ± 800 (41)	620 ± 340 (35)	1000 ± 566 (13)

[a]Numbers in parentheses are the number of patients evaluated.

Humoral immunity as measured by EAC lymphocyte rosette formation showed no change in absolute numbers in either group before and after irradiation. Serum immunoglobulins (Table 3) also demonstrated no change pre and postirradiation. Of interest was the unexpected observation that patients in either group did not respond to immunization with pneumococcal polysaccharide vaccine during irradiation, suggesting that irradiation alters the normal ability to recognize and/or process a new antigen for permanent antibody production.

TABLE 3. Serum immunoglobulin level (mg/dl)

	Preirradiation	Postirradiation
IgG	1110 ± 490	1158 ± 587
IgM	172 ± 85	147 ± 61
IgA	275 ± 113	272 ± 114

No response to immunization with PPS 7, 12, 14, 18.

Evaluation of cellular immunity (Table 4) showed essentially normal values for each group pretreatment and marked decrease in numbers for both groups postirradiation ($P < .01$). The serial results of lymphocyte function are shown in Table 5. Before treatment, our patient populations are comparable and demonstrate no abnormal function. Postirradiation, a marked decrease in function is noted for both tests, with a quicker recovery in the thymosin-treated patients. This difference is statistically significant for both PHA stimulation and MLC data, with recovery and retention of normal effect in the thymosin-treated patients.

TABLE 4. Total E cell count (E rosette formation)
(Normal > 1200)[a]

	Preirradiation	Postirradiation	1 Year
Thymosin F5	1224 ± 578	578 ± 273	793 ± 446
Control	1258 ± 226	433 ± 249	739 ± 383

[a]Mean ± S.D.

TABLE 5. Lymphocyte function (cellular immunity)

	Preirradiation	Postirradiation	1 Year
	PHA Stimulation (normal > 22,000)		
Thymosin F5	25,294	10,377	21,782
Control	24,126	7,146	12,364
	MLC (normal > 5,000)		
Thymosin F5	11,655	5,466	7,990
Control	12,044	3,888	6,270

p = < .05

We now have 33 evaluable head and neck patients treated with
thymosin fraction V and 42 comparable control patients. As noted
previously, there is no difference in stratification between the two
groups in regard to significant prognostic variables. With a minimum
follow-up interval of eight months and a median of two years, the
disease-free interval is shown in Figure 1. Thymosin patients have a
64% (21/33) disease-free interval compared to the control group's 45%
(19/42), demonstrating an increase favoring the thymosin group
($p < .08$). Of interest is that patients do equally well for the first
six months before the curves separate and the difference becomes
apparent. Because patients who relapse can be salvaged by other
modalities, more time must elapse before a definitive statement can be
made regarding survival.

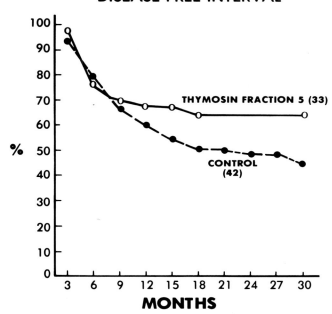

DISEASE FREE INTERVAL

FIG. 1.

DISCUSSION

Our results demonstrate that localized irradiation (5000-6000 rads)
produces secondary suppression of cellular immunity. Although the
exact mechanism for this effect remains unclear, it probably results
from irradiation of large blood volumes during treatment. Stjernsward
et al. (13) support this hypothesis in showing a minimal effect in

irradiated brain tumor patients who have a low blood flow per minute. Serum inhibitory factors or activation of suppressor cells may also contribute in some malignancies where in vitro depression has been noted (1,6).

Various authors have reported patients with squamous cell carcinoma of the head and neck as having abnormal numbers of T cells and/or decreased PHA stimulation or MLC function (3,8,9,12,14). These reports have usually examined patients with one test and have utilized different methodologies. Most reports have lacked serial studies to document the kinetics of immunologic recovery. In contrast, our patients are normal before treatment and only after irradiation do we demonstrate the marked immunosuppression noted by others. Our results demonstrate in the thymosin-treated patients the recovery of PHA stimulation and MLC function. This data and that of Raben et al. (10) suggest an increased proportion of "null cells" (lymphocytes with no surface marker) postirradiation which may be matured by thymosin into mature functioning cells. The demonstrated difference in relapse-free interval in this study indicates that when thymosin is used as adjuvant therapy after eradication of the majority of disease, an increase in disease control may result. Further investigation in head and neck and other forms of cancer to determine the optimum dose of thymosin which will yield the greatest biologic effect is clearly warranted.

REFERENCES

1. Bieber, M.D., Fuks, Z., and Kaplan, H.S. (1977): Clin. Exp. Immunol., 29:369-375.
2. Costanzi, J.J., Galiano, R.G., Delaney, F., et al. (1977): Cancer, 40:14-19.
3. Deegan, M.J., Coulthard, S.W., Qualman, S.J., et al. (1977): Cancer Res., 37:4475-4481.
4. Goldstein, A.L., Low, T.L.K., McAdoo, M., et al. (1977): Proc. Natl. Acad. Sci., 74:725-729.
5. Hardy, M.A., Dattner, A.M., Sarkar, D.K., et al. (1976): Cancer, 37:98-103.
6. Idestrom, K., Petrini, B., Blomgren, H., et al. (1979): Int. J. Radiat. Oncol. Biol. Physics, 5:1761-1766.
7. Kenady, D.E., Chreitien, P.B., Potvin, C., et al. (1977): Cancer, 39:642-652.
8. Mason, J.M., Kitchens, G.G., Eastham, R.J., et al. (1977): Arch. Otolaryngol., 103:223-227.
9. Olkowski, Z.L., and Wilkins, S.A. (1975): Am. J. Surg., 130:440-444.
10. Raben, M., Walach, N., Galili, U., et al. (1976): Cancer, 37:1417-1421.
11. Schaefer, L.A., Gutterman, J.U., Hersh, E.M., et al. (1979): Cancer Immunol. Immunother., 1:259-264.
12. Stefani, S., Kerman, R., and Abbate, J. (1976): Am. J. Roentgenol., 126:880-886.
13. Stjernsward, J., Jondal, M., Vanky, F., et al. (1972): Lancet, 1:1352-1356.
14. Wanebo, J.H., June, M.Y., Strong, E.W., et al. (1975): Am. J. Surg., 130:445-451.

15. Wara, D.W., Goldstein, A.L., Doyle, N.E., et al. (1975): New Eng.
     J. Med., 292:70-74.
16. Wara, W.M., Phillips, T.S., Wara, D.W., et al. (1975): Am. J.
     Roentgenol., 123:482-485.
17. Wara, D.W., and Ammann, A.J. (1978): Trans. Proc., 10:203-208.
18. Wara, W.M., Ammann, A.J., and Wara, D.W. (1978): Cancer Treat.
     Rep., 62:1775-1778.
19. Wara, W.M., Wara, D.W., Ammann, A.J., et al. (1979): Int. J.
     Radiat. Oncol. Biol. Phys., 5:997-1001.

ACKNOWLEDGEMENTS

   This work was supported by National Cancer Institute Grant CB 64004-
31 and the Division of Research Resources Clinical Research Center.

*Lymphokines and Thymic Hormones: Their
Potential Utilization in Cancer Therapeutics,*
edited by A. L. Goldstein and M. A. Chirigos,
Raven Press, New York © 1981.

In Vivo Release of Lymphokines and Their Relation to Cell-Mediated Immunity

Samuel B. Salvin

*Department of Microbiology, School of Medicine, University of Pittsburgh,
Pittsburgh, Pennsylvania 15261*

The early work on the induction of lymphokines was carried out in vitro by exposure of sensitized lymphoid cells to specific antigen (1,2,3,4,5). Subsequently, lymphokines were also induced in vitro by exposure of normal unsensitized cells to such mitogens as Concanavalin A or phytohemagglutinin. Such experiments, however, did not provide evidence for the possible role of these lymphokines in vivo (a) in the development of cell-mediated immunity in the intact animal, afflicted with malignant or infectious disease, or (b) in the possible cell interactions that result in cell-mediated immunity. Questions may therefore be asked as to whether lymphokines are non-essential soluble by-products in the development of cell-mediated immunity or whether they are active, essential ingredients of the immunity process. Are all lymphokines produced within a given animal on a given stimulus? Are these lymphokines produced in vivo in a particular sequence, or are they produced simultaneously? Are these lymphokines produced by the same or different lymphoid cells?

The release of lymphokines has been demonstrated in vivo in a number of species, including man, calf, guinea pig, rat, and mouse. For example, in mice, migration inhibitory factor (MIF) and Type II interferon (IFN γ) were induced by intravenous infection with living Mycobacterium bovis strain BCG, and three weeks later, by intravenous challenge with old tuberculin (OT) (6). More recently, either dead cells of BCG or a cell-wall antigen from BCG[1] emulsified in Drakeol-Tween 80 has been used for sensitization (7). Four hours after the animals had been sensitized and challenged, they were exsanguinated. This time sequence has been found to result in the release of maximum activities of MIF and IFN γ into the circulation. Such MIF induced in vivo reached titers as high as 1:512 to 1:1024 dilution of serum, whereas maximum titers in in vitro-induced supernatants were only 1:2 to 1:4.

---

[1] Cell-wall antigen was obtained from Dr. Edgar Ribi, Rocky Mountain Laboratory, Hamilton, Montana.

Success has also been obtained in causing the release of MIF into the circulation of rats (8) and in the body fluids or circulation of guinea pigs (9,10,11). MIF has been demonstrated in the circulation of humans with a variety of lympho-proliferative diseases such as non-Hodgkins lymphoma, Hodgkin's Disease, chronic lymphocytic leukemia, multiple myeloma, and Sezary syndrome (12). In patients with rheumatoid arthritis, MIF has been demonstrated in the synovial fluids (13,14).

MIF has been released in vivo in mice after stimulation with other antigens, such as Nocardia asteroides and Candida albicans (7). A variety of fractions of BCG and other mycobacteria have induced the release of MIF in vivo into the circulation. In these experiments, the mice were sensitized and challenged intravenously.

Thymus-derived lymphocytes are necessary for the in vivo release of MIF and IFN γ. This conclusion is based on the observations that neither neonatally thymectomized mice nor athymic nude mice would release detectable titers of MIF into their circulations after they had been sensitized and challenged (15). Also, adult mice that had been thymectomized, lethally irradiated with 900 rads, and then inoculated with normal bone marrow cells did not release MIF on sensitization and challenge with BCG and OT, respectively. However, when thymic cells were added to the bone marrow suspension, mice were then capable of releasing MIF into the circulation on appropriate challenge (15,16). Thus, T-lymphocytes seem to be an essential component for the release of such lymphokines as MIF and IFN γ into the circulation.

Three types of experiments were conducted to indicate that a correlation existed between the in vivo capacity to release lymphokines and the capacity to develop cell-mediated immunity. In the first set of experiments, mice were sensitized with cell-walls in Drakeol-Tween 80 emulsion either intravenously or subcutaneously. Three weeks later, they were challenged intravenously with OT and exsanguinated four hours later. Those animals that had been sensitized subcutaneously did not release detectable amounts of MIF into their circulation. However, they did develop striking footpad reactions (Table 1).

TABLE 1. Lymphokine (MIF) release and footpad reactions in mice sensitized with 300 µg cell walls in Drakeol-Tween 80 emulsion via one of two routes.

Route	Titer of MIF	Footpad reaction (% increase 24 hours after injection of antigen)
i.v.	128	9
s.c.	0	33
Control	0	2

In contrast, those mice that had been sensitized intravenously did not develop marked delayed footpad reactions, but did release MIF into the circulation in high titers. Mice in the latter group had increased resistance to aerosol challenge with virulent <u>Mycobacterium</u> <u>tuberculosis.</u>

In a second set of experiments, mice were sensitized intravenously with various fractions of BCG. Two groups of mice were sensitized with a particular fraction of BCG: one group was challenged intravenously with OT and exsanguinated, in order to determine whether that fraction could sensitize the mice and result in the release of MIF into the circulation; the other group was challenged intranasally with an aerosol of virulent <u>Mycobacterium</u> <u>tuberculosis</u> (H37Rv). The number of units of living tubercle bacilli in the lungs was determined quantitatively. Animals that had been sensitized with those fractions (as cell-wall skeleton or PPD) that did not result in the capacity to release MIF <u>in vivo</u> also did not show enhanced resistance to the tubercle bacillus on challenge. Like the control animals, they had approximately 10^7 units of bacteria in their lungs. In contrast, fractions such as those containing a combination of cell-wall skeleton, P^3 (which is a trehalose mycolic acid ester) and PPD developed the capacity to release MIF into the circulation and also showed a 1,000-fold decrease in the number of living tubercle bacilli in the lungs (7). These experiments were carried out in outbred Swiss Webster mice (Table II).

TABLE 2. Correlation between <u>in vivo</u> release of MIF and cell-mediated resistance to challenge with virulent <u>M.</u> <u>tuberculosis</u> (H37Rv)[a].

Sensitizing antigen	Titer of MIF	Number of viable bacteria per lung
CWS	0	1.5×10^6
CWS + P3	0	1.0×10^6
CWS + P3 + PPD	32	3.6×10^3
P3 + PPD	32	3.5×10^3
Control	0	7.0×10^6

[a] Reproduced in part from Salvin, S. B., <u>et al.</u>, <u>J. Immunol.</u> 114: 354-359, 1975.

In a third group of studies involving inbred strains of mice, the MIF-activity released into the blood varied greatly from strain to strain. Some were "high responders"; others, "low responders" (17). Some of the high and low responder strains were challenged with a weak pathogen, <u>Candida</u> <u>albicans</u>, either intraesophageally, in which case the fecal pellets were cultured quantitatively for the number of living units of Candida albicans, or intravenously, in which case the kidneys were cultured quantitatively. Strains, such as DBA/2J and C57Bl/10SNJ, that could release high titers of MIF into the circulation in vivo also showed a high degree of resistance to challenge with Candida albicans. In contrast, those strains, such as DBA/1J and C3H/HeJ, which released low or non-detectable titers of MIF into the circulation were highly susceptible to infection with Candida albicans.

The capacity of a given inbred strain of mouse to release MIF in vivo into the circulation did not necessarily correlate with the capacity of that strain to release such other lymphokines as mitogenic factor, lymphotoxin, or chemotactic factor (Table 3).

TABLE 3. Activities of four different lymphokines released in vivo into the circulation of five inbred strains of BCG-sensitized mice[a].

Strain	H-2	MIF[b]	CF[b]	MF[b]	LT[b]
A/J	a	256		3.6 ± 0.3	84.4 ± 4.4
C57Bl/10SNJ	b	256	1.81 ± 1.2	2.3 ± 0.6	N.D.
C57Bl/KsJ	d	256	-4.7	1.1 ± 0.3	-3.5 ± 9.2
CBA/CaJ	k	8-16	3.0 ± 0.9	3.4 ± 0.7	39.1 ± 6.7
C3H/HeJ	k	4	$.68 \pm 0.68$	2.3 ± 0.5	N.D.

[a] Reproduced in part from a manuscript just submitted for publication.

[b] MIF: migration inhibitory factor; CF: chemotactic factor; MF: mitogenic factor; and LT: lymphotoxin.

Although the capacity of a given strain to release a given pattern of lymphokines is genetically determined, it is not known what pattern of lymphokines, if any, is associated with cell-mediated resistance against a given microorganism or foreign or malignant cells.

In summary, lymphokines can be induced to be released in vivo to any one of several antigens. Secondly, a correlation exists between the capacity to form MIF and the capacity to develop cell-mediated resistance. Thirdly, the capacity of a given strain to release MIF or IFN γ does not correlate necessarily with the capacity of that strain to release other lymphokines into the circulation.

REFERENCES

1. Holst, P. M. (1922): Tubercle, 3:249-256.

2. Rich, A. R. and Lewis, M. R. (1932): Bull. Johns Hopkins Hosp., 50:115-131.

3. George, M. and Vaughan, J. H. (1962): Proc. Soc. Exp. Biol. Med., 111:514-521.

4. David, J. R., Al-Askari, S., Lawrence, H. S., and Thomas, L. (1964): J. Immunol., 93:264-273.

5. Bloom, B. R. and Bennett, B. (1966): Science, 153:80-82.

6. Salvin, S. B., Youngner, J. S., and Lederer, W. H. (1973): Infect. Immun., 7:68-75.

7. Salvin, S. B., Ribi, E., Granger, D. L., and Youngner, J. S. (1975): J. Immunol., 114:354-359.

8. Ruscetti, S. K., Gill, T. J., Salvin, S. B., Hermann, J., and Bailie, C. W. (1976): Intern. Arch. Allergy and Appl. Immunol., 52:417-421.

9. Yamamoto, K. and Takahashi, Y. (1971): Nature(London) New Biology, 233:261-263.

10. Yoshida, T. and Cohen, S. (1974): J. Immunol., 112:1540-1547.

11. Van Maarsseveen, A. C. (1977): Immunology, 32:893-898.

12. Cohen, S., Fisher, B., Yoshida, T., and Bettigole, R. E. (1974): New Eng. J. Med., 290:882-886.

13. Stastny, P., Rosenthal, M., Andreis, M., Cooke, D., and Ziff, M. (1975a): Ann. N. Y. Acad. Sci., 256:117-131.

14. Stastny, P., Rosenthal, M., Andreis, M., and Ziff, M. (1975b): Arthr. Rheum., 18:237-243.

15. Salvin, S. B., Sonnenfeld, G., and Nishio, J. (1977): Infect. Immun., 17:639-643.

16. Sonnenfeld, G., Salvin, S. B., and Youngner, J. S. (1977): Infect. Immun., 18:283-290.

17. Neta, R. and Salvin, S. B. (1980): Cell. Immunol., 51:173-178.

*Lymphokines and Thymic Hormones: Their
Potential Utilization in Cancer Therapeutics,*
edited by A. L. Goldstein and M. A. Chirigos,
Raven Press, New York © 1981.

In Vivo Induced Immune Interferon: Relation to Other Lymphokines and Effect on Growth of Tumor Cells

Ruth Neta

Department of Microbiology, University of Notre Dame, Notre Dame, Indiana 46556

The discovery that autochtonous tumors may induce in the host cell-mediated immune reactions directed against themselves (4,6,13), has challenged immunologists into developing tools for prevention and control of malignant growth. However, despite numerous reports on successful treatment of tumors in experimental animals with a number of immunopotentiating agents (5,7,8), the incidence of successful immunotherapy of tumors in human patients remains quite low. Apparently, means for controlling of the flexible immune system remain to be developed. It is now recognized that every immune response represents a dynamic equilibrium of helper and suppressor functions. At present, the ability to stimulate various arms of the immune response preferentially is limited. It also remains to be determined what balance of responses is necessary for the rejection of tumors by the host's immune system. One way to obtain such knowledge may involve studies on the lymphokines and on their role in tumor therapy.

Since lymphokines are thought to be the soluble mediators of cell-mediated immunity, treatment with lymphokines (LK) may present an effective tool in tumor therapy. If successful, such treatment would have an advantage of allowing the selection of lymphokines most active in tumor rejection and elimination of lymphokines harmful to host defenses.

1. Inhibition of tumor growth by LK-containing serum

Lymphokines were induced into the circulation of tuberculous mice after intravenous challenge with old tuberculin (OT) (14). Sensitization of the mice was carried out by intravenous inoculation of either viable BCG or cell walls of BCG in Drakeol-Tween 80 emulsion. The tumor that was studied most extensively was a 3-methylcholanthrene induced sarcoma (MC-36) in C_3H mice (15). Solid tumor fragments were implanted subcutaneously into the abdominal area of mice. Within 24 hours after the implantation the lymphokine containing serum (LK-serum) or the control serum was inoculated subcutaneously into the tumor or the tumor implant site. Such inoculation was carried out daily with a standard dose of LK-serum containing 300 units of IFNγ. (Table 1).

Table 1

Inhibition of MC-36 sarcoma by LK-containing sera

Expt	Duration (days)	Tumor mass (mm^3) in mice given		Percent inhibition
		Control sera; mean $\pm$ SE[a]	LK-containing sera; mean $\pm$ SE[a]	
1	30	(6) 998$\pm$159	(8) 18$\pm$38	99.8
2	31	(6) 780$\pm$450	(4) 22$\pm$63	97.2
3	28	(16) 1,322$\pm$243	(14) 52$\pm$54	97.0
4	32	(15) 624$\pm$177	(13) 24$\pm$62	96.3
5	31	(12) 858$\pm$520	(11) 6$\pm$58	99.3
Average volume of tumor mass		(55) 916$\pm$310	(50) 24$\pm$55	98

[a]Number of mice in parentheses.

[b]Data reproduced from Ref. 15.

The effect of such treatment on tumor growth was dose dependent. Lower doses merely inhibited the growth of tumors, while higher doses caused elimination of tumors as indicated by the finding that upon termination of the treatment recurrence of tumor growth was not detected (9).

These results raised a question concerning the mechanism of the tumor rejection, namely whether the LK-serum had a direct cytotoxic effect on tumor cells and/or whether it was effective by mobilizing the host's defenses.

To determine the mechanisms involved in such rejection, in vitro and in vivo studies were carried out (16). Several cell lines from homologous and heterologous species were lysed on an addition of the LK-serum. Established monolayers of MC-36 mouse sarcoma, of human HeLa cells, and of rat Kirsten virus induced sarcoma, were lysed on addition to the culture medium of 1-2% LK-serum.

In another series of experiments the role of LK-serum in activation of PE macrophages was examined. The addition of 10^6 macrophages or of 0.5% LK-serum separately had little effect on the growth of the monolayers. However, the addition of 10^6 macrophages and 0.5% LK-serum in combination resulted in lysis of cell monolayers.

The in vivo effect of the LK-serum was studied by preparing histologic sections from the site of LK-serum inoculation. Such examination revealed extensive cellular infiltration and vacuolization. Thus, the results provide evidence that a direct lytic effect on tumor cells and

Table 2

Cytotoxicity and IFNγ in sera of sensitized and challenged C57BL/KsJ mice at times after challenge

Time after challenge (hours)	5% serum			2.5% serum			IFN titer
	Total # of colonies	# of colonies > 20 cells	# of colonies > 50 cells	Total # of colonies	# of colonies > 20 cells	# of colonies > 50 cells	
Control	175.0±25.3	67.8±5.3	23.7±6.1	168.2±22.3	58.3±11.3	32.0±7.8	< 100*
2	187.3±27.4	31.3±8.1	3.3±1.2	172.7±21.0	65.3±10.3	28.7±3.3	1200
4	177.3±23.4	22.7±7.1	4.3±0.9	178.7±165	48.7± 7.9	14.0±4.0	110,000
8	55.3±65	2	0.6	128.7± 5.2	16.6± 4.6	4.7±1.7	11,000
24	0.7	0	0	72.7± 5.5	3.1	1.0	150

Groups of 7-10 mice sensitized intravenously with CW/Dr and challenged 3 weeks later with 50 mg OT were bled at times after challenge. Control sera were obtained from normal mice of the same strain challenged with 50 mg OT and bled 4 hours later. Cytotoxicity and IFN were assayed as described.

*Ten units of IFN in this assay are equivalent to 1 unit of standard reference IFN.

(Data reproduced from Ref. 10)

the mobilization of host's defenses may be the basis for tumor inhibition and elimination.

When type I interferon (IFN α + β) was used in parallel experiments, the doses of this IFN required to similarly suppress tumor growth were many folds higher than the doses of IFNγ (15,3). Preparations of IFNγ have been also shown to be more potent than those of IFN α + β in the immunomodulatory action (17). Is such higher potency of IFNγ due to much higher specific activity of this substance or is it due to an interaction of this interferon with other lymphokines present in the preparation? A direct answer to this question is not possible, since purified IFNγ is not available at the present time. However, there is some evidence to indicate that the cell receptors for interferon may be the same for different types of interferons. The genetic locus controlling the expression of such receptors has been mapped to chromosome 21 in humans (18) and 16 in mice (2). Cells from patients with Down syndrome trisomic for chromosome 21 have similarly increased sensitivity to the three known types of interferon (1).

The conditions for induction of IFNγ, which include stimulation of lymphoid cells with specific antigen or T-cell mitogen, are also the conditions that stimulate the release of other lymphokines. However, at the present state of the art a rigorous separation of IFNγ from other lymphokines has not been achieved.

2. Separation in vivo of cytotoxic from IFNγ activity

The finding that strains of mice vary greatly in the release of IFNγ and MIF (11) and in the release of other lymphokines (12) may serve as a means for separation of lymphokines from one another or for elimination of certain lymphokine activities from a mixture.

Two approaches were developed to initiate the possible separation.
1. Activities of six different lymphokines were compared in the sera of 16 strains of mice.
2. The same strains of mice were bled at different times after challenge to determine if the times for the optimal release of different lymphokines within the strain may vary.

The pattern of the presence of different lymphokines vary from strain to strain (11,12). In addition, although the titers of IFNγ and MIF vary in parallel in the sera of different strains, with the maximal titers in high- and in low-responder mice occurring at 4 hours after challenge, similar pattern was not observed for the presence of cytotoxic activity (10).

The cytotoxicity was measured by the colony inhibition of rat prostate tumor cells. In this assay the lytic effect expressed by the reduction in the number of colonies could be separated from the proliferation inhibitory effect expressed by the differential count of colonies of various sizes. Sera from A/J mice, high-responders in the release of IFNγ, and from CBA/CaJ and Balb/cByJ mice, low-responders in the release of IFNγ, were highly cytotoxic (100% cytotoxicity of 2.5% serum concentration) at 8 and 12 hours after challenge. In contrast, sera

from C57Bl/KsJ mice with high titers of IFNγ had no cytotoxic activity
(Table 2). The highest cytotoxicity in the serum of this strain was
detected at 24 hours after challenge. Sera with high titers of IFNγ had
proliferation inhibitory activity. These results indicate that it is
possible in the in vivo system to separate the sera with IFNγ from those
with cytotoxic activity.

Additional evidence for the separate appearance of the cytotoxic
and IFNγ activity was obtained when the release of IFNγ in Swiss Webster
mice was regulated with complete Freund's adjuvant to either enhance the
production of IFNγ or suppress it (9). Despite a thousand fold difference in the titer of IFNγ marked differences in the cytotoxicity were
not observed (Table 3).

Table 3

Cytotoxic effect of LK-sera from Swiss Webster mice on rat
prostate tumor cells

Interferon titer	Cytotoxicity (% inhibition) with	
	5% serum	2.5% serum
450,000	46+19	29+6
4,200	54+12	15+2
21,000	47+11	17+3
500	41+13	21+2

The colonies were counted after 5 days incubation at 37⁰. The numbers
of colonies grown in control serum were 251+33 in 5% and 248+18 in 2.5%.

This result was not due to the lack of sensitivity of the cytotoxicity
assay, since a two-fold dilution of the sera resulted in an average reduction in the cytotoxic activity by a factor of 2.4. It is, therefore,
possible that the mechanisms controlling the release or the activity of
the two lymphokines may be separate.

3. Inhibitor to IFNγ in sera of low responders

In view of the observed variations in the presence of individual
lymphokine activities, the question arises whether such lymphokines are
selectively not produced or whether their activity was not detected because of some inhibitory factor(s) in the sera. To examine the latter
possibility, sera from strains which are low-responder in the production
of IFNγ were mixed with sera from high-responder strains (Table 4).

The inhibitory activity was detected in the sera of sensitized and
challenged low-responder mice. These results make the attempts to study
in vivo separation of the mechanisms of the release of different lymphokines more difficult. However, the variations in the expression of
lymphokine activities in different sera may present a means to study the
role of treatment with certain combinations of lymphokines in therapy of

Table 4

Suppressor Factor in Sera of Low-responder Strains

Donor Strain	IFNγ titer			Reduction ratio
	Background	Donor	Mixture[a]	
-	>1,000,000	-	-	-
BALB/cByJ (LK)[b]	>1,000,000	<100	22,000	>45.5
BALB/cByJ (con.)[c]	>1,000,000	<100	135,000	> 7.4
AKR (LK)	>1,000,000	850	22,000	>45.5
AKR (con.)	>1,000,000	<100	220,000	> 4.5

[a]Serum from background Swiss Webster mice was admixed with serum from a donor strain in 1:1 ratio

[b](LK) serum obtained from sensitized mice challenged with OT

[c](Con) serum obtained from normal mice challenged with OT
        (Reproduced from Ref. 9)

tumors.

It is quite apparent that the presence of the lymphokines in the blood of sensitized and challenged animals in various titers may not be indicative of the responsiveness of other lymphoid tissues to an *in vitro* challenge with mitogens or specific antigens. However, the presence of such lymphokines in the blood mirrors the immunological events in the circulation of sensitized and challenged animals. The correlation of the observed differences in the titers of various lymphokines with (a) variations in resistance of different mice strains and (b) effectiveness of passive transfer of LK-sera in protection against tumors or infections, may lead to determination of the role for individual lymphokines or groups of lymphokines in resistance.

References

1. Epstein, L. B., and Epstein, C. J. (1976) J. Infect. Dis. (Suppl.) 133, A-56-62.
2. Epstein, L. B., Cox, D. R., and Epstein, C. J. (1980) Ann. N.Y. Acad. Sci., 350, 171-175.
3. Gresser, I., and Bourali, C. (1970) J. Natl. Cancer Inst., 45, 365-375.
4. Foley, E. J. (1953) Cancer Res., 13, 835-837.
5. Halpern, B. N., Biozzi, G., Stiffel, C., and Mouton, D. (1966) Nature (London) 212, 853-854.
6. Klein, G., Sjogren, H. O., Klein, E., and Hellstrom, K. I. (1960) Cancer Res., 20, 1561-1572.
7. Mathe, G., Pouillart, P., and Lapeyraque, F. (1969) Brit. J. Cancer, 23, 814-824.
8. Mathe, G., Halle-Pannenko, O., and Bourut, C. (1972) Eur. J. Clin. Biol. Res., 17, 997-1000.

9. Neta, R. (1981) Cell. Immunol., <u>59</u> in press.
10. Neta, R. (1981) J. Interferon Res., in press.
11. Neta, R., and Salvin, S. B. (1980) Cell. Immunol., <u>51</u>, 173-178.
12. Neta, R., Salvin, S. B., and Sabaawi, M., submitted for publication.
13. Prehn, R. T., and Main, J. H. (1957) J. Natl. Cancer Inst., <u>18</u>, 769-778.
14. Salvin, S. B., Youngner, J. S., and Lederer, W. H. (1973) Infec. Immun., <u>7</u>, 68-75.
15. Salvin, S. B., Youngner, J. S., Nishio, J., and Neta, R. (1975) J. Natl. Cancer Inst., <u>55</u>, 1233-1236.
16. Salvin, S. B., Nishio, J., and Neta, R. (1976) Proc. Eleventh U.S.-Japan Tuberculosis Conference, Tokyo, Japan, pp. 221-229.
17. Sonnenfeld, G. (1980) Lymphokine Reports, <u>1</u>, 113-131.
18. Tan, Y. H., Tishfield, J., and Ruddle, F. H. (1973) J. Exp. Med., <u>137</u>, 317-330.

Lymphokines and Thymic Hormones: Their Potential Utilization in Cancer Therapeutics, edited by A. L. Goldstein and M. A. Chirigos, Raven Press, New York © 1981.

The Use of Liposomes as Carriers for Lymphokines to Achieve Activation of Tumoricidal Properties in Murine Macrophages and Destruction of Pulmonary Metastases

I. J. Fidler and W. E. Fogler

Cancer Metastasis and Treatment Laboratory, Frederick Cancer Research Center, Frederick, Maryland 21701

INTRODUCTION

Among the many biological responses to lymphokines (2), the activation of tumoricidal properties in mononuclear cells may be instrumental in augmenting host defense against neoplastic disease. The lymphokine component responsible for the activation of tumoricidal properties in macrophages has been designated as macrophage-activating factor (MAF). Evidence that tumoricidal macrophages may be effective in controlling cancer metastasis has come from studies in which macrophages activated in vitro were injected systemically into syngeneic mice bearing pulmonary metastases (3,4,7,18). However, this approach to therapy has a serious limitation because it requires the transfusion of large numbers of histocompatible or autologous macrophages. A more feasible regimen would be to deliver activating stimuli to the mononuclear phagocyte in situ since murine macrophages from the tumor-bearing host are responsive to lymphokine-mediated activation (5,17,22,25). Therapeutic use of MAF is hindered, however, by the lack of purified preparations of this mediator and the inability of lymphokine preparations rich in MAF activity to render macrophages tumoricidal in situ when injected systemically. In the last few years, increasing attention has been given to the potential value of liposomes, concentric phospholipid vesicles separated by aqueous compartments, as carriers of agents in the treatment of a variety of diseases, including cancer (12). Lymphokines rich in MAF activity can be encapsulated within liposomes and can then render mouse peritoneal macrophages (PEM) or rat alveolar macrophages (AM) tumoricidal in vitro at concentrations up to $1-2 \times 10^4$ times lower than unencapsulated (free) MAF added to the culture medium (27,31). These findings raised the question of whether liposome-encapsulated lymphokines could induce nonspecific activation of macrophages and the reticulo-endothelial system in vivo, thus offering a useful therapeutic regimen toward inhibition or destruction of cancer metastases. Liposomes are an attractive vehicle for the in situ delivery of MAF to macrophages for several reasons. Unlike activation by free MAF, which requires its binding to a receptor on the macrophage surface (26), liposome-encapsulated MAF can activate macrophages lacking functional receptors for MAF (22,27). Moreover, liposome-encapsulated MAF can induce the activation of macrophages that are completely refractory to activation by free MAF (22,25,28). The majority of systemically injected liposomes are taken up by macrophages (16) and, although this represents a major obstacle to the "targeting" of liposomes to other cell types, the uptake of liposomes by macrophages offers a means of enhancing uptake of agents that stimulate macrophage activity. Finally, liposomes in themselves represent a nontoxic and nonimmunogenic form of adjuvant therapy (1).

In this paper we present our observations on the in situ activation of tumoricidal properties in murine macrophages following the intravenous administration of liposomes containing lymphokines and the effectiveness of this approach for the treatment of spontaneous pulmonary metastases.

MATERIALS AND METHODS

Animals

Specific-pathogen-free mice of the inbred strain C57BL/6N and F344 strain rats were obtained from the Frederick Cancer Research Center's Animal Production Area.

Cell Cultures

The B16-BL6 variant line of the C57BL/6 melanoma has been adapted to grow in vitro. Following implantation at a subcutaneous (sc) site, this tumor metastasizes to the lungs and lymph nodes in about 90% of mice (14,23). All monolayer cultures were maintained in Eagle's minimal essential medium supplemented with 5% fetal bovine serum, vitamin solution, sodium pyruvate, nonessential amino acids, and L-glutamine (complete minimal essential medium, CMEM). The components of this medium were obtained from Flow Laboratories, Rockville, MD. All cultures were incubated at 37°C in a humidified atmosphere containing 5% CO_2. All cultures were free of Mycoplasma, reovirus type 3, pneumonia virus of mice, K virus, Theiler's encephalitis virus, Sendai virus, minute virus of mice, mouse adenovirus, mouse hepatitis virus, lymphocytic choriomeningitis virus, ectromelia virus, and lactate dehydrogenase virus (MA Bioproducts, Walkersville, MD).

Lipids and Other Materials

Purified egg phosphatidylcholine (PC) and beef brain phosphatidylserine (PS) were purchased from Avanti Biochemicals (Birmingham, AL). All lipids were shown to be chromatographically pure by thin layer chromatography and were stored in a nitrogen atmosphere at -70°C in chloroform in sealed ampules until use. [4-^{14}C]cholesterol (specific activity 54 mCi/mmole) was purchased from New England Nuclear (Boston, MA). Bovine serum albumin (BSA), Fraction V, was purchased from the Sigma Chemical Co. (St. Louis, MO) and labeled with carrier-free [^{125}I]Na (Amersham Corp., Arlington Heights, IL), as described previously (11). [^{125}I]-labeled BSA was dialyzed against phosphate-buffered saline (PBS) at 4°C until no radioactivity was detected in the dialysate. The specific activity of [^{125}I]-labeled BSA preparations ranged from 5 to 10 cpm/mg protein.

Preparation of Lymphokines

Cell-free supernatants rich in MAF activity were harvested from cultures of rat lymphocytes stimulated in vitro with concanavalin A bound to Sepharose beads (Con-A Sepharose, Pharmacia, Piscataway, NJ), as described previously (29). Spleens from normal F344 rats were collected aseptically, minced in cold Hanks' balanced salt solution (HBSS) and pressed through a 60-mesh stainless steel wire sieve (E-C Apparatus Corp., St. Petersburg, FL). The resulting suspensions were then passed over sterile gauze and centrifuged. The cell pellets were resuspended in CMEM. The viability of the mononuclear cells was >90% as determined by the trypan blue exclusion test. The cells were diluted in CMEM to 10^7 viable cells/ml. Con-A Sepharose was washed three times with HBSS and then added to the mononuclear cell cultures at a final concentration of 100 µg bound Con-A Sepharose/ml. The cultures were then incubated for 48 hr on a gently rocking platform in a 37°C incubator. Following incubation, the suspensions were centrifuged for 20 min at 5000 RPM. Rat normal lymphocyte supernatant fluids (NRSUP) were obtained from similarly treated lymphocytes without Con-A Sepharose stimulation. Cell-free supernatants filtered through a 0.22 µm Millipore membrane were stored at -70°C until use. Lymphokines rich in MAF were shown to be endotoxin-free by the Limulus amebocyte lysate assay (Associates of Cape Cod, Woods Hole, MA). For descriptive convenience and brevity, cell-free culture supernatants that are rich in MAF activity will be referred to simply as MAF throughout the remainder of this paper.

Preparation of Liposomes

Multilamellar vesicles (MLV) composed of PS/PC (3:7 mole ratio) were prepared by mechanical vortex shaking, as described previously (27). In certain experiments, $[4-^{14}C]$cholesterol was added to the initial phospholipid mixture to give a final specific activity of 0.1 µCi/ µmole lipid. For encapsulation of rat NRSUP, MAF or $[^{125}I]$BSA within MLV, phospholipids (20-50 µmoles) were first evaporated to dryness under nitrogen, resuspended in the material to be encapsulated (1-5 ml) and then vortex shaken to form MLV. Nonencapsulated material was separated from liposomes by centrifugation for 20 min at 37,000 x g, and the pelleted liposomes were resuspended in HBSS for injection into animals. Capture of $[^{125}I]$BSA in liposomes was calculated as described elsewhere (27). The internal volume of the MLV was determined to be 3.4 ± 0.5 µl per µmole phospholipid.

In Vivo Activation of Macrophages with Lymphokines Encapsulated in Liposomes

Four days after intraperitoneal (ip) injection of 2.0 ml thioglycollate, mice were injected ip or intravenously (iv) into the lateral tail vein with 5 µmole of MLV containing either MAF or rat NRSUP. The MLV were suspended in HBSS and the inoculum volume was 1.0 ml for the ip and 0.2 ml for the iv injections. Control experiments included the ip injection of 5 µmole of MLV containing PBS but suspended in 1.0 ml of either MAF or rat NRSUP. We have used PS/PC MLV as carriers for MAF because they are not toxic at the dose used here (15) and are arrested efficiently in the lungs following iv injections (8,9). Mice were killed 24 hr later, and their macrophages were harvested as described below. In some experiments the prior injection of thioglycollate was omitted.

Preparation and Purification of Murine PEM and AM Cultures

All PEM were harvested by lavage with Ca^{2+}-, Mg^{2+}-free HBSS without heparin. AM were harvested by a tracheobronchial lavage method described fully elsewhere (31). Routinely, cell populations were suspended in serum-free CMEM and plated into Microtest II wells (Falcon Plastics, Oxnard, CA) at a concentration of 1×10^5 cells per well. Forty min after plating at 37°C, the wells were rinsed and refed with CMEM. The cellular composition of the resulting monolayers was examined and determined to be macrophages, both morphologically and by the carbon particle phagocytosis test. These cells were then used for the in vitro assay.

Macrophage-Mediated Cytotoxicity Assay (In Vitro)

Macrophage-mediated cytotoxicity was assessed by a radioactive release assay as described previously (29). Following an activation period in vivo, the cultures were washed with media, and 5×10^3 ^{125}I-iododeoxyuridine ($[^{125}I]IUdR$)-labeled target cells were added to each well in 0.2 ml medium containing 5% fetal bovine serum. Target cells alone were always plated as an additional control. Twenty-four hr after the addition of target cells, the cultures were washed and refed to remove nonplated cells. Adherent target cells were lysed at 24 or 72 hr after plating with 0.1 ml of N NaOH. The lysate was adsorbed on cotton swabs, placed directly into 12 X 75 mm tubes and monitored for radioactivity in a gamma counter. The percent cytotoxicity in the macrophage assays was computed by the following formula:

$$\frac{\text{cpm of target cells with normal macrophages} - \text{cpm of target cells with activated macrophages}}{\text{cpm of target cells with normal macrophages}} \times 100$$

The statistical significance of differences between groups was determined by the Student's two-tailed t-test.

Determination of the In Vivo Uptake of Liposomes by PEM

Four days after the ip injection of 2.0 ml thioglycollate (Baltimore Biologicals, Cockeysville, MD), C57BL/6 mice were injected ip with $[^{125}I]BSA$ encapsulated within varying concentrations of liposomes containing $[4-^{14}C]$cholesterol in the lipid membrane. The initial ratio of $[4-^{14}C]/[^{125}I]$ was 3.51. Mice were killed 4 hr after liposome injection, and their PEM were harvested. The PEM were washed, suspended in serum-free media and plated into 200-mm^2 wells (Falcon Plastics, Oxnard, CA) at a concentration of 1×10^6 cells/well. Forty min after plating at 37°C, the adherent cells were rinsed, lysed with 1 ml of 0.1 N NaOH and monitored for radioactivity in a gamma or liquid scintillation counter.

Regression of Spontaneous Metastases Following the Systemic Injection of Liposomes Containing Lymphokines

C57BL/6 mice were injected sc in the footpad with 3×10^4 viable B16-BL6 tumor cells. Four weeks later, when the tumors reached 10-12 mm in diameter, the mice were anesthetized by methoxyflurane inhalation, and the tumor-bearing leg, including the popliteal lymph node, was amputated at midfemur. Liposome treatment began 3 days later, and each treatment consisted of an i.v. injection in the tail vein of MLV (5 µmoles phospholipids) suspended in 0.2 ml of HBSS. The MLV consisted of PS and PC at a 3:7 mole ratio and contained either MAF or HBSS (empty liposomes). The latter liposomes were suspended in PBS containing MAF. Additional controls included mice given iv injections of HBSS or free MAF. Treatments were given twice weekly for 4 weeks. Mice were killed two weeks after the final treatment or were observed for survival analysis. Pulmonary metastases in each animal were counted under a dissecting microscope by two independent observers. All suspected pulmonary and extrapulmonary metastases were confirmed by microscopic examination of fixed histological sections.

RESULTS

The in vitro cytotoxicity mediated by murine macrophages was assayed against the B16-BL6 melanoma since this tumor was also used in the therapy studies reported below. PEM, harvested from mice 24 hr after the ip injections of liposome-encapsulated MAF, were cytotoxic to the B16-BL6 (32% specific cytotoxicity, $p < 0.01$, Table 1). In contrast, AM harvested from the same donors (given ip injections) were not cytotoxic to tumor targets. On the other hand, 24 hr following the iv injection of liposome-encapsulated MAF, AM harvested from the injected donors were tumoricidal (25% specific cytotoxicity, $p < 0.01$), but PEM were not. The in situ activation of AM or PEM required the injection of MLV containing MAF. Control injections of MLV containing rat NRSUP failed to activate AM or PEM (Table 1). Furthermore, control ip injections of free rat NRSUP, free MAF or liposomes containing HBSS ("empty") suspended in either MAF or rat NRSUP also failed to render PEM tumoricidal (Table 1). Only liposome-encapsulated MAF rendered macrophages tumoricidal. This clearly demonstrates that the in situ activation of murine macrophages by liposome-encapsulated MAF was not caused by a liposome-mediated alteration in the macrophages, which enhanced their responsiveness to MAF to a level where MAF molecules leaking from MLV could induce activation by binding to the macrophage surface. It is also important when comparing PEM activation by liposome-encapsulated MAF and free MAF to recognize that the total amount of MAF encapsulated within liposomes injected ip was far lower than the amount of free MAF (5 µmole of MLV contained approximately 17 µl of encapsulated material).

To quantitate liposome-macrophage interaction in situ, we injected [^{125}I]BSA encapsulated in varying concentrations of MLV that contained [$4-^{14}$C]cholesterol in the lipid membrane (as an independent marker) into the peritoneal cavity of mice stimulated with thioglycollate. The degree of macrophage activation by liposome-encapsulated MAF was correlated with the total volume transferred to macrophages by liposomes (Table 2). Increasing the amount of injected MLV (0.5 to 5 µmoles) led to a direct increase in the amount of [^{125}I]BSA transferred to PEM. These data suggested that increasing the amount of injected MLV increased the transfer of MAF to macrophages in situ. Indeed, the level of cytotoxicity generated in PEM was found to be proportional to the internal volume of liposomes transferred to the macrophages (Table 2).

TABLE 1. Compartmental activation of tumoricidal properties in murine PEM and AM following ip or iv injection of liposome-encapsulated lymphokines

Treatment of donors[a]	Treatment route	Macrophage population		Radioactivity (cpm) in live target cells on day 3[b]
		PEM	AM	
None, tumor cells alone	--	--	--	1095 + 52
Free NRSUP	ip	+		1113 + 30
Free NRSUP + "empty" liposomes[c]	ip	+		1116 + 78
Liposomes-NRSUP[d]	ip	+		1011 + 86
	ip		+	1006 + 57
	iv	+		1092 + 53
	iv		+	1168 + 42
Free MAF	ip	+		1047 + 10
Free MAF + "empty" liposomes[c]	ip	+		1056 + 41
Liposomes-MAF[d]	ip	+		687 + 39 (32)[e]
	ip		+	1111 + 58
	iv	+		1094 + 29
	iv		+	876 + 21 (25)[e]

[a]Four days following the ip injection of 2.0 ml thioglycollate, C57BL/6 mice were injected iv or ip with the indicated material in an inoculum volume of 0.2 or 1.0 ml, respectively. AM or PEM were harvested 24 hr postinjection and macrophage cultures were prepared as described under Materials and Methods. Three mice per group.

[b]5×10^3 target cells labeled with [^{125}I]IdUrd were plated onto macrophage monolayers. The cultures were maintained in CMEM and refed 24 h after addition of the target cells. Results represent mean + SD of triplicate cultures.

[c]MLV (5 μmol total phospholipid) containing HBSS suspended in 1.0 ml of NRSUP or MAF.

[d]MLV (5 μmol total phospholipid) containing either NRSUP or MAF.

[e]Percentage of cytotoxicity, compared with the control macrophages (P < 0.001).

TABLE 2.   <u>In vivo uptake of liposomes containing lymphokines by murine PEM and corresponding activation of tumoricidal properties</u>

Total phospholipid (µmol) injected[a]	PEM $[^{14}C]$/ $[^{125}I]$ratio[b]	Liposome internal volume transferred (µl)/10^6 PEM[c]	Percentage cytotoxicity[d]
5.0	2.15	0.47	45
2.5	2.90	0.28	20
1.0	3.35	0.06	12
0.5	2.82	0.04	0

[a]Four days after ip injection with 2.0 ml thioglycollate, C57BL/6 mice were injected ip with MLV containing $[4-^{14}C]$chol in the lipid membrane and $[^{125}I]$BSA in the aqueous interior in an inoculum volume of 1.0 ml. PEM were harvested 4 hr later and processed as described in Materials and Methods. Five mice per group.

[b]Ratios are normalized by defining original $[^{14}C]$/$[^{125}I]$ as 1.0 so that the ratio of the two labels present in PEM can be calculated by dividing the percentage of total $[^{125}I]$ radioactivity present in the same group. The results represent mean values of five determinations. Variations from the mean did not exceed 10%.

[c]Obtained by multiplying the ratio of total $[^{125}I]$ radioactivity/ 10^6 PEM by the capture volume of the phospholipid preparation as described in Materials and Methods. The results represent mean values of five determinations. Variations from the mean did not exceed 10%.

[d]Four days after ip injection with 2.0 ml thioglycollate, C57BL/6 mice were injected ip with MLV containing MAF. PEM were harvested 4 hr later and processed for the cytotoxicity assay following an additional 20 hr incubation as described in Materials and Methods.

The level of macrophage cytotoxicity obtained in vitro following the injection of liposome-encapsulated MAF was dependent on the time of macrophage harvest (Table 3). Maximal activation of PEM was achieved by 24 hr following the ip injection of liposome-encapsulated MAF (32% cytotoxicity), and by 48 hr the activity declined to 19% cytotoxicity. By 72 hr, no demonstrable macrophage-mediated cytotoxicity was apparent. These data indicate that the tumoricidal state induced in macrophages by liposome-encapsulated lymphokines fades over a defined time interval (72 hr) and suggests that for a sustained level of macrophage cytotoxicity, multiple treatments with liposome-encapsulated MAF are required.

Progressively growing tumors have been reported to depress various aspects of macrophage function (19-21). It was important, therefore, to determine if liposome-encapsulated lymphokines could render macrophages tumoricidal in the tumor-bearing host. As shown in Table 4, the ip injection of liposomeencapsulated MAF into mice bearing the sc B16-BL6 tumor rendered resident peritoneal macrophages tumoricidal (cytotoxicity range 25-28%). Control injections consisting of PBS or liposome-encapsulated rat NRSUP into mice did not activate resident peritoneal macrophages.

TABLE 3. Duration of tumoricidal activity of PEM following the ip injection of lymphokines encapsulated within MLV

Treatment of donors[a]	Time of harvest (hr) after ip injection of liposomes	Radioactivity (cpm) in live target cells on day 3[b]
None, tumor cells alone	--	1869 + 26
HBSS	24	1927 ∓ 27
Liposome-NRSUP[c]	24	1853 ∓ 70
Liposome-MAF[c]	24	1317 ∓ 18 (32)[d]
None, tumor cells alone	--	2287 ∓ 75
HBSS	48	2266 ∓ 13
Liposome-NRSUP[c]	48	2232 ∓ 47
Liposome-MAF[c]	48	1844 ∓ 35 (19)[d]
None, tumor cells alone	--	1719 ∓ 31
HBSS	72	1742 ∓ 14
Liposome-NRSUP[c]	72	1609 ∓ 196
Liposome-MAF[c]	72	1698 ∓ 91

[a]Four days after ip injection with 2.0 ml thioglycollate, C57BL/6 mice were injected ip with the indicated material in an inoculum volume of 1.0 ml PBS. PEM were harvested as indicated, after injection, and macrophage cultures were prepared as described in Materials and Methods. Three mice per group.

[b]5×10^3 B16-F10 labeled with $[^{125}I]$IUdR were plated onto macrophage monolayers as described in Materials and Methods. Results are mean cpm $\pm$ standard deviation from triplicate cultures.

[c]MLV composed of PS/PC (3:7 mole ratio) containing the indicated material in 5 μmoles total phospholipid.

[d]Percentage of cytotoxicity compared with control macrophages ($P < 0.005$).

The observations on the activation of tumoricidal properties in murine AM by the systemic administration of liposome-encapsulated MAF were extended to investigations of its potential to the therapy of spontaneous pulmonary metastases (Table 5). The B16-BL6 tumors, without therapy (HBSS control mice), produced spontaneous pulmonary metastases in 44 of 48 control mice with a median of 29 metastases per mouse (range 0 - 107). The multiple injections of free MAF or MLV containing HBSS ("empty") suspended in MAF did not influence the incidence or extent of the metastasis. In contrast, multiple iv injections of liposome-encapsulated MAF significantly decreased the incidence and median number of metastases.

In addition to reducing the metastatic burden, therapy with liposome-encapsulated MAF also significantly enchanced long-term survival in mice bearing metastases produced by the B16-BL6 melanoma growing at a "primary site." As shown in Table 6, 7 of 10 mice injected iv with liposome-encapsulated MAF were still alive when the experiment was terminated after 190 days, whereas virtually all animals in the control groups were dead by day 70 (40 days after amputation of the primary tumor). Since the median life span of mice injected with the minimum tumorigenic dose (10 B16-BL6 cells) is 40-50 days (13,30), animals that survived at least 190 days can be considered to be disease-free.

TABLE 4. In vivo activation of murine resident peritoneal macrophages in mice bearing a progressively growing sc tumor following the ip injection of lymphokines encapsulated within MLV

Treatment of donors[a]	Tumor size (cm)	Radioactivity (cpm) in live target cells on day 3[b]
None, tumor cells alone	--	2544 + 14
HBSS	--[c]	2624 + 103
Liposome-NRSUP[d]	--[c]	2318 + 44
Liposome-MAF[d]	--[c]	1980 + 39 (24)[e]
HBSS	1.05	2609 + 33
Liposome-NRSUP[d]	0.85	2416 + 62
	1.30	2459 + 51
Liposome-MAF[d]	0.90	1831 + 47 (28)[e]
	1.40	2111 + 19 (27)[e]
	2.25	1908 + 39 (25)[e]

[a]Three weeks following sc inoculation with 5×10^4 B16-F10, C57BL/6 mice were injected ip with the indicated material. PEM were harvested 24 hr after injection, and cultures were prepared as described in Materials and Methods.

[b]5×10^3 B16-F10 labeled with [^{125}I]IUdR were plated onto macrophage monolayers as described in Materials and Methods. Results are mean cpm + standard deviation from triplicate cultures.

[c]Normal host.

[d]MLV composed of PS/PC (3:7 mole ratio) containing the indicated material in 5 μmoles total phospholipid.

[e]Percentage of cytotoxicity compared to target cells alone (P < 0.005).

TABLE 5.   Inhibition of established B16-BL6 pulmonary metastases in C57BL/6 mice after the multiple iv injections of liposome-encapsulated lymphokines

Treatment group	Pulmonary metastases[a]		
	Negative mice/total	Median	Range
PBS control mice	4/48	29	0-107
Free MAF	4/20	16	0-38
Free MAF + "empty" liposomes[b]	8/26	20	0-65
Liposome-MAF[c]	18/24[d]	0	0-10

[a]5×10^4 viable B16-BL6 cells were implanted in the footpad of syngeneic C57BL/6 mice. Tumors (0.9-1.2 mm in diameter) were amputated 4 weeks later. Therapy commenced 3 days following surgery and consisted of iv injection of the indicated material, twice weekly for 4 weeks. Mice were killed 2 weeks after the last treatment and necropsied. Lung metastases were determined microscopically.

[b]MLV (5 μmol total phospholipid) containing HBSS suspended in 0.2 ml MAF.

[c]MLV (5 μmol total phospholipid) containing MAF.

[d]Incidence of metastasis differed significantly from other groups (P < 0.001 Chi square analysis).

TABLE 6.   Eradication of established B16-BL6 pulmonary metastases in C57BL/6 mice by the iv injection of liposomes containing lymphokines

Treatment Group	Percent survival on day:[a]			
	40	60	90	190
PBS control mice	100	60	0	0
Free MAF	100	50	0	0
Free MAF + "empty" liposomes[b]	100	50	10	10
Liposome-MAF[c]	100	80	70	70

[a]5×10^4 viable B16-BL6 cells were implanted in the footpad of syngeneic C57BL/6 mice. Tumors (0.9-1.2 mm in diameter) were amputated 4 weeks later. Therapy commenced 3 days following surgery and consisted of iv injection of the indicated material, twice weekly for 4 weeks. Ten mice per grup.

[b]MLV (5 μmol total phospholipid) containing HBSS suspended in 0.2 ml MAF.

[c]MLV (5 μmol total phospholipid) containing MAF.

DISCUSSION

The present results indicate that multiple systemic treatments of mice with liposome-encapsulated MAF are associated with the regression of well-established pulmonary and lymph node metastases originating from a syngeneic melanoma growing sc. Injections of unencapsulated (free) MAF were not effective in treatment of metastasis. At the time of surgical resection of the "primary tumor," i.e., just before the start of liposome therapy, many individual metastases were grossly visible, confirming that the tumor burden in lung and lymph node metastases could have exceeded 5×10^6 cells (6). Since, in this tumor system, the median life span of mice inoculated with as few as 10 viable tumor cells has been shown to be 40-50 days (13,30), it is significant that 70% of mice treated with liposome-encapsulated MAF survived at least 190 days. This suggests that tumor burden in the surviving mice must have been reduced to less than 10 viable cells.

The mechanisms(s) responsible for destruction of established metastases following the systemic administration of liposome-encapsulated MAF probably involve the activation of macrophages to become tumoricidal. This is supported by evidence that macrophages activated in vitro inhibit experimental metastases when injected into the tumor-bearing host (3,4,7,18) and that tumoricidal activity of liposome-encapsulated MAF is reduced in vivo when animals are treated with agents that impair macrophage function (24). We also found (as have others, 8,10) that liposome-encapsulated MAF can render murine AM and PEM tumoricidal following iv and ip administrations, respectively. Unencapsulated (free) MAF failed to activate either macrophage population.

Although the preceding experiments illustrate the feasibility of using liposome-encapsulated material(s) to stimulate macrophage antitumor activities, the use of lymphokine preparations in this work introduces several problems. Apart from the fact that we do not have a quantitative assay for MAF activity and that there is significant variation of MAF activity between different preparations, the presence of a number of biological mediators other than MAF, including mitogenic, angiogenic and vascular permeabilizing factors, complicates the evaluation of observed host responses. It would thus be desirable, and probably mandatory for studies in man, that future efforts to stimulate macrophage function by liposome-encapsulated agents employ material(s) of defined composition and purity.

REFERENCES

1. Allison, A.C. (1979):J. Reticuloendothel. Soc., 26:619-630.
2. Cohen, S., Pick, E., and Oppenhein, J.J., editors (1979): Biology of the Lymphokines. Academic Press, New York.
3. Den Otter, E., Dullens Hub, F.J., Van Lovern, H., and Pels, E. (1977):In: The Macrophage and Cancer, edited by K. James, B. McBride, and A. Stuart, pp.119-140. Econoprint, Edinburgh.
4. Fidler, I.J. (1974): Cancer Res., 34:1074-1078.
5. Fidler, I.J. (1975): J. Natl. Cancer Inst., 55:1159-1163.
6. Fidler, I.J. (1980): Science, 208:1469-1471.
7. Fidler, I.J., Fogler, W.E., and Connor, J. (1979):In: Immunobiology and Immunotherapy of Cancer, edited by W. Terry and T. Yamamura, pp.361-372. Elsevier North Holland, Amsterdam.

8. Fidler, I.J., Raz, A., Fogler, W.E., Kirsh, R., Bugelski, P., and Poste, G. (1980):Cancer Res., 40:4460-4466.
9. Fidler, I.J., Raz, A., Fogler, W.E. and Poste, G. (1980):In: Recent Results in Cancer Research, edited by G. Mathe and F.M. Muggia, pp.246-251. Springer-Verlag, Berlin.
10. Fogler, W.E., Raz, A., and Fidler, I.J. (1980):Cell. Immunol., 53:214-219.
11. Greenwood, F.C., Hunter, W.M., and Glover, J.S. (1963):Biochem. J., 89:114- 123.
12. Gregoriadis, G., and Allison, A.C., editors (1980):Liposomes in Biological Systems. John Wiley & Sons, Chichester.
13. Griswold, D.P., Jr. (1972):Cancer Chemotherapy Reports, 3:315-323.
14. Hart, I.R. (1979):Am. J. Pathol., 97:587-600.
15. Hart, I.R., Fogler, W.E., Poste, G., and Fidler, I.J. (1981): Cancer Immunol. Immunother., (in press)
16. Kimelberg, H.K. and Mayhew, E. (1979):CRC Crit. Rev. Toxicol., 9:25-44.
17. Kripke, M.L., Budmen, M.B., and Fidler, I.J. (1977):Cell. Immunol. 30:341-352.
18. Liotta, L.A., Gattazzi, C., Kleinerman, J., and Saidel, G. (1977): Brit. J. Cancer, 36:639-641
19. Melchner, H. and Hilgard, P. (1979):Europ J. Cancer, 15:779-783.
20. Normann, S.J. and Cornelius, J. (1978):Cancer Res., 38:3453-3459.
21. Normann, S.J., Schardt, M., and Sorkin, E. (1979):J.N.C.I., 63:825-832.
22. Poste, G.(1979):Am. J. Pathol., 96:595-608.
23. Poste, G., Doll, J., Hart, I.R. and Fidler, I.J. (1980):Cancer Res., 40:1636-1644.
24. Poste, G. and Fidler, I.J. (1981):In:The Study of Drug Activity and Immunocompetent Cell Functions, edited by C. Nocolau and A. Paraf, (in press) Academic Press, New York.
25. Poste, G. and Kirsh, R. (1979):Cancer Res., 39:2582-2590.
26. Poste, G., Kirsh, R., and Fidler, I.J. (1979):Cell. Immunol., 44:71-87.
27. Poste, G., Kirsh, R., Fogler, W.E., and Fidler, I.J. (1979):Cancer Res., 39:881-891.
28. Poste, G., Kirsh, R., Raz., A., Sone, S. Bucana, C., Fogler, W.E. and Fidler, I.J. (1980):In:Liposomes and Immunobiology, edited by B. Tom and H. Six, pp.93-107. Elsevier North Holland, New York.
29. Raz, A., Fogler, W.E. and Fidler, I.J. (1979):Cancer Immunol. Immunother. 7:157-163.
30. Schabel, F.M., Jr., Griswold, D.P. Jr., Laster, W.R., Jr., Corbett, T.H. and Lloyd, H.H. (1977):Pharmacol. Ther. [A], 1:411-435..
31. Sone, S., Poste, G., and Fidler, I.J. (1980):J. Immunol., 124:2197-2202.

Lymphokines and Thymic Hormones: Their
Potential Utilization in Cancer Therapeutics,
edited by A. L. Goldstein and M. A. Chirigos,
Raven Press, New York © 1981.

In Vivo Biological Studies with Lymphoblastoid Lymphokines

Ben W. Papermaster, C. Dean Gilliland, John E. McEntire,
Ned D. Rodes, and Pamela A. Dunn

Cancer Research Center, Columbia, Missouri 65201

Preliminary studies reported from our laboratories in the past with lymphokine preparations derived from the cultured human lymphoblastoid cell line, RPMI 1788, have demonstrated that concentrated preparations of cultured supernatant containing various lymphokine activities are capable of producing local tumor regression in humans and in mice (9-14). In addition, skin reactions produced in both the guinea pig (10) and in man (16) have been indicative of host ability to develop inflammatory reactions at the site of injection. These reactions are superficially typical of recall sensitivity to microbial antigens, but unlike delayed type hypersensitivity (DTH) reactions, a skin test reaction to lymphokines reaches peak size by six to 12 hours after injection (2,10). The histological picture also differs from DTH reactions with fewer lymphocytes in the inflammatory infiltrate as discussed by Hamblin et al (6). Patients with advanced tumors fail to give a skin test reaction to lymphokines and are generally incapable of mounting a strong host response to the tumor. Indeed, a negative lymphokine skin test has been interpreted as a grave sign for host response to tumor burden (10,16).

Studies of a similar type have been repeated by D. Dumonde and his colleagues in London (2) and are reported at this workshop. We report here our experience with subcutaneous injection of material prepared as in Figure 1 and described in detail by McEntire et al (8) at this workshop. We have used this preparation predominantly in our preliminary clinical and mouse tumor studies, and Figure 2 demonstrates an isoelectric focusing analysis comparing it with human leukocyte interferon prepared by K. Cantrell, Helsinki, Finland and supplied to us by Drs. Evan Hersh and J. Gutterman. As can be seen from the electrophoresis gel, the predominant contaminants involve serum proteins which are involved in the production of the material and are not removed during harvesting of these types of fractions. Whether or not the serum proteins present in the production of interferon contribute significantly to biologic or any toxic effects will be known only after highly purified interferon now available from recombinant E. coli (15) has been tested.

Supported by NCI grants CA 26224, CA 29145 and CA 15740, DHHS; Fraternal Order of Eagles, Order of the Eastern Star, and the A.P. Green Foundation.

In order to determine the response to increasing doses of the lymph-okine preparations outlined in Figures 1 and 2, a Phase I dose response study was initiated at the Ellis Fischel State Cancer Hospital, under the supervision of Dr. N. D. Rodes. The preparation used in the study was prepared as described by McEntire (8) at this workshop and as in Figure 1. Lyophilization and resuspension in pyrogen-free saline at 17 mg/ml in 2 ml vials gives a yield of approximately 25 vials per original liter of culture supernatant. Preclinical testing for endo-toxin by the limulus technique (7) and for presence of microorganisms, mycoplasma, and acute and subacute toxicity in mice, rats, guinea pigs, and dogs was carried out as required in the Federal Register (3), and all tests for toxicity and contamination were negative. In vitro lymphokine biological activities were measured by assays for MIF, endotoxin, chemotaxis, macrophage activation, and in vitro and in vivo induction of mouse NK cell activity (5). Inflammatory response measure-ments in guinea pigs and patients and correlation of lymphokine skin reactions with microbial antigen recall reactions were carried out and have been previously reported (16).

Patients with Stage III and IV metastatic cancer were placed on protocol following evaluation for skin reactivity to microbial antigens (mumps, PPD, SKSD, and Dermatophytin) and lymphokines. Blood was obtained for prestudy hemogram and basic chemistries. Injections were carried out on an increasing dosage basis from approximately four to 2000 guinea pig skin test units of material injected in a single dose study. Volumes of lymphokine preparation from 0.1 to 10 ml were in-jected subcutaneously in one to four different sites. Peripheral blood was monitored for neutrophil phagocytic function, NK cell, E-rosette levels, and blood chemistries. No signs of clinical toxicity or distur-bances in blood chemistry values referable to lymphokine injections were noted. The stimulation effect of lymphokine administration on blood cell, NK cell reactivity, and neutrophil phagocytosis was more pronounced in doses between 30 and 100 guinea pig test units than at higher levels. These preliminary data would suggest that both NK cell and phagocytic activity were partially suppressed at higher dose levels. The highest levels studied were comparable to the administration of 10^0 to 10^7 interferon units as calculated by concentration of similar volumes from the NAMALWA cell line (4), which has been used for clinical trials in England. More complete information is in preparation (17).

Studies of biologic activity in tumor-bearing mice with the prepara-tion shown in Figures 1 and 2 were carried out for evaluation of the adjuvant effect of lymphokines when combined with chemotherapy. Both human and mouse (13) sources of lymphokines were employed. Syngeneic DBA/2 mice were used in a study of the L1210 tumor. Tumors were ob-tained from the National Cancer Institute, courtesy of the Division of Cancer Treatment, NCI. The effect of intraperitoneally administered lymphokine preparation on the growth of ascites form of the L1210 lymphoma was studied. We reasoned that a fast-growing tumor, such as the L1210, would readily enable us to determine whether an additional therapeutic effect over that supplied by chemotherapy alone would be noticeable following administration of lymphokines. Figure 3 shows the dose response curve to IP-injected L1210 tumor cells in DBA/2 mice. The slope is approximately -1 (-.91), with the 95% confidence limits shown in dotted lines. A log increment increase in cell dose reduces median survival by approximately one day. The generation time of the

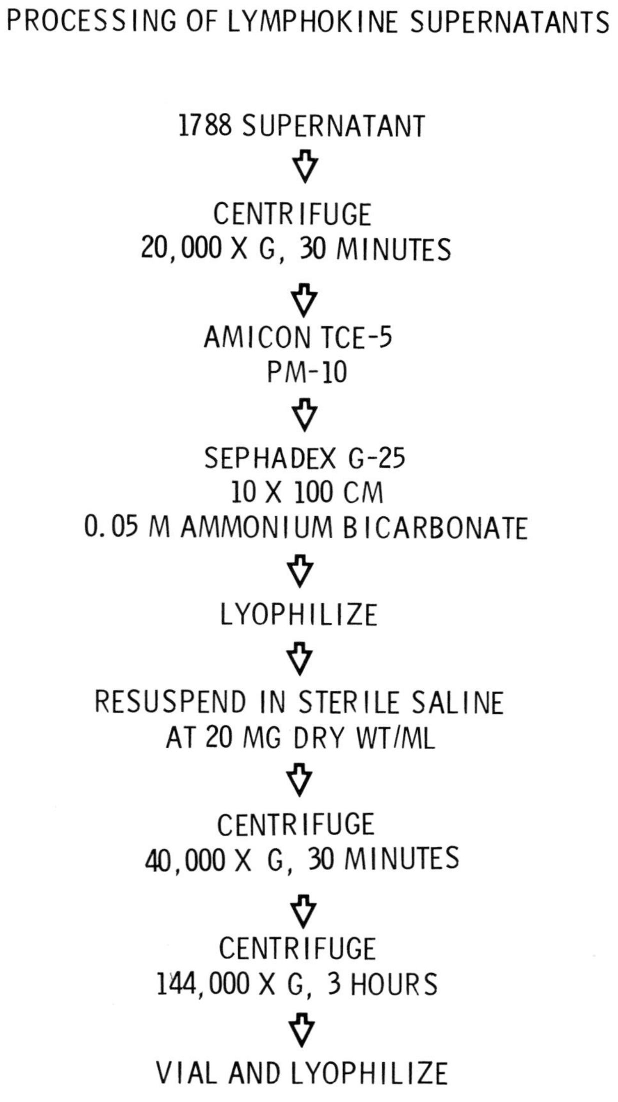

PROCESSING OF LYMPHOKINE SUPERNATANTS

1788 SUPERNATANT

CENTRIFUGE
20,000 X G, 30 MINUTES

AMICON TCE-5
PM-10

SEPHADEX G-25
10 X 100 CM
0.05 M AMMONIUM BICARBONATE

LYOPHILIZE

RESUSPEND IN STERILE SALINE
AT 20 MG DRY WT/ML

CENTRIFUGE
40,000 X G, 30 MINUTES

CENTRIFUGE
144,000 X G, 3 HOURS

VIAL AND LYOPHILIZE

FIG. 1. Preparation of crude lymphokine from RPMI 1788 culture supernatant. Samples are prepared as above in volumes of 16-20 L daily. For detailed procedures, see McEntire, this publication (8).

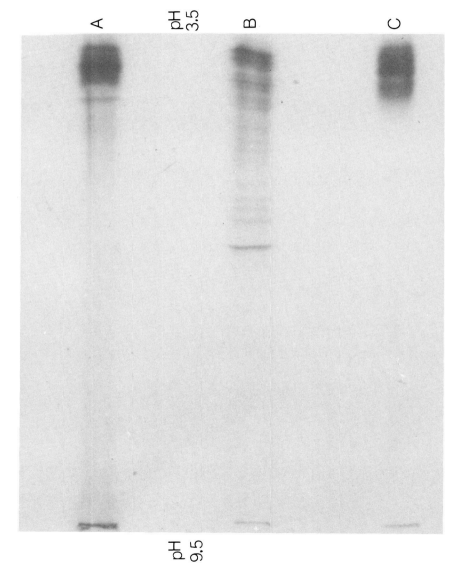

FIG. 2. Isoelectric focusing of the lymphokine fraction from RPMI 1788 (Fig. 1) and a leukocyte interferon preparation. Samples were focused on a 3.5 - 9.5 PAG plate (LKB). Samples are: A, crude lymphokine; B, interferon; C, human albumin standard. Note the heterogeneity of the preparations and the predominance of albumin in both the human leukocyte interferon (B) and lymphokine (A) preparations.

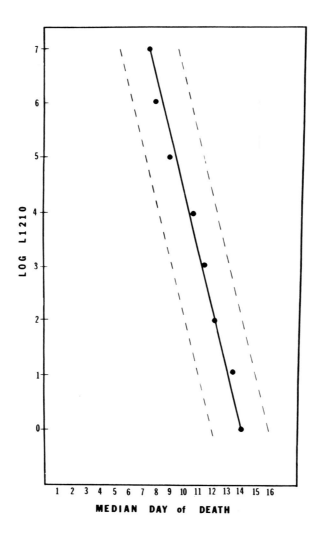

FIG. 3. Dose response to inocula of L1210 cells. The solid line is the regression of log dose versus survival determined by best fit analysis on data base of 550 animals. The broken lines are 95% confidence limits. Dose range studied varied from 10^0 - 10^7 cells injected I.P.

tumor was calculated to be 0.33 days. The effect of lymphokines administered alone is indifferent from the control growth of tumor (Table 1, experiment 133, and references 9 and 13). Likewise, there is little or no effect of the vehicle control (9,13).

When the drug MeCCNU[2] is used as the chemotherapeutic agent,[3] there is a prolongation of survival time and when the drug is used in combination with lymphokines, there is not only proglongation of survival time, but an increase in the number of survivors. A crucial test of survival is the response to a subsequent challenge of 10^5 injected tumor cells. All animals receiving doses as high as 10^6 to 10^7 cells were dead by day eight after injection. Studies were carried on with animals receiving 10^7 tumor cells and the effects of various dosages of the drug and times of injection of lymphokines after the receipt of drugs (Tables 1 through 4). In general, we were not able to determine a dose response relationship between increases in volume of lymphokines administered and survival. Furthermore, the dose response between the amount of drug administered and the survival time or survivors in these studies was not clear-cut and did not follow a linear relationship. Greater detail on these experiments is presented elsewhere (5).

A small amount of the TCA soluble extract (8) was available for preliminary experiments with the L1210 tumor. The results shown in Table 5 suggest that the lymphokine activity in the acid soluble fraction retains the ability to promote adjuvant immunostimulatory activity as in the cruder fraction described above. However, larger numbers of experiments would have to be performed (as in Tables 1-3) when material becomes available before firm conclusions can be drawn.

---

[2] 1-(2-chloroethyl-3-(4-methylcyclohexyl)-1-nitrosourea, NSC 95441

[3] Obtained from the National Cancer Institute

TABLE 1. Survival of Mice Treated with Mouse Lymphokines One Day After MeCCNU

Experiment	Treatment	MDD	%ILS	Survivors/ Total	Challenge[a] Survivors/ Total
130	None	7	--	0/10	
	30 mg/kg[b]	13	85.7	0/10	
132	None	7	--	0/10	
	30 mg/kg	16	178.0	2/10	0/2
133	None	8	--	0/10	
	30 mg/kg	12	50.0	0/10	
	30 mg/kg + LK[c]	14	75.0	0/10	
	LK only	7	--	0/6	
134	None	6	--	0/10	
	30 mg/kg	16	167.0	4/10	0/4
	30 mg/kg + LK	16	167.0	8/30	4/8

TABLE 2. Survival of Mice Treated With Human Lymphokines One Day After MeCCNU

Experiment	Treatment	MDD	%ILS	Survivors/ Total	Challenge[a] Survivors/ Total
136	None	8	--	0/10	
	30 mg/kg[b]	15	87.5	1/9	0/1
	30 mg/kg + LK	17	113.0	5/9	5/5
138	None	7	--	0/10	
	30 mg/kg	10	42.8	0/10	
	30 mg/kg + LK[c]	13	85.7	3/20	2/3

[a]Mice reinjected with 10^5 L1210 cells

[b]Dose-single injection of drug on day 2 after cell implant of 10^7 cells

[c]Lymphokines were injected daily for 10 days at approximately three units (0.1 ml) per dose

TABLE 3. Survival of Mice Treated With Human Lymphokines at Various Intervals After MeCCNU

Experiment	Treatment	MDD[f]	%ILS[f]	Survivors/ Total	Challenge Survivors/ Total
138	None	8	--	0/10	
	30 mg/kg[d]	15	87.5	1/9	0/1
	30 mg/kg + 1[e]	17	113.0	5/9	5/5
	30 mg/kg + 4	19	137.5	2/9	2/2
	30 mg/kg + 7	15	87.5	7/9	7/7
139	None	7	--	0/10	
	30 mg/kg	10	42.8	0/10	
	30 mg/kg + 1	13	85.7	3/20	2/3
	30 mg/kg + 7	13	85.7	0/20	
140	None	7	--	0/18	
	30 mg/kg	15	114.3	2/40	0/2
	30 mg/kg + 7	15	114.3	8/40	6/8

[d]Dose-single injection of drug on day 2 after cell implant of 10^7 cells

[e]Day after drug treatment at which lymphokine injections were begun as in Tables 1 and 2. Lymphokines were injected daily for 10 days at approximately 3 units (0.1 ml) per dose.

[f]MDD = median day of death; ILS = increased life span

TABLE 4. Summary of Cumulative Survival Parameters in Mice Bearing Ascites L1210 and Treated by MeCCNU Followed by Lymphokines

Treatment	Survivors/Total	% Survivors	Challenge[g]
None	0/88	0	
Drug alone (30 mg/kg)	9/109	8.2	0/9
Drug + LK[h]	33/147	22.4	25/33

[g]Mice were challenged IP with 10^5 L1210

[h]$\chi^2 = 9.02$, $p < .005$

TABLE 5.   Preliminary Results Utilizing TCA Soluble Fraction of LK 1788
           Treating Male DBA/2J Mice Inoculated With 10   L1210

Group	Animals	Median Survival Time	Long Term Survivors (60/d)
Medium control	10	16	0/10
Lymphokine only	10	15	0/10
MeCCNU (40 mg/kg)	10	24	0/10
MeCCNU (40 mg/kg) + TCA medium control	10	24	0/10
MeCCNU (40 mg/kg) + TCA fraction (8)	10	24	3/10

Long term survivors represent those mice surviving for longer than 60 days after implant of tumor.

SUMMARY AND DISCUSSION

These preliminary results suggest that the preparations of lymphokines described herein are non-toxic in the amounts tested in humans and mice. Efficacy has been preliminarily tested only in a mouse model, DBA/2 strain, bearing the L1210 lymphoma.

Indeed, there were relatively few survivors with the high inoculum of tumor cells (10^7) and the doses of drug alone (8.2%) or with lymphokines as an added adjuvant (22.4%). The tumor grows extremely rapidly in the DBA/2 mouse, which is highly susceptible to additional toxic effects of MeCCNU and MeCCNU and lymphokines combined. However, one striking observation is apparent, and that is, when these results are summarized, as in Table 4, the results show a statistically significant difference between animals treated with drug only and drug plus lymphokines. Not only was there a larger number of survivors in the lymphokine/drug-treated groups, but also the only animals surviving challenge with additional 10^5 L1210 cells were lymphokine/drug group. These results confirm the important adjuvant effects in the administration of immunomodulators following chemotherapeutic, cytoreductive therapy, as suggested by Chirigos et al (1). In a tumor growing as fast as L1210, it may be difficult to dissect the best therapeutic regimens. In addition, the time of administration may not have been optimal in these experiments. Nevertheless, the results do suggest the need for continuing study of similar types of models; and when these results are put into perspective with other chemoimmunotherapeutic studies (1,18), it is clear that lymphokines may act as an important immunostimulator and adjuvant to chemotherapy. The studies of Fidler and colleagues (18) also support the importance of an adjuvant concept for lymphokines.

Fidler has documented the increased effectiveness of immunostimulator agents when encapsulated in liposomes (this symposium and reference 18). In addition, the overall stimulation of the immune system obtained during lymphokine administration may act to develop antigen-sensitive T cells and stimulate growth such that permanent immunity to the tumor develops.

REFERENCES

1. Chirigos, M.A., Pearson, J.W., and Pryor, J. (1973): <u>Cancer Res.</u>, 33:2615-2621.
2. Dumonde, D.C., Wolstencroft, R.A., Panayi, G.S., Matthew, M., Morley, J., and Howson, W.T. (1969): <u>Nature</u>, 224:38-42.
3. <u>Federal Register</u>, Vol. 38, No. 223 (1973): 610.11-610.12.
4. Finter, N.B., and Fantes, K.N. (1980): In: <u>Interferon 2 1980</u>, edited by I. Gresser. Academic Press, New York.
5. Gilliland, C.D., McEntire, J.E., Woods, W.L., Tyrer, H.T., and Papermaster, B.W. (1981): In: <u>Cellular Responses to Molecular Modulators</u>. Academic Press, New York, in press.
6. Hamblin, A.S., Wolstencroft, R.A., Dumonde, D.C., den Hollander, R., Schuurs, A.H.W.M., Backhouse, B.M., O'Connell, D., and Paradinas, F. (1978): In: <u>Developments in Biological Standardization</u>, edited by International Association of Biological Council, pp. 335-344. S. Karger, Basel.
7. Jorgensen, J.H., and Smith, R.F. (1973): <u>Appl. Microbiol.</u> 26:43-48.
8. McEntire, J.E., Dunn, P.A., and Papermaster, B.W. (1981): In: <u>Proceedings of the International Workshop on Lymphokines and Thymic Factors</u>. Raven Press, New York. (Article included in this publication.)
9. Papermaster, B.W., Gilliland, C.D., McEntire, J.E., Smith, M.E., and Buchok, S.J. (1980): <u>Cancer</u> 45:1248-1253.
10. Papermaster, B.W., Holterman, O.A., Klein, E., Djerassi, I., Rosner, D., Dao, T., and Costanzi, J.J. (1976): <u>Clin. Immunol. Immunopathol.</u> 5:31-47.
11. Papermaster, B.W., Holterman, O.A., Klein, E., Parmett, S., Dobkin, D., Laudico, R., and Djerassi, I. (1976): <u>Clin. Immunol. Immunopathol.</u> 5:48-59.
12. Papermaster, B.W., Holterman, O.A., Rosner, D., Klein, E., Dao, T., and Djerassi, I. (1974): <u>Res. Commun. Chem. Pathol. Pharmacol.</u> 8:413-416.
13. Papermaster, B.W., McEntire, J.E., Gilliland, C.D., Buchok, S.J., and Smith, M.E. (1980): In: <u>Biochemical Characterization of Lymphokines</u>, edited by A.L. de Weck, F. Kristensen, and M. Landy, pp. 193-198. Academic Press, New York.
14. Papermaster, B.W., McEntire, J.E., Gilliland, C.D., Dunn, P.A., Rodes, N.D., Lopatin, E., and Smith, M.E. (1981). In: <u>Cellular Responses to Molecular Modulators</u>. Academic Press, New York, in press.
15. Pestka, S., McCandliss, R., Maeda, S., Levy, W.P., Familletti, P.C., Hobbs, D.S., Moschera, J., and Stein, S. (1981): In: <u>Cellular Responses to Molecular Modulators</u>. Academic Press, New York, in press.

16. Rios, A., Hersh, E.M., Gutterman, J.U., Mavligit, G.M., Schimer, H., McEntire, J.E., and Papermaster, B.W. (1979): <u>Cancer</u> 44:1616-1621.

17. Rodes, N.D., McEntire, J.E., Dunn, P.A., Oxenhandler, R., Gay, C., Kardinal, C.G., and Papermaster, B.W., in preparation.

18. Sone, S., and Fidler, I.J. (1981): <u>Cell. Immunol.</u> 57:42-50. See also Folger, W.E., and Fidler, I.J. (1980): <u>Cell. Immunol.</u> 53:214-219.

Lymphokines and Thymic Hormones: Their Potential Utilization in Cancer Therapeutics, edited by A. L. Goldstein and M. A. Chirigos. Raven Press, New York © 1981.

Short-Term and Long-Term Administration of Lymphoblastoid Cell Line Lymphokine (LCL-LK) to Patients with Advanced Cancer

D. C. Dumonde, Melanie S. Pulley, Anne S. Hamblin, *A. K. Singh, †Barbara M. Southcott, †D. O'Connell, §F. J. Paradinas, **M. R. G. Robinson, ‡Carol C. Rigby, §§F. den Hollander, §§A. Schuurs, §§H. Verheul, and §§Elenie van Vliet

*Departments of Immunology and *Haematology, St. Thomas' Hospital, London SE1; Departments of †Radiotherapy and §Histopathology, Charing Cross Hospital, London W6; **Pontefract General Infirmary, Yorkshire; ‡Institute of Urology, London WC2, England; and §§Organon Scientific Development Group, Oss, The Netherlands*

SUMMARY

LCL-LK isolated from supernatants of human lymphoblast cultures, containing a range of lymphokine activities, were given by both local and systemic injection to patients with advanced carcinoma.

Three breast carcinoma patients received lymphokine injections into dermal metastases and 6 prostatic carcinoma patients had intralesional injections. Systemic injections were given to 11 patients with breast carcinoma, 2 patients with prostatic carcinoma and 1 patient with Ewing's sarcoma. Nine of the patients received regular intravenous injections for more than 2 months; and 3 breast carcinoma patients received intravenous injections over about a 2-year period.

Intravenous injection produced a pyrexia, maximal at 2 - 4 hours post-injection; a neutrophil leucocytosis maximal at 2 - 4 hours; a lymphopenia maximal at 4 hours; and a rise in plasma cortisol (assessed in 1 patient) maximal at 2 - 4 hours. Intradermal testing produced a dose-related erythema, maximal at 12 - 24 hours post-injection, from which an 'effective dose' was derived to compare with the dose required to effect given changes in other parameters. The response to repeated systemic injection was evaluated and findings included a marked rise in K-cell activity (assessed in 1 lymphopenic patient). Histological examination of lymphokine skin tests, injected breast metastases and prostatic carcinoma following lymphokine injection, showed a mixed cellular infiltration and tumour cell necrosis.

This study showed that lymphokines, administered both locally and systemically, were well tolerated. No short-term or long-term toxicity was observed over a 2-year period of systemic administration. The effects of LCL-LK seem to relate to host defence mechanisms yet the interferon system is not apparently involved. In demonstrating that long-term administration of LCL-LK to cancer patients is without attributable toxicity, this study provides biological response data on which to base more definitive protocols for evaluation of lymphokines in cancer research therapy. More detailed information is being published separately.

BACKGROUND, RATIONALE AND OBJECTIVES OF STUDY

Background and rationale

The background to this work arose from investigations in the 1960's of the role of lymphocyte activation products in the expression of experimental delayed hypersensitivity (3,8,11,12). In 1969 the generic term 'lymphokine' (13) was coined in order to communicate the broader concept that non-antibody protein products of lymphocyte activation may themselves activate and regulate cellular systems controlling a wide variety of immunological and inflammatory processes relevant to host defence, including mechanisms restricting the spread of tumours (5,13). It soon became clear that lymphokines fulfilled many of the criteria anticipated of autopharmacological mediators of the cellular immune response (14,16) including the ability to induce paracortical lymph node hyperplasia (22); and on this basis it was suggested that the lymphokine field might find therapeutic application in human diseases involving disordered cellular immunity (15,17). The recognition that human lymphoblasts in larger-scale culture could also generate soluble lymphokine-like substances (LCL-LK) invited consideration of the potential of LCL-LK's in therapeutic investigation of host:tumour relationships (18,21,26,27).

The rationale for giving LCL-LK systemically to tumour-bearing patients was reinforced by six lines of investigation. First, that patients with progressive neoplasia frequently develop depression of cellular immune status which is a bad prognostic sign (4) and that such patients may have serum factors blocking lymphocyte function (4) or expression of lymphokine activity (19). Second, that lymphokines can directly inhibit the growth, migration or metabolism of tumour cells in vitro (6) and can activate the tumouricidal capacity of cultured macrophages (25). Third, that lymphokines augment the metabolic, chemotactic and immunological reactivity of white cell populations in ways which would seem relevant to the containment of metastatic disease (7). Fourth, that injection of lymphokine into mice augments tumour regression induced by chemotherapy (28). Fifth, that local injection of LCL-LK into human metastatic nodules causes their clinical regression (27). Sixth, that some bacterial preparations which may induce regression or limit the spread of human tumours may well act by enhancing local or systemic cellular immune mechanisms in vivo (1,23).

Objectives

(1) To confirm and extend knowledge of the biological and histopathological effects of injecting LCL-LK directly into recurrent, metastatic or inoperable tumour;

(2) To determine whether LCL-LK injections could be tolerated in advanced patients without acute toxicity;

(3) To investigate the clinical, haematological, biochemical and immunological responses of patients with advanced cancer to the repeated systemic injection of LCL-LK;

(4) To determine whether patients with advanced cancer could be maintained in the long-term (ie up to 2 years) on systemic injections of LCL-LK without adverse toxicity.

Clinical setting

With ethical permission it was decided to begin this study by investigating some 20 patients in depth under circumstances of individual care and informed consent. We chose patients principally with advanced cancer of the breast and prostate for two reasons: (a) on the basis of other published experience of intra-lesional injection of LCL-LK into metastatic breast carcinoma (26,27); and (b) on the basis of our own experience of injecting BCG recurrently into carcinomatous prostate (28). All patients had metastatic or inoperable local tumour spread; and by virtue of persistent or recurrent disease, despite previous treatment (eg surgery; irradiation; chemotherapy; endocrine therapy) were placed in the category of 'irreversible neoplastic disease'. All patients were hospitalized for an initial period and, where appropriate, for extended intervals during their longer-term maintenance on LCL-LK. This allowed for the highest standards of individual medical and nursing care; for haematological and clinical chemistry investigations; for some immunological monitoring; and for excision biopsy of lesions and for clinical photography. Where clinically indicated, conventional treatment modalities (eg local irradiation; cytotoxic/hormonal treatment; nutritional supplementation; antibiotics; analgesics, etc) were not withheld.

The purpose of this preliminary study was therefore to gain as much information as ethically possible on the response to LCL-LK, in a heterogeneous group of advanced cancer patients, so as to provide us with a body of experience on which to base the design of future protocols and phase I studies. This report summarises our experience with 20 patients during the period November 1977-February 1981.

MATERIALS, PATIENTS AND METHODOLOGY

Nature of LCL-LK preparations

Cell culture and supernatant processing
Human lymphoblasts (RPMI-1788) were precultured in RPMI-1640 medium with the addition of 1% AB/A human plasma until the cells reached 10^6/ml, when they were recultured for 48 hours in the absence of plasma. Supernatants were inactivated with β-propiolactone and then ultra-filtered through hollow fibre cartridges to obtain a fraction between (nominally) 100,000 and 5,000 D. The concentrates were dialysed, lyophilized, re-dialysed, filtered (0.2 μm) into vials and again lyophilized. Four preparations were thus prepared (3582,4362,4882,5792). A plasma protein control (blank) preparation (5794) was produced in exactly the same way as the LCL-LK preparation but without using the cell line.

Control tests and partial characterization
All reactants were tested for sterility; the cell line for mycoplasma; the human plasma for HBsAg, mycoplasma, endotoxin and pyrogenicity; the culture medium for endotoxin; the supernatant (just before ultrafiltration) for β-hydroxypropionic acid; and the concentrate for endotoxin, protein content and leucocyte migration inhibition activity (LIF) (9). Further control tests on the vialed product included animal toxicity, pyrogenicity and sterility studies, as well as estimates of the solubility, pH, protein, salt and water content.

Properties of LCL-LK

Lymphokine activities found in these preparations were LIF, as judged by migration inhibition under agarose in a block designed assay (9,10); macrophage migration inhibition factor (MIF), similarly judged; macrophage activating factor (MAF), judged by increased ^{3}H-glucosamine uptake in vitro and increased Listeria clearance in mouse spleen; lymph node activating factor (LNAF) judged by increased lymph node (24) and spleen weight in mice; and skin-inflammatory factor (SIF). Lymphocyte mitogenic activity, lymphotoxin activity and increased natural killer (NK) cell activity of lymphocytes from human cancer patients (20) had also been found in some preparations.

Patients and lymphokine administration

The 20 patients included 11 with breast cancer; 8 with prostatic cancer; and 1 with a metastatic Ewing's sarcoma who had been extensively treated by chemotherapy and radiotherapy.

Breast cancer

Aged 46 - 75; inoperable local disease at stage T4 with involvement of regional lymph nodes. Nine also had distant metastases. All patients had poorly differentiated tumour and had been treated with various combinations of surgery, radiotherapy, chemotherapy and hormone therapy; however these patients had all previously stopped these forms of therapy prior to commencing lymphokines.

Prostatic cancer

Aged 52 - 83; primary tumour stage T2 - T4 with involvement of regional lymph nodes in 2 patients. Five patients also had distant metastases. All patients had poorly differentiated tumour; and had been treated with various combinations of surgery, hormone therapy, chemotherapy and radiotherapy. All patients had stopped treatment before receiving lymphokine.

Schedules of LCL-LK administration

(a) Intralesional injection. A total of 11 nodular skin metastases in 3 patients with breast carcinoma were given several (1 - 6) injections of one of 3 LCL-LK preparations; individual nodules received 0.5 - 19.0 mg of LCL-LK. Six prostatic carcinoma patients received 3 - 5 injections each of one of 2 LCL-LK preparations on alternate days into the prostate; individual tumour sites received 3.0 - 7.0 mg of LCL-LK.

(b) Systemic injection (Table 1) The accompanying table sets out the courses and quantities of 4 LCL-LK preparations used for injecting 14 patients by intravenous (I/V) or intramuscular (I/M) routes. Table 1 shows that long-term courses of LCL-LK were given to 3 patients for a period of 17 - 25 months and a fourth patient over a 9-month period. In most of the patients, escalating doses of LCL-LK were first given daily or thrice weekly to determine a maximum tolerated maintenance dose.

Investigative methods

Acute clinical, haematological and biochemical monitoring

Temperature, pulse and blood pressure were monitored immediately before lymphokine injection and at $\frac{1}{2}$-hourly intervals for 6 hours or until asymptomatic, after injection. The time of onset and duration of other responses (eg rigors) were noted. Full blood counts, including

TABLE 1. Schedules of LCL-LK administered systemically

| Patient (disease) | LK-prep (#) | Injection schedules | | | Total dose (mg) |
		Course	Duration	Study period	
ECo (breast)	3582	2 IV inject.	4D	1W	9.0
AC (breast)	4362	Daily : IV x 5	1W		
	4882	Daily : IV x 10	2W	25M	36.0 (4882)
	4882	Weekly : IV x 30	30W		16.0 (5792)
	5792	Weekly : IV x 87	87W		
IW (breast)	4882	3 x weekly : IV x 6	2W		
	4882	Weekly : IV x 26	26W	17M	13.9 (4882)
	5792	Weekly : IV x 20	20W		31.8 (5792)
	5792	Weekly : IM x 14	14W		
IB (breast)	4882	3 x weekly : IV x 9	3W		
	4882	Daily : IV x 10	2W		
	4882	Weekly : IV x 25	25W		19.0 (4882)
	5792	Weekly : IV x 19	19W	22M	42.3 (5792)
	4882	Daily : IM x 5	1W		
	5792	Weekly : IM x 13	18W		
MC (breast)	4882	Weekly : IV x 15	15W	4M	1.2
SW (breast)	4882	3 x weekly : IV x 12	4W	2M	2.8
	4882	Weekly : IV x 4	4W		
MV (breast)	4882	3 x weekly : IV x 15	5W	4M	1.3 (4882)
	5792	Weekly : IV x 8	8W		3.3 (5792)
HA (breast)	5794[a]	Daily : IV x 5	1W		
	5792	Daily : IV x 5	1W		3.6 (5794)
	5792	Weekly : IM x 7	7W	9M	68.8 (5792)
	5792	Daily : IV x 10	2W		
	5792	Weekly : IV x 26	26W		
YC (breast)	5792	Daily : IV x 15	3W	2M	22.1
	5792	Weekly : IV x 4	4W		
ECa (breast)	5792	Daily : IV x 10	2W	3M	6.0
	5792	Weekly : IV x 8	8W		
AH (prostate)	5792	Daily : IV x 5	1W	1W	0.3
HC (prostate)	5792	Daily : IV x 10	2W	2W	1.4
MO (Ewing's)	5792	Daily : IV x 4	1W	1W	0.6
CW (prostate)	5792	Weekly : IV x 3	3W	3W	0.2

[a] Medium control ('blank') preparation.   IV = intravenous
                                             IM = intramuscular

differential WBC, were examined at zero time and at 4 and 24 hours post-injection.

In patients AH and CW (Table 1) the time course of changes in white cell count were examined at hourly intervals. In patient CW, levels of plasma cortisol, growth hormone, prolactin, glucose and acute-phase reactants (C-reactive protein; α_1-acid glycoprotein) were also examined during the first 24 hours. Clinical chemistry monitoring also included electrolyte levels, and other tests of renal and hepatic function.

Immune status, white cell function and skin reactions
Levels of complement, immune complexes, autoantibodies and interferon
were examined in both the acute response and after longer-term lymphokine
administration. Tests of WBC function (eg LIF-activity and lymphocyte
transformation) were performed on occasion. In patient MO (Table 1)
lymphocyte populations were examined by rosetting techniques and surface
immunofluorescence; K-cell activity and polymorph phagocytic capacity
were also examined. Patients were skin tested with several doses of
corresponding lymphokine as well as with a recall antigen (PPD) in
relation to short-term and long-term schedules.

Histopathology of injected lesions and skin reactions
Excision biopsy of metastatic breast nodules was undertaken 1 - 7 days
after the last injection of lymphokine; nodules were examined histologically for leucocytic infiltration and tumour cell necrosis. Prostatic
needle biopsies were done 2 days, 2 weeks and 4 weeks after the course
of intra-prostatic injections. Biopsies of skin tests were taken at
intervals during the 48 hours after intradermal lymphokine and were compared histologically with the evolution of the tuberculin reaction.

Methods of comparing responses
Pairs of the following variables were examined for possible relationships: (i) extent of maximum temperature rise (ΔT° C); (ii) percentage
of change in polymorph count at 4 hours (%ΔPMN); (iii) percent change in
lymphocyte count at 4 hours (%ΔL). The effective dose needed to produce
defined areas of erythema (ED) was compared to that required to effect a
given degree of inhibition of leucocyte migration as well as other
criteria of lymphokine activity (see also Table 2).

RESPONSE TO INTRA-LESIONAL INJECTION OF LYMPHOKINE

Dermal metastases: in breast carcinoma

Ulceration was seen in 7 out of 11 nodules that had been injected
with lymphokine and flattening or reduction in diameter in 7 of these
nodules. Tumour cell necrosis was seen in 9 of the nodules, associated
with a cellular infiltrate mainly consisting of polymorphs and macrophages. This necrosis was confluent rather than patchy and in one
nodule (12.5 mg LK-4362 by 4 injections) there was vacuolation of the
tumour cells producing a ballooning effect. Numerous polymorphs were
seen to have phagocytosed cellular debris. The tumour cell change was
more marked when there were closely packed tumour cells instead of a
predominantly fibrous tissue architecture. No macroscopic change or
tumour cell necrosis was seen in a control nodule given 6 saline
injections.

Intra-lesional: prostatic carcinoma patients

All 6 patients had a marked pyrexia with a similar time course to
that in the breast cancer patients, except it was of a longer duration.
Rigors occurred as the temperature rose. No consistent pattern of
changes in WBC counts at 4 hours post-injection was apparent apart from
a transient decrease in lymphocyte count after the majority of injections.
A diminution in the size of tumour was obtained in one patient (DH)
and 3 patients showed tumour cell necrosis which was associated with an

inflammatory cellular infiltrate in which mononuclear cells appeared to
predominate. Two patients developed herpes labialis whilst under treatment; however, all patients wished to continue LCL-LK injections so as
to complete the course. There was no clinical evidence of micturition
abnormality or local discomfort which could be attributed to lymphokine
injection. Three patients volunteered a decrease in severe metastatic
bone pain, either during or shortly after the course of LCL-LK; one
patient still remaining pain-free 18 months later (Feb 1981). The longer
duration of the pyrexia after intra-lesional injection was probably due
to the time necessary for absorption into the systemic circulation.
This study has shown indications that intra-lesional injections may be
useful where a localised tumour is easily accessible.

SHORT-TERM RESPONSES TO SYSTEMIC LYMPHOKINE

Clinical and haematological responses

The characteristic response to a first intravenous (I/V) injection of
(20 - 100 μg) LCL-LK consists of transient pyrexia, polymorph leucocytosis
and lymphopenia during the first 6 - 7 hours. The rise in temperature
(latency 0.5 - 1.5 hrs) is frequently accompanied by mild rigors and
occasionally by nausea and vomiting. Maximal temperature rise occurs
usually 2 - 4 hours after I/V injection. The peak of granulocytosis
occurs between 2 and 4 hours whereas the lowest lymphocyte counts are
usually found around 4 hours after I/V injection (Fig 1). Granulocytosis
affects the neutrophils selectively; blood levels of monocytes, basophils
and eosinophils appear unchanged. By 24 hours the white count usually
reverts to pre-injection values. At 4 hours there is usually a slight
fall (< 20%) in the platelet count. There are no short-term changes in
the red cell count, haematocrit or erythrocyte sedimentation rate.

The study of short-term responses to repeated LCL-LK injection daily
or on alternate days, in escalating doses reveals that both the height
of the pyrexia and the extent of white count changes can be related to
the dose of LCL-LK given I/V. This also applies to the duration of
pyrexia (though not to its latency). A maximum tolerated dose of I/V
LCL-LK is usually one which produces a 2^{O} C pyrexia and which has varied
from 200 μg - 3 mg according to preparation and patient. On repeated
daily or alternate-day injection of doses producing $\geqslant 1^{O}$ C pyrexia or
$\geqslant 20\%$ leucocytosis or lymphopenia, there is some evidence of 'tolerance'
of pyrexial and white-count changes; but there is no evidence of
'sensitization' to either response. Intravenous injections of sufficient
LCL-LK at weekly intervals usually elicit reproducible responses within
individual patients given individual LCL-LK preparations. A 'shift to
the left' sometimes accompanies polymorph leucocytoses of > 50% suggesting increased cellular recruitment from bone marrow.

Correlations
More detailed analysis of temperature and white count changes
revealed associations between the extent of maximum temperature rise at
any time between 1 - 7 hours and (a) the extent of granulocytosis at 4
hours with LK-5792; and (b) the extent of lymphopenia at 4 hours with
LK-4882. However, at 4 hours post-injection, the extent of granulocytosis did not correlate with the extent of lymphopenia; this is
probably because they may run a different time course. Further observations suggest that where the white count is depressed and/or where the

patient has received recent chemotherapy or extensive irradiation, a pyrexial response to LCL-LK may not be accompanied by granulocytosis or lymphopenia. We conclude that transient pyrexia, granulocytosis and lymphopenia are physiologically-linked responses of the host to I/V LCL-LK but that there are circumstances in which the white cells may be 'unresponsive'.

Changes in blood chemistry and endocrinology

Liver function, renal function, serum enzymes, electrolytes

Tests of liver function (ie total protein, albumin, bilirubin and the enzymes γ-glutamyl transferase, aspartate amino-transferase, alanine amino-transferase, alkaline phosphatase) were done at 0, 4 and 24 hours after lymphokine injection in some of the breast and prostatic carcinoma patients. Renal function was examined at the same times by looking at urea and creatinine levels; and routine electrolytes included calcium and phosphate. However, no change considered to be significant was observed in the blood chemistry.

Plasma cortisol and other hormones

In one patient (CW) levels of cortisol were studied at hourly intervals for 6 hours and at 24 hours after I/V injection of 100 μg LK-5792 on 2 occasions. On the second occasion levels of growth hormone, prolactin and glucose were also measured as indicators of a non-specific 'stress' reaction. The injections were given at 1.00 pm so the levels would be assessed during a period when they would not rise due to the inherent diurnal variation of the patient.

Plasma cortisol rose to levels more than twice that of the peak early morning level at 2 – 4 hours post-injection and then decreased (Fig 2). No increase in growth hormone, prolactin or glucose, considered to be significant, were found. These findings were associated with a maximal increase in temperature at 3 – 4 hours post-injection, together with a granulocytosis and a lymphopenia, both maximal at 5 hours (Fig 2). Injection of plasma protein control produced no changed in hormone levels (or white count) on a subsequent occasion in the same patients.

Acute phase reactants

Levels of the acute-phase reactants C-reactive protein (fast to rise and fall) and α_1-acid glycoprotein (slow to rise and fall) were studied in patient CW. They were measured at hourly intervals for 6 hours and at 12, 24, 48, 72 and 96 hours after injection of 100 μg LK-5792 on the same 2 occasions as the plasma cortisol was measured.

An increase in the C-reactive protein above normal levels (5 – 10 mg/l) was evident at 12 hours post-injection and a maximal level was reached at 24 hours of 25 – 30 mg/l. It returned to normal by 72 hours. Only a slight increase in the α_1-acid glycoprotein was detected, present only in the 24 hour sample. The injection of plasma protein control in CW produced no changes in acute-phase reactant levels.

Conclusions

The failure to elicit short-term changes in blood chemistry that are associated with toxicity, indicates that the lymphokine is not acutely toxic.

There is normally an inverse relationship between the diurnal variation of endogenous plasma cortisol with lymphocyte levels; and exogenous

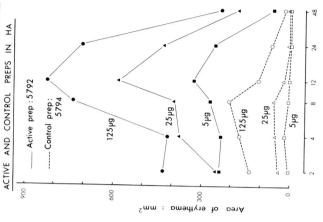

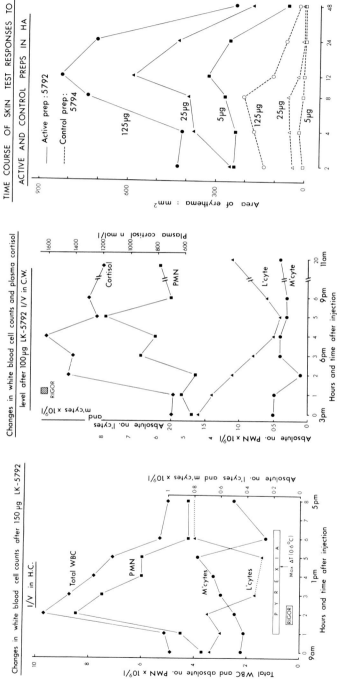

FIG 1. Shows time-course of changes in peripheral blood white cell count after injection of 150 μg LK-5792 I/V. Duration of pyrexia and rigors are indicated; maximum pyrexia: 0.6° C.

FIG 2. Shows time-course of changes in plasma cortisol after injection of 100 μg LK-5792 I/V. Time-course of white count changes are indicated; there was a short rigor at 1 hr.

FIG 3. Shows time-course of skin-test responses to intradermal injection of LK-5792 (125, 25, 5μg) and its plasma protein control (5794) at similar doses (see also Table 2).

pharmacological doses of glucocorticoids are known to cause transient
lymphopenias in man (30). Administration of lymphokine-containing
(Con A)-generated supernatants from human peripheral blood leucocytes,
have been found to increase corticosterone levels in rats, reaching a
maximum 1 - 2 hours after injection (2). The marked elevation of plasma
cortisol seen in CW 2 - 4 hours after LCL-LK injection, with no significant increases of other indicators of a non-specific 'stress' reaction,
indicates that the lymphokine is having a primary effect on the adrenal-
pituitary axis. This warrants further investigation, including study of
the time-course of the early cortisol and lymphocyte responses.

The increase in C-reactive protein indicated that activation of systemic inflammatory mechanisms was taking place after lymphokine injection.

Effects on immune status and white-cell function

Serum interferon levels

These were measured by the Department of Microbiology, London School
of Hygiene and Tropical Medicine (Prof A J Zuckerman). No appreciable
interferon levels were found in any of the wide variety of serum samples
tested in relation to single and repeated injections of LCL-LK
(ie < 6.3 U/ml). Furthermore the cell line used (RPMI-1788) was not
known to produce interferon. It was concluded that the reaction of the
patients was not due to interferon.

Sero-immunology

No change in the following parameters was found that could be attributed to lymphokine injection: serum immunoglobulins (IgG; IgA; IgM);
complement screens (CH50; alternate pathway haemolysis; C3; C4); immune-
complex activity in serum (C1q-binding; PEG-precipitation); anti-
bacterial antibody titres (streptococcal; salmonella; treponemal); or
autoantibody titres (antiglobulins; anti-nuclear and tissue antibodies).

Effects on white-cell function

Attempts were made to determine whether there was increased responsiveness of the patients' granulocytes to the LIF activity of LCL-LK
preparations, or increased lymphocyte transformation to phytomitogens
or recall antigens, which could be attributed to intravenous injection
of LCL-LK; to date, no obvious trend has emerged. Most of the patients
were anergic to tuberculin PPD when first skin-tested but no conversion
of tuberculin reactivity was observed. One patient (with a Ewing's
tumour) presented with depressed K cell activity following intensive
chemotherapy and irradiation. After 3 daily intravenous injections of
LCL-LK, K-cell activity (against group O Rhesus positive red blood cells
coated with human Anti-D) rose from 2.5% to 23% (at a 2.5:1 effector:
target cell ratio) and EAγ-rosetting lymphocytes rose from 12% to 32%,
despite the fact that no significant changes in total or differential
white counts were observed. More definitive studies of white-cell
function are now incorporated into an investigative protocol (see below).

Route of administration

The majority of systemic injections were given I/V rather than I/M
as a lower dose was required to produce the same extent of pyrexia,
with the maximum rise in temperature usually at least 1 hour earlier.
There was also less variation in the time-course of the haematological

responses which made for easier assessment. The shorter duration of
pyrexia with I/V administration would be valuable if treatment was given
in an out-patient clinic. However I/M injection was not unduly painful
and may be more appropriate where lymphokine is given outside the clinic.

Compliance of patients to repeated systemic injection in short-term courses of LCL-LK

Against a background of informed consent and individual patient
management, only 1 of 14 patients receiving repeated systemic injections
of LCL-LK withdrew. Where rigors, nausea, vomiting and sweating
occurred these were remarkably well tolerated; some patients volunteered
feelings of lassitude afterwards but by the subsequent day most patients
(not pre-terminal) experienced feelings of well-being. This was
especially true of the 4 patients maintained on a long-term schedule of
LCL-LK injections (see below).

INTRADERMAL INFLAMMATORY RESPONSES TO LCL-LYMPHOKINE

During the course of this study we obtained a large body of data
concerning the time-course, clinical appearance, histopathology and
dose-related responses of inflammatory skin reactions in the forearms
of patients given intradermal (I/D) injections of the different LCL-LK
preparations.

Clinical appearance; time-course; histopathology

An early phase of vasodilatation begins 10 - 20 min after I/D injection
and after 2 - 4 hours there is increasing central induration, areas of
erythema reaching maxima between 12 - 24 hr (unlike responses in guinea
pig skin maximal at 6 hours). The time course of reactions produced by
fivefold dilutions of LK-5792 are shown in Fig 3. At higher doses or
with more potent LCL-LK preparations there is central haemorrhage at
24 hours and the skin reaction site is still visible after 5 - 7 days as
a purple flat area with central discolouration. Histopathology reveals
an early phase of predominantly polymorphonuclear cell infiltration (at
4 hr) followed by perivascular mononuclear cell accumulation (at 24 hr);
and mononuclear cells predominate in later (48 - 72 hr) reactions. The
phenomenon of sustained erythematous inflammation (SIF activity) is a
characteristic feature of human skin reactions to LCL-LK; and dose
response studies reveal that human skin is about 100 times more responsive than guinea pig skin.

By plotting areas of erythema against log dose LCL-LK we record
effective LK doses required to give areas of erythema equivalent to 10,
20, 30, 40 mm diameter at defined times after skin testing eg 'ED$_{30}$' at
24 hr, or at the time of maximum response (ie areas of 79, 314, 707,
1257 sq mm). By multiple skin testing, 2 or 3 different LCL-LK preparations can be compared on a given patient; and the sustained skin
reaction can be used to assay the activity of physicochemical fractions
of a given LCL-LK.

Clinical significance of SIF activity

The majority of our patients with a large tumour load (or with recent
exposure to irradiation/chemotherapy) are Mantoux-negative yet they

retain the ability to give prominent and sustained inflammatory responses to intradermal lymphokine. This implies integrity of whatever cellular responses are involved in the sustained skin reaction, and provides one response parameter for in vivo study. Three patients lost their skin reactivity to LCL-LK as they entered the pre-terminal phase and the predictive value of skin testing merits further evaluation. It is likely that the skin reaction to crude LCL-LK is due to heterogeneity of lymphokines and to activation of several endogenous pathways involved in leucocyte:endothelial interaction in vivo. Because Man is 100 times more responsive than the guinea pig to the SIF activity of LCL-LK, and because 24-hour skin reactions are readily attainable in Man (unlike the guinea pig), we feel that particular significance should be placed upon the phenomenon of sustained intradermal inflammation in Man (12). It therefore seem appropriate to evaluate the 24-hour skin reaction as a 'model' of the host response to intra-lesional injection of lymphokine; to determine whether it has correlative or prognostic significance; to undertake biochemical and pharmacological characterization of the active factor(s); and to determine the relationship between erythema-inducing and other biological activities of LCL-LK fractions.

NUMERICAL EVALUATION OF LYMPHOKINE ACTIVITIES AND PATIENT RESPONSES

A principal reason for undertaking this 'open' study with 'crude' LCL-LK was to obtain experience of patient responses and lymphokine activities so as to determine what associations might profitably be evaluated in the design of future protocol procedures.

Pyrexial and leucocytic responses

In view of the diurnal variations in body temperature we consider that a pyrexia in the 6 hours following I/V LCL-LK (given say at 10 am) is only 'significant' if greater than $0.3 - 0.5^{\circ}$ C (the maximum 'response' to 5 ml NaCl I/V). Likewise, in view of diurnal variations in white count and technical variations in reproducibility we regard as 'significant' alteration of total or differential white counts > 20%. To accommodate the additional features of timing and tolerance, we are now evaluating in each new patient, on an escalating I/V schedule (daily or thrice weekly), the smallest LCL-LK dose required to effect (within 6 hours) a rise in temperature (ΔT) of 1.5° C (TD_{15}); a rise in granulocytes of 50% (PD_{50}); and a fall in lymphocytes of 50% (LD_{50}). For each new patient and for each LCL-LK preparation the numerical values of these doses are recorded (in μg LCL-LK) and a unitage is assigned for that LK:patient combination (in effective doses/mg LK protein).

Skin-inflammatory (SIF) and LIF responses

Likewise we are now evaluating the LK dose required to elicit 24 hr erythematous responses equivalent to 20 mm diameter (314 mm^2) and 30 mm diameter (707 mm^2) by interpolation from dose-response skin tests (ED_{20}; ED_{30}) as well as the LK dose (in μg) required to elicit erythematous responses at the time of maximum skin test area. In evaluating the results of LIF assays we record the dose of LK required (in μg) in the Clausen test (ie in a standard preincubation volume: see refs 9,10) to effect 30% inhibition of migration of human granulocytes (MI_{30}) from normal healthy subjects and from patients. Both SIF and LIF data are plotted semi-logarithmically and a unitage is assigned for both criteria (in effective doses/mg LK protein).

TABLE 2.   Illustrative evaluation of protein/endotoxin effects

Test	Index	LK-5792	5794 (blank)
24-hr erythema in Man (30 mm diam)	ED_{30}	20 - 125 µg	≫ 125 µg[a]
LIF activity on human granulocytes (30% inh.)	MI_{30}	40 - 50 µg	> 1 mg[a]
Pyrexia (1.5°C rise in 6 hrs after I/V LK)	TD_{15}	50 - 250 µg	> 2.5 mg[b]
PMN-leucocytosis (increase of 50%)	PD_{50}	20 - 200 µg	> 2.5 mg[b]
Lymphopenia (50% drop in lymphocyte count)	LD_{50}	50 - 200 µg	> 2.5 mg[b]
Listeria clearance (100-fold decrease in recovery from mouse spleen)	ID_{100}	< 200 µg[c]	≫ 200 µg[b]
Increased spleen weight (30% in mice)	SD_{30}	∿ 200 µg[c]	≫ 200 µg[b]
Lymphocyte proliferation in mouse lymph nodes (10-fold increase)	ND_{10}	< 150 µg[c]	≫ 150 µg[b]
Lowry protein (referred to albumin)		1 mg/mg	1 mg/mg
Limulus endotoxin (≡ E coli 0111-B4)		10 ng/mg	20 ng/mg

[a]Values obtained by extrapolation;   [b]Highest dose tested;

[c]Listeria clearance, spleen weight and Mackaness test (24) undertaken in mice by the Dutch Institute of Public Health, Bilthoven.

Illustrative evaluation of protein/endotoxin effects

Table 2 illustrates one application of this numerical approach: to ascertain how far contamination of a crude LCL-LK preparation by plasma protein or endotoxin-like activity could account for the biological and clinical effects observed. The preparation LK-5792 was tested against a 'blank' preparation (5794) in which 1% human AB plasma in RPMI-1640 was processed in exactly the same way as the LCL-LK. The 'blank' preparation had the same content of plasma protein and twice the concentration of endotoxin-like activity as did the putatively active LCL-LK. However, as Table 2 shows, the biological and clinical effects of LK-5792 are not simply ascribable to its content of plasma protein or to endotoxin; this adds further weight to the view that the observed effects are due primarily to lymphokine activity.

Other clinical, immunological and biochemical effects

On an escalating dose schedule, we are now attempting to evaluate lymphokine doses which produce other host responses. Illustrative acute response parameters are: (a) significant (eg 100%) rise in plasma cortisol level during the 6 hours after injection; and (b) significant duration of rigor (eg 30 min). Where host responses may take longer to become manifest (eg improvement in white-cell function) it may still be possible to evaluate the dose of lymphokine required to effect this. For example, where white-cell function has become depressed due to recent radiotherapy or chemotherapy, it may be useful to record the amount of lymphokine which, when given over a specified time-interval, normalises white-cell function parameters (eg NK-cell and K-cell activity; phagocytic capacity).

Evaluation of variations between patients' responses
and between lymphokine preparations

Data now available indicates that variations between the biological activities of different batches of LCL-LK (in vitro and in vivo) outweigh variations between individual patients in response to any given preparation. These batch variations cannot be accounted for by gross differences in protein content or endotoxin-like activity, nor by gross differences in chromatographic or electrophoretic profiles of individual preparations.

LONG-TERM ADMINISTRATION OF LYMPHOKINE

Four advanced breast carcinoma patients received systemic lymphokine injections for 9 months or longer (see Table 1). Three of these patients received almost continuous courses for a period of approx. 2 years:- 25 months (AC); 17 months (IW); 22 months (IB). At the time of starting lymphokine it was accepted that these patients were unresponsive to other forms of treatment. However, during long-term administration of lymphokine, the patients received short courses of Tamoxifen (all 4 patients); methotrexate (AC; IW; IB) and local radiotherapy (HA). During this time the clinical condition of these patients remained remarkably stable for long periods and with only slow deterioration at other times. The general condition of the patients was improved as evidenced by return of appetite, cessation of weight loss and increase in activity level; their psychological state appeared much improved. The condition of AC remained static while on weekly I/V injections of LK-5792 for a period of 6 months until she started to deteriorate 3 months before her death. IW remained relatively stable while receiving weekly I/V injections, until 5 months before death. IB had a badly ulcerated *en cuirasse* tumour which at 9 months after commencing I/V lymphokine, showed objective regression. (She was receiving weekly I/V LK-4882 at this time.) The regression continued until 13 months, when the ulcer was healed apart from one small area and there was a decreased induration of the remaining tumour. Throughout this time IB volunteered feelings of well-being. She then gradually deteriorated for the next 10 months when she died. After commencing I/V lymphokine the condition of HA remained static for 2 months but then like the other patients she deteriorated only very gradually until she died 7 months later.

Changes in the size and appearance of these tumours were supported by a photographic record; and the prevalence of bony metastases was recorded on bone scans. Routine biochemical estimations at monthly intervals revealed no changes in electrolytes or evidence of renal or hepatic toxicity. Elevated alkaline phosphatase in IW and IB reflected the progression of bony metastases. Repeated skin testing with lymphokine and one recall antigen (PPD) revealed a decreased reactivity to lymphokine in IB when pre-terminal, in accord with other patients in the study. None of these patients acquired a positive skin test to PPD.

This long-term study shows that systemic lymphokine can be given for at least 2 years without evidence of attributable toxicity and with no problems of patient compliance.

INDICATIONS OF CLINICAL BENEFIT

This study was not designed to examine the potential clinical efficacy of LCL-LK preparations in tumour-bearing patients; for all such patients had been placed in the category of 'irreversible neoplastic disease'. However, the following evidence was obtained of improvement in clinical condition:

(a) reduction in extent of an *en cuirasse* breast tumour (IB);
(b) reduction in palpable size of a prostatic tumour (DH);
(c) decrease of metastatic bone pain in 3 patients with prostatic carcinoma (JB; WJ; JR);
(d) tumour-cell necrosis after intra-nodular injection in 3 breast cancer patients (ECo; AC; IW) and after intra-lesional injection in 3 prostatic cancer patients (DH; WJ; JR).

At present we conclude that it is worthwhile and ethically justifiable to continue this work in advanced cancer, against the background of informed consent and of careful and compassionate management of individual patients.

EMERGENCE OF PROTOCOL DESIGN

On the basis of this experience we are now formulating protocols for evaluating specific effects of systemically-administered LCL-LK in advanced cancer patients which might be relevant to both Phase I and Phase II trials in less advanced patients. A first protocol has been devised with the objective of measuring biological activity of any specified batch of LCL-LK in terms of effective doses giving standard acute responses (see above) and longer-term changes in white-cell function. Patients in this first 'activity' protocol will have carcinoma of the breast and will be post-menopausal, unresponsive to chemotherapy and/or radiotherapy, not having received chemotherapy for 2 months or radiotherapy for 6 months. The protocol will compare active and control (blank) preparations by administering each to 7 patients in a double blind group comparison. Injections will be given 5 days per week for 3 weeks, initially by escalating doses. Acute clinical and haematological responses will be assessed after each injection; tests of WBC function and sero-immunology assessed weekly; and cell mediated immunity to recall antigens, assessed before and after the course. Ethical management and informed consent will be mandatory.

Examples of other protocols are:

(1) Protocol for evaluating any effects of plasma protein or endotoxin in given LK preparation;

(2) Protocols for evaluating LK effects on WBC-function in patients given recent chemotherapy or irradiation;

(3) Protocol for evaluating short-term changes in hormone levels;

(4) Protocol for evaluating systemic effects of LK on WBC function in patients also receiving intra-lesional BCG.

When this 'quality assurance' information, together with toxicity (phase I) data, is available for LCL-LK, we envisage two principal approaches to phase II studies in breast carcinoma:

(a) Single-blind efficacy study of 20 - 40 high risk ($T_{1-3}/N_1/M_0$) patients after surgery/DXT against a similar number receiving control ('blank') preparations; and

(b) Single-blind efficacy study in 20 - 40 'first-time' recurrences ($T_{1-4}/N_1/M_0$) against a similar number receiving control ('blank') preparations.

CONCLUSIONS

In realizing that this preliminary study over a 5-year period has revealed the need to properly structure a multidisciplinary approach to the host response to lymphokines in cancer, the following conclusions would seem justified:-

(1) Repeated LCL-LK administration to tumour-bearing patients is safe and is well tolerated locally and systemically without adverse toxicity;

(2) Host responses relate to LK-activity rather than to contaminants in LCL-LK preparations (plasma protein; endotoxin);

(3) Nature of host responses appear relevant to both inflammatory and host-defence mechanisms and can be evaluated quantitatively;

(4) Mechanistic views may be testable in animal models;

(5) Relationships can be evaluated between effects of LCL-LK on WBC-function ex vivo and other criteria of LK activity and host response;

(6) Realistic protocols can be established to investigate specific questions about LCL-LK activities in cancer research therapy;

(7) Larger-scale (eg 100 L) batch culture capability may circumvene some problems of LK-standardization inherent in protocol design;

(8) Selective local and systemic administration allows a balanced approach in evaluating host responses to both crude and purified LK's;

(9) Long-term administration of (LCL) LK to (tumour-bearing) patients is no longer the 'pipe-dream' that we had 10 years ago (15); and

(10) Careful patient selection, monitoring and management provides the basis for evaluating LCL-LK's as 'biological response modifiers' in relation to human cancer.

Acknowledgements We are grateful to Mr G Carter and Mr B Muller, Department of Chemical Pathology, Charing Cross Hospital, London, for endocrine and acute-phase reactant estimations.

REFERENCES

1. Baldwin,R.W.(1978): Develop. Biol. Standard., 38:3.

2. Besedovsky,H.O., del Rey,A., and Sorkin,E.(1981): J.Immunol., 126:385.

3. Bloom,B.R., and Bennett,B.(1966): Science, 153:80.

4. Borsos,T., and Rapp,H.(1972): Immunology and Carcinogenesis. National Cancer Institute Monograph, Number 35.

5. Burnet,F.M.(1968): Nature, 218:426.

6. Cohen,M.C., Goss,A., Yoshida,T., and Cohen,S.(1978): J.Immunol., 121:840.

7. Cohen,S., Pick,E., and Oppenheim,J.J.(1978): Biology of the lymphokines. Academic Press, New York.

8. David,J.R.(1966): Proc.Nat.Acad.Sci.(Wash), 56:72.

9. Den Hollander,F.C., van Lieshout,J.I., and Schuurs,A.H.W.M.(1980): In: Biochemical Characterization of Lymphokines, edited by A.L.de Weck, F.Kristensen, and M.Landy, p.109. Academic Press, New York.

10. Den Hollander,F.C., van Lieshout,J.I., and Schuurs,A.H.W.M.(1981): Immunopharmacology, (in press).

11. Dumonde,D.C.(1967): Brit.Med.Bull., 23:9.

12. Dumonde,D.C., Howson,W.T., and Wolstencroft,R.A.(1968): In: Immuno- pathology, Vth International Symposium, Punta Ala, 1967, edited by P.A.Miescher, and P.Grabar, p.263. Grune and Stratton Inc., New York.

13. Dumonde,D.C., Wolstencroft,R.A., Panayi,G.S., Matthew,M., Morley,J., and Howson,W.T.(1969): Nature, 224:38.

14. Dumonde,D.C.(1971): In: Immunopathology, VIth International Symposium, Grindlewald, 1970, edited by P.A.Miescher, p.289. Grune and Stratton, New York.

15. Dumonde,D.C., and Maini,R.N.(1971): Clin.Allergy, 1:123.

16. Dumonde,D.C., Kelly,R.H., and Wolstencroft,R.A.(1973): In: Microenviron- mental aspects of Immunity, edited by B.D.Jankovic, and K.Isakovic, p.705. Plenum Publishing Corporation, New York.

17. Dumonde,D.C., Kelly,R.H., Preston,P.M., and Wolstencroft,R.A.(1975): In: Mononuclear Phagocytes, edited by R.van Furth, p.675. Blackwell Scientific Publications, Oxford.

18. Dumonde,D.C., Pulley,M.S., O'Connell,D., Southcott,B.M., Robinson,M.R.G., Paradinas,F.J., Rigby,C.C., den Hollander,F.C., Schuurs,A., and de Bruin,R.W.(1980): Int.J.Immunopharmacol., 2(3):190(abstr.)

19. Favila,L., Jimenez,L., Castro,M.E., Garcia-Garcia,G., Gutierrez,A., and Pulida,I.(1978): J.Nat.Canc.Inst., 60:1279.

20. Goupner,A., Misep,G.L., Gouveia,G., Ribears,P., and Mathé,G.(1981): In: New Trends in Human Immunology and Cancer Immunotherapy, edited by B.Serron and R.Rosenfeld, p.901. Doin publications, Paris.

21. Hamblin,A.S., Wolstencroft,R.A., Dumonde,D.C., den Hollander,F.C., Schuurs,A.H.W., Backhouse,B.M., O'Connell,D., and Paradinas,F.(1978): Develop.Biol.Standard., 38:335.

22. Kelly,R.H., Wolstencroft,R.A., Dumonde,D.C., and Balfour,B.M.(1972): Clin.Exp.Immunol., 10:49.

23. Klein,G.(1978): In:Manipulation of the Immune Response in Cancer, edited by N.A.Mitchison, and M.Landy, p.339. Academic Press, New York.

24. Mackaness,G.B., Auclair,D.J., and Lagrange,P.H.(1973): J.Nat.Canc.Inst. 51:1655.

25. McDaniel,M.C., Laudico,R., and Papermaster,B.W.(1976): Clin.Immunol. Immunol., 5:91.

26. Papermaster,B.W., Holtermann,OA., Klein,E., Djerassi,I., Rosner,D., Dao,T., and Costanzi,J.J.(1976): Clin.Immunol.Immunopathol., 5:31.

27. Papermaster,B.W., Holtermann,O.A., McDaniel,M.C., Klein,E., Djerassi,I., Rosner,D., Dao,T., and Costanzi,J.J.(1976): Ann.N.Y.Acad,Sci., 276:584.

28. Papermaster,B.W., McEntire,J.E., Gilliland,C.D., and Buchok,S.J.(1980): In:Biochemical Characterization of Lymphokines, edited by A.L. de Weck, F.Kristensen and M.Landy, p.193. Academic Press, New York.

29. Robinson,M.R.G., Rigby,C.C., Pugh,R.C.B., Vaughan,L.C., and Dumonde,D.C. (1976): Clin.Exp.Immunol., 26:137.

30. Thomson,S.P., McMahon,L.J., and Nugent,C.A.(1980): Clin.Immunol. Immunopathol., 17:506.

Subject Index